THERAPEUTIC RIDING II
STRATEGIES FOR REHABILITATION

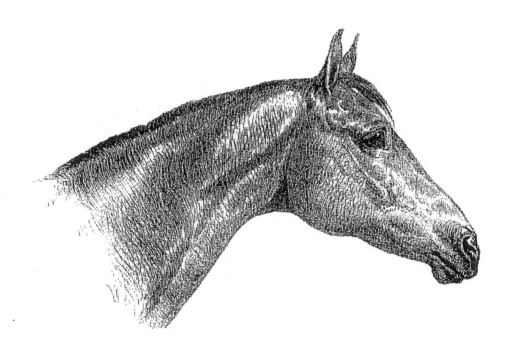

COVER ACKNOWLEDGEMENT

Cover photographs are by courtesy of Colleen Zanin, occupational therapist and founder of the Old Dominion School of Therapeutic Riding. A treatment in progress led by Angela Dusenbury, physical therapist and her treatment team. The child is Ellen Rickerson. This team also appears on page 264.

THERAPEUTIC RIDING II
STRATEGIES FOR REHABILITATION

Edited by

Barbara Teichmann Engel, M.Ed., O.T.R

Illustrators
Stephanie C. Woods, B.F.A.
&
Barbara T. Engel, M.Ed., OTR

Published by
Barbara Engel Therapy Services
Durango, Colorado USA

It is expected that the content of this book will be used by those who are qualified to apply the methods discussed or those who will seek the training to effectively use the knowledge that the many contributors have provided to the reader.

Then dynamic field of the horse as a partner in treatment has a strong foundation but will only expand with experience, questions, search for new methods and the validation of its practice

No warranty, expressed or implied, is made regarding the content of this book by the editor , publisher, consultants, reviewers, or contributors The book has been developed independently with out the assistance of grants, sponsors or support of any organization. No endorsement has been made or received from and foundation or organization.

The opinion or experiences expressed in the article of the text are those of each author or contributor and do not necessarily represent the views of the editor, reviewers, or that of any organization. It is the intent of this text to present to the reader many view points from those who have had extensive experience in the field. The text is intended to expand the views of those in the field and to challenge present knowledge and to enrich the reader's base of knowledge

Copyright © 1997 by Barbara T. Engel
Second printing 3/2000
Third Printing 8/2003
Fourth Printing 8/2005
Fifth Printing   6/2007
Sixth Printing 7/2010

Library of Congress **Catalog Card Number: 97-090342**
ISBN 10: 0-9633065-6-1
ISBN 13: 978-0-9633065-6-2

Manufactured in the United States of America   Printed in the USA

Publisher: Barbara Engel Therapy Services
          10 Town Plaza, #238, Durango, Colorado 81301 USA
          FAX: 973-563-9599; E-mail engelbt@bu.edu   Phone- 970-563-5617

CONTRIBUTORS

ACKNOWLEDGMENTS

PREFACE

CROSS REFERENCE OF
THERAPEUTIC RIDING I STRATEGIES
IN INSTRUCTION
AND
THERAPEUTIC RIDING II STRATEGIES
IN REHABILITATION

TABLE OF CONTENT

*This book is dedicated in the memory of my husband
Edward "Jay" Engel
Without his tolerance, support and help
this manuscript would not have been possible..*

Barbara T. Engel, B.S., M.Ed., OTR - EDITOR
Pediatric occupational therapist retired, private practice and consultant since 1976; administrator-18 years; university and clinical instructor-24 years; extensive work experience in pediatrics, rehabilitation medicine and psychiatry; 20 yrs training with sensory integration international, cerebral palsy treatment methods, NDT, CST and hippotherapy; consultant and lecturer in therapeutic riding- hippotherapy since 1981. Registered by the American Hippotherapy Association with advanced training in Germany. Hippotherapy Curriculum Development Committee. Editor of eight therapeutic riding books and co-author of one. Recipient of the NARHA prestigious James Brady Professional Achievement Award. Active member of NARHA, US Dressage Federation, US Combined Training Association, the AHSA, and our local Dressage & CT club. Was a Pony Club DC. Member of AVA, FRDI. President/owner of a publishing company. She trains with her Lipizzan stallion and her Lipizzan/Andalusian mare in classic dressage, breeds her horses with her trainer and coaches a vaulting team on her farm in Ignacio Colorado.

CONTRIBUTORS

Ellen Adolphson, PT
Bryn Mawr Rehabilitation Hospital equine-assisted therapy practitioner since 1985, advanced hippotherapy course in Germany, Hippotherapy Curriculum Development Committee.

Elizabeth Baker, PT
Physical Therapy supervisor, Children's Hospital, Wrentham State school, physical therapist Greenlock Therapeutic Riding Center, advanced hippotherapy course in Germany, Hippotherapy Curriculum Development, Committee. Board member of American Hippotherapy Association, Medical Committee of NARHA, hippotherapy practitioner since 1985. Life-long equestrian.

Joann Benjaman, PT
NDT, Feldenkrais practioner, practioner of hippotherapy-14 yrs.; Board of directors and consultant to therapeutic riding programs. AHA Board of Directors, NARHA medical committee; sports rider.

Barb J. Brock, MA, Re.D.
Associated professor recreational management, Eastern Washington University, researcher & programmer for physically disabled adult population; doctoral dissertation - Effect of therapeutic horseback riding on physically disabled adults-Indian University, and video.

Lois J. Brockmann, RPT
NDT pediatric certified, SI trained; hippotherapy since 1988, Special Olympics-1992; therapeutic riding -1992; NARHA registered instructor, registered with AHA; presenter at 9th FRDI congress; owns and events her horse.

John Brough, OTR
Principal, Windward Preparatory School; founder with Nancy Winters of Wayne Dupage Riding and Hunt Club Program; past NARHA VP & chair of medical research committee.

Hana May Brown, PT
Registered with AHA; minor in psychology and teacher of special needs children; hippotherapy in PT practice; NARHA registered instructor; owner/director of Ride On inc.; horse manager and trainer; fund raiser and grant writer since 1983; conferences presentor; author of articles.

Ann Cole, MS, RN, CS
Ms in psychiatric nursing; psychotherapist; centered riding instructor-level 2; psychiatric clinical nurse specialist for infectious disease group practice- univ hospital; author, lecturer.

Karen DePauw, Ph.D
Associate Dean Graduate School, Professor Physical Education Sport Leisure Studies, Washington State University. Author and lecturer on therapeutic riding research and disabled sports and adaptive physical education.

Susanna von Dietze, PT
Physical therapist. Involved in therapeutic riding and hippotherapy since childhood, accomplished dressage rider, dressage judge; author of *Balance in der Bewegung: der sitz des reiters;* conference presenter, specialist in the riding seat.

Ruth Dismuke-Blakely, MS/CCC-SLP.
Director-THNM/Skyline Therapy Services-full-time multi-discipline hippotherapy/rehabilitation program; researcher, lecturer, and leader in equine-assisted therapy; life long equestrian-rider/trainer of American Quarter Horses. AHA board member.

Sandy Dota
American Judging Association certified judge; therapeutic riding instructor; Somerset Hills Handicapped Riders Club; NARHA board of directors; since 1985--faculty for NARHA workshops, lecturer; international riding competitor in para-Olympic games.

Jane Copeland Fitzpatrick, BS, MA, PT
MA psychology; NDT certified; executive director & physical therapist at Pegasus Therapeutic Riding Inc, since 1982; physical therapist Westport board of education; Hippotherapy Curriculum Committee; AHA board member, NARHA committees, past treasurer & board member Delta Society. Who's Who of American Women, American Society of Assoc. Executives, APTA, FRDI.

Nora Fischback, BA
Program director Special Equestrian Riding Therapy; behaviorist, tutors children with behavior problems.

Ronald Fischback, BA, MS, PhD
Associate professor Cal State Univ Northridge; owner/director of "Steps to Independence Through Education"; president of Special Equestrian Riding Therapy, board member;

Linda Frease, BFA, MHS/OT, OTR/L
Cheff Center instructor program, Loudoun County 4H therapeutic riding instructor and volunteer, research study- evaluation tool, registered with AHA; school occupational therapist,

Gertrude Freeman, BS, MA, PT.
Professor Emeritus-Department of Physical Therapy, School of Allied Sciences, AHS, UTMB, University of Texas Medical Branch; consultant and member of Curriculum Development Committee; consultant to Hope Arena Therapeutic Riding Program, Galveston TX. Charter member AHA, board member 5 yrs.; researcher.

Miguel Gallardo
Founder of Sic Xirio Farm School in Spain. Degree in educator. Director of school. Presentor at many conferences.

Barbara Glasow, PT
NDT trained; private pediatric practice; combines neuro-developmental treatment approach, sensory integration, motor control/ motor learning and manual therapy techniques (cranial sacral therapy, myofascial release techniques, strain counterstrain and muscle energy techniques) in her practice; therapeutic riding since 1975; forerunner in the development of hippotherapy, remedial vaulting, and teaching sports riding in a therapeutic manner in U.S.; given workshops throughout the U.S. & Canada since 1978; studied hippotherapy in Germany in 1982 & 1987; presented papers at International Congresses on Therapeutic Riding; wrote the script for Winslow Unlimited's videotape, "Challenged Equestrians", therapist consultant for Winslow Unlimited from 1975-1987 and Easter Seal -Riding Instruction for Special Equestrians from 1987 to present; was the hippotherapy consultant for the National Hippotherapy Curriculum Development Committee, board of directors for the American Hippotherapy Association since 1992; member of AHA education committee; AHA faculty; recipient of NARHA James Brady Professional Achievement Award in 1990.

Hilda Gurney, BS, FEI (S) judge
Dressage trainer, breeder in Moorpark CA; six time USET grand prix champion; US Olympic Team medalist in dressage; an "S" judge; clinic instructor.

Victoria Haehl, MS, PT, BS
NDT certified (adult), consulting--All Seasons Riding Academy and other Bay Area therapeutic riding centers; member-NAHRA, Bay Area Equines for Sports & Therapy.

Gloria Hamblin BS, RTR
Therapeutic Recreation; prior program director Equestrian Therapy for Handicapped Riders, since 1975; director head instructor; Cheff Center certified; prior--RTR at Woodview Calabassas psych hospital-adolescent unit; 5 years international equestrian therapeutic riding coach; equestrian competitor.

Kyle Hamilton, MS, PT
Physical therapist; MS in sports science; experience with therapeutic riding since 1985. *Contributor to The Horse, The Handicapped, The Riding Team.*

Arthur S. Hansen, DDS
Active member of the dental association; rider; volunteer, NARHA member, past board member of National Center for Equine Facilitated Therapy.

Gundula Hauser, PT
Head person of school for mentally handicapped & bodily injured children; Vice President of Austrian Kurtorium fur Hippotherapie Heilpadagogisches Voltigieren/Rieten u Behindertenreiten; responsible for education of professionals teaching remedial educational vaulting and riding; hippotherapy and vaulting practioner since 1983.

Barbara Heine, PT (Australia)
Executive director of the National Center for Equine Facilated Therapy; registered with AHA; 7 years hippotherapy; board member and committees of AHA; certified 1B1 level dressage with Am Riding Instructor certification program, NARHA registered instructor, competitor, trainer in dressage and eventing.

Judy Hilburn , OTR
Private Practice; sensory integration certified; 1987 in equine-assisted therapy; advanced hippotherapy course in Germany; member Hippotherapy Curriculum Committee; dressage rider.

Carol Huegal, PT, BHS
Private practice, hippotherapy since 1990, AHA registered therapist; NARHA registered instructor; owner -It's GREAT; clinical instructor- OT/PT students; vice-pres. Univ Hunter Jumper Club; 4-H leader.

Ho Ming Hsia, BA, DC
Born in China where he studied Mandarin Acupuncture. Doctor of chiropractic instructor at university; private practice.

Carolyn Jagielski, MS, PT
NDT certified; physical therapist; High Hopes Therapeutic Riding; past NARHA medical and accreditation committee.

Antonio Kröger, Physiologist
Headmast of special education school, member German Kuratorium für hippotherapie heil-padagogisches voltigieren/reiten u. behindertenreiten; responsible for the education of and professional teaching of remedial vaulting; international lecturer and researcher, author of many papers, video on remedial vaulting, vaulting practioner.

Elizabeth Atwood Lawrence, V.M.D., PhD.
Professor of environmental studies; veterinary anthropologist--Tufts University School of Veterinary Medicine. Specializing in research, writing and teaching human/horse relationships. Author: *Redeo: An Anthropologist Looks at the Wild and the Tame*; *Hoofbeats and Society: Studies of Human-Horse Interactions*; *Horses in Society*

Molly Lingua-Mundy, PT
Advanced Hippotherapy Course in Germany. Member-Hippotherapy Curriculum Committee. Life long equestrian

Beatriz Marins, MS, OT, ST
Practioner of hippotherapy in Brazil since 1992; post graduate in neurology; Brazil assoc of OT; NARHA member; AHA member; works with developmental and orthopedic clients.

Virginia G. Mazza, BA, MS
Special education teacher--21 Years; member--NAHRA, Delta Society, O.C.D.A., U.S.E.T.; presenter: Winslow Therapeutic Riding seminars; president and on Board of Directors: Special Olympics: head equestrian coach and judge for 18 years.

Peggy H. McClure, BA, MBA, MS/CCC-SLP
Therapeutic riding since 1991, Special Olympics coach, speech pathologist-Albuquerque public schools and Los Lunas Center for persons with developmental disabilities, competitors and active members US Dressage Federation and local groups

Nancy H. McGibbon, MS, PT
Therapeutic riding/hippotherapy since 1973;.director of therapy services therapeutic Riding of Tucson; 1st president of AHA and board of directors; national and international lecturer and instructor; advanced hippotherapy course in Germany; member, hippotherapy curriculum

Chris McParland, BS
Adaptive physical education specialist--credential general secondary; Cheff Center certified instructor; NAHRA master instructor; director/instructor Project R.I.D.E. & Elk Grove unified school district; 13 years therapeutic riding instructor; co-author: *Aspects and Answers*; NAHRA's President's Award; NARHA board.

Linda Mitchell, BS, MS, PT
Special education; physical therapist; NDT certified; advanced hippotherapy course in Germany; member- Hippotherapy Curriculum Committee; therapy services coordinator UCP; NARHA member; board member AHA; owner Work Walk equine assisted therapy.

Joanne Henry Moses, Ph.D
Founder, Clinical and executive director of Tucson Animal Assisted Psychotherapy Associates, Inc.-1986- the 1st outpatient equestrian psychotherapy program in AZ to qualify for Title XIX-Behavioral Health Licence. Teaching since 1955 at St. Micheal's Indian Mission. Member-International Transnational Analysis Assoc., specialized in geriatric psychotherapy.

Craig Nettleton, Ph.D
Equine-assisted psychotherapy since 1992, parent of hippotherapy client, psychologist - Skyline Therapy Services, St. Joseph Rehabilitation Hospital, and the Child & Family Center outpatient ADD Clinic.

Eva Phelps
NARHA certified instructor.

Sandra Rafferty, MS,OTR
Special education; Therapeutic Horsemanship, St. Louis, MO; riding instructor; teacher of therapeutic riding since 1975. registered with AHA; NARHA member, registered instructor, coach for the para-olympic team.

Barbara Rector, BA, MA
Co-founder, head instructor and executive director of TROT, certified riding instructor, equine facilitated psychotherapist and program coordinator of STIRRUP; Breath work certification student with the GROF's program; founding board member of Flagstaff Equine Therapeutic Enterprises; advisory board of National Center for Equine Facilitated Therapy, Woodside, CA; member of NAHRA medical/educational research committee; 20 years experience therapeutic riding; developing handbook of equine experiential learning.

Marcee Rosenzweig, Bsc, PT
Consultant to CANTRA & Ontra, Hippotherapy Development Committee Member, hippotherapy course instructor, 10 years experience in horse therapy programs; NAHRA member

Samuel B. Ross Jr., PhD, BA, MA, EED (Hon)
Past executive director of Green Chimneys Children's Services, 40 years as executive director of a residential school with farm and horseback riding program; Delta Society board member; NARHA member.

Pegi Ryan
Director and instructor of the Helen Wood Animal Care and Education Center & the Therapeutic Riding Program.

Michaela Scheidhacker, MD
Psychiatrist using riding therapy, author of many papers, researcher and presenter in Germany and at International congresses.

Patricia J. Sayler, MA
MA - personality and social psychology; Director - therapeutic riding services, Easter Seal Society of Lehigh Valley & the Poconos, head instructor for Easter Seal (R.I.S.E.); NAHRA Medical Committee, accreditation committee, accreditation task force. NARHA faculty - Hippotherapy Workshops, NAHRA General & Instructor's Courses, NARHA accreditation site visitor; member - AHA & EFMA.

Anita Shkedi, HV,SRN,RSCN obs,TRI
Founder-instructor Therapeutic Riding Club of Israel; director/instructor of certification course through Wingate Institute for physical education; lecturer on therapeutic riding internationally, coach international equestrian team from Israel.

Nancy Spencer
Specialist in equine kinesiotherapy through exercise and education; equine sports physiology since 1978; video - Basic Equine Stretching; clinician in equine kinesio-therapy.

Jan Spink, MA
Founder/director of New Harmony Foundation, 30 years riding experience- hunters, jumpers, dressage, combined training, 18 years field work-lecturing/education with national & international presentations on therapeutic riding, created "developmental vaulting" which later evolved into the treatment method known as "Developmental Riding Therapy" of D.R.T, helped input hippotherapy knowledge from Germany & co-presented first U.S. workshops.

Katherine Splinter, MOT, OTR/L
Assistant professor & level II fieldwork coordinator, Eastern Kentucky University at Richmond, KY; therapeutic riding since 1981, hippotherapy since 1995; NARHA medical committee, registered with AHA; president-board of directors, Central Kentucky Riding for the Handicapped; instructor & therapist.

Jill A. Standquist, OTR/L
Pediatric private practice, NDT certified, certified ski instructor for disabled, advanced hippotherapy course in Germany, member Hippotherapy Development Committee, 8 yrs occupational therapist Pegasus Therapeutic Riding Program, NARHA

Ingrid Strauss, MD
Physician. Held a leading position at the clinic of Dr. Heinz May in Germany. Head of Kuratorium für Therapeutisches Reiten, authored many papers and book contributions, lecturer and presentor at national and international conferences. Since 1975 developed physiotherapeutic treatment with the horse - leader in the use of the horse in therapy . Authored *Hippotherapy: Neurophysiological Therapy on the Horse* - 1995.

Gigi Sweet, BA, M.Ed.
Arizona teaching and supervisory certificate, director of instruction Therapeutic Riding of Tucson, therapeutic riding since 1976. NARHA accreditation committee and workshop faculty; raises and shows Appaloosas horses.

Ann Viviano, OTR, MS/CCC-SLP
NDT advanced course, certified SI & Praxis tests, NARHA registered instructor, hippotherapy 4 years and certified in hippotherapy. Occupational therapist and speech-language pathologist in pediatric rehabilitation.

Walsh, Mary-Beth, BS, PT
Physical therapist-Georgetown University Hospital, BS-Biology, BHSAI Instructor, Lift Me Up Riding Program; 3 years experience therapeutic riding; instructs and treats able bodied riders with low back pain with proper exercises.

Beth Standford Werkheiser, PT
Physical therapist in therapeutic riding and hippotherapy, national and international presentor, lecturer, consultant; past NARHA board member; NDT certified; private pediatric practice and physical therapist at Flying High Equestrian Therapy Inc.

Jill Wham, Dip OT/NZ, OTR
Occupational therapist in New Zealand, therapist with riding program; presentor at international congress.

Amy Wheeler, BS, MS, PT
MS in neurological physical therapy; therapeutic riding since 1983; NARHA advanced instructor, registered with AHA, board of directors AHA , life long equestrian.

Nina Wiger, MA
Microbiology; independent instructor Dressage, vaulting, horse trainer, remedial vaulting, Horsepower, Calif Carousel; 4-H Vaulters, national AVA training clinics; part of NCEFT when remedial & therapeutic vaulting introduced.

Collen Zanin, M. Ed,OTR
Pediatrics, certified therapeutic riding instructor, NDT certified; BHSAI; founder Old Dominion School of Therapeutic Horsemanship Inc, member Wildbad Germany Hippo-therapy Curriculum Development Committee; advanced hippotherapy course in Germany.

Kate Zimmerman, PT, BS, MBA
Director of rehabilitation San Francisco General Hospital; taught 4 years at All Seasons; set up & taught at ran Rehab Ranch, 4 years at All Seasons.

ACKNOWLEDGMENTS

The sixty-two individuals who contributed to this text, from many countries, will be commended for their thoughts and expertise. They gave priority time to assist in making this text informative and to help the reader with the learning process. Many thanks to each of you.

I want to acknowledge Jeanne Moody and Linda McLaughlin of Durango for their fine work in editing this manuscript.

Joann Benjamin must be acknowledged for her comments, corrections and especially her prompt assistance. One can always count on dear Joann.

Most of all I want to thank Jay Engel for taking on all the horse and farm jobs so that I was able to devote my time to the revision of the manuscripts.

Barbara T. Engel

THERAPEUTIC RIDING II
STRATEGIES IN REHABILITATION

CONTENTS

Chapter 7

THE THERAPIST

Chapter 8

THE THERAPY HORSE

Chapter 9

THE THERAPY ENVIRONMENT

Chapter 10

TREATMENT PROCEDURES

Chapter 11

HANDLING THE THERAPY HORSE DURING TREATMENT SESSIONS

Chapter 12

MOUNTING THE CLIENT ASTRIDE THE HORSE

Chapter 13

IMPROVING THE CLIENT'S POSTURE

Chapter 26
DEVELOPMENTAL RIDING THERAPY

Chapter 27

Therapeutic Riding I & II - Strategies for Instruction & Strategies for Rehabilitation
A Cross Reference of Author and Articles

INTRODUCTION

While the use of the horse as a therapeutic modality to treat individuals with disabilities had its formal beginnings in the early 1970s in Germany, Austria and Switzerland, textbooks for therapist education were slow to evolve. The first such text, ***Therapeutisches Reiten*** - Medizin, Pädagogik, Sport, by Wolfgang Heipertz, et. al.[1] was published in Germany in 1977, and translated into English in 1981.[2] This text was a very basic one, covering all of the aspects of therapeutic riding, not just the medically therapeutic modalities. It filled a void. In 1993, Jan Spink published her books ***Developmental Riding Therapy*** - A Team Approach to Assessment and Treatment[3] and its companion book, ***The Therapy Horse*** - A Model for Standards and Competencies.[4] These books, plus a handful of others, formed a good base for the education of the therapists wishing to incorporate the use of equines into their overall treatment approach.

Still, what was missing was one text that covered many aspects of this complex discipline - the use of the horse to treat individuals with disabilities. This is such a text. Barbara Engel, as an occupational therapist registered with the American Hippotherapy Association and a therapist with many years of experience using horses for treatment, as a teacher teaching other therapists about hippotherapy, and as an involved and concerned international educator, saw the need for such an all-encompassing work. She began the odious and difficult task of compiling and editing a multi-author potpourri for the inquiring therapist.

The result is a very in-depth publication that addresses many of the complicated scenarios a therapist using the horse might encounter:
- insights into the therapy horse
- the treatment environment
- treatment plans in this unusual setting
- handling the horse during therapy
- methods and techniques for mounting and improving the posture of the client in hippotherapy
- assessment and evaluation of the client
- sensory- perceptual motor processing.
- psycho-social approaches in the hippotherapy setting
- and, thoughts from and about the physical, occupational, and recreation therapist who work in equestrian therapy.

---

[1] Therapeutisches Reiten - Medizin, Pädagogik, Sport., Wolfgang Heipertz, Christine Heipertz-Hengst, Antonius Kröger, Werner Kuprian, Kurt Zinke, Franckshs Reiterbibliothek, Stuttgart, 1977.

[2] Therapeutic Riding in Medicine, Education and Sport., W. Heipertz, et. al., translated by M. Takeuchi, GRAD Inc., Riverside Dr., Ottawa, Canada K1V 8W6, 1981.

[3] Developmental Riding Therapy, Jan Spink, M.A., Therapy Skill Builders, Tucson, AZ 85733, 1993.

[4] The Therapy Horse, Jan Spink, M.A., Barbara Engel Therapy Services, Durango, Co., 1993.

We owe a debt of gratitude to this conscientious and hard-working editor for putting together such a wide selection of readings, which not only answer many of our most critical questions about using horses to treating people with disabilities, but also challenges us to think more carefully and creatively about the best ways to make use of this valuable treatment option.

Good luck to each reader. Nothing is more gratifying to the treatment therapist than to see a strategy help a client. The horse, when correctly partnered with a knowledgeable therapist, can bring about huge success. So once again, in history, the horse receives accolades, accolades that are well-deserved. What a magnificent animal, and what a wonderful new use of his talents.

And finally a word of caution to each reader - though the horse is a warm and friendly beast, and one that can melt our hearts and help motivate patients where nothing else has worked, he is still a potential danger. The

horse deserves our respect and thorough understanding. Therapy using the horse is not to be undertaken lightly and without rigorous training. The therapist using the horse should be a competent horse person, possess sound basis riding and horse handling skills, understand the unique temperament of the horse, and be able to assess a variety of horses not only for soundness but also for appropriate therapeutic application. A tall order, indeed!

Jean M. Tebay, MS, Director
Therapeutic Riding Services
Baltimore, MD
July, 1997

PREFACE

Therapeutic Riding II Strategies in Rehabilitation contains the essays related to intervention in occupational and physical therapy, speech and language pathology, psycho-social re-education, education, and recreation. The manuscript is a revision and enlargement of the "therapy and intervention sections" of ***Therapeutic Riding Programs: Instruction and Rehabilitation***. Forty-two percent of the articles are new and many of the old articles have been revised. ***Therapeutic Riding I Strategies in Instruction*** and ***Therapeutic Riding II Strategies in Rehabilitation*** are intended to be a set. The information on the horse, the disabilities, equipment and other information will be found in *Therapeutic Riding* I. It is intended that you have access to both volumes

It is hoped that this manuscript will aid the reader in furthering the education process in equine-assisted therapy, hippotherapy, psycho-social facilitation, and educational intervention. There are a number of articles that are not included in this manuscript due to the busy schedules of those potential authors. Their expertise will be missed. Hopefully they will share their knowledge in future publications. Many have presented at conferences but have not published their papers thus their contributions are not accessible.

The field of hippotherapy and equine facilitated psychotherapy is very young. There is much to be learned. Hopefully those of you who continue in the field will explore and search for what is really contributing to the rehabilitation process with the horse. A number of factors have been identified, but isn't there more going on? I think so.

We often "lean" on the information from others. This limits the rehabilitation of future clients. Certain terms and phrases are often repeated by therapists. Are you really sure that only a horse of 14 plus hands is appropriate for all therapy? Is this because you heard it or read about it or has your knowledge come from experience? Are you knowledgeable about the gaits of many breeds of horse and know what matches your client? I wonder. The Germans and Swiss seem to have discovered otherwise. If you are teaching or writing on this subject, have you actually ridden many breeds to gain this knowledge? Some therapists think only the pelvis is mobilized on the horse. They certainly have limited experience riding a horse for when I ride, my whole body is involved. It is not the therapist-teacher-instructor's responsibility to test out information to accurately inform others? I believe it is, if information is to be presented accurately.

This will be the last revision of this book by this editor. There is one more book on the addenda focused on occupational therapy. It is time for me to partially change my focus from work orientation to less stressful activities. Though my interest in the development of the field of therapeutic horseback riding - especially hippotherapy and equine-assisted therapy - will continue, my major focus will turn to my horses. I have an exceptional young Lipizzan stallion with whom I plan to pursue musical dressage to take advantage of his dancing gaits. In addition we now have a Haflinger mare who has produced an exceptional filly - whose grand sire was a Lipizzan from the Spanish Riding School. She favors her sire and will need attention to bring her along. And of course my two Haflinger mares cannot be ignored along with the kids that ride them. I look forward to many hours of working with my Lipizzan stallion, Pluto Lynda and mare Salina, and my Lipizzan/Andalusian stallion Fabio and mare Majoria. I am sure I will learn a great deal from them. Certainly, I will learn from them the sensitive union of horse and rider and how hippotherapy truly work.

With the complection of the sister volume *Therapeutic Riding I Strategies in Instruction* later this year, I will turn over the difficult and immense task of editing future manuscripts of this nature to a younger and experienced therapist and instructor. I wish you well. The task must continue if education in this field is to progress to a higher level of professionalism - a place where it belongs.

Barbara Teichmann Engel
July, 1997
March 2000

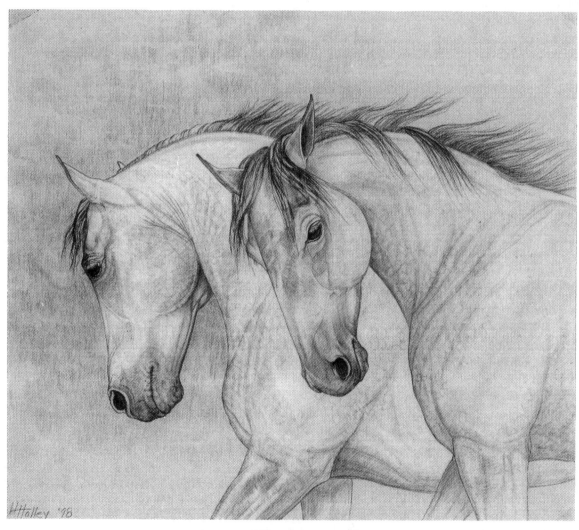

PLUTO LYNDIA (BO) AND SALINA
full registered Lipazzaners
Art work by Heidi Holley of Bayfield, Colorado

XXX

CHAPTER 1

AN INTRODUCTION TO THERAPEUTIC HORSEBACK RIDING

FOUR THERAPEUTIC ASPECTS OF HORSEBACK RIDING FOR THE DISABLED

Jane Copeland Fitzpartick, M.A., P.T.

Therapeutic riding in the United States evolved from two directions -- the adapted sports model practiced in the British Riding for the Disabled programs, and the more clinical model of the Germans and Swiss that emphasizes treatment. The philosophical backgrounds of these two models differ in that the British model promotes mental and physical well-being through riding as a recreational sport, while the German and Swiss clinical model relies on a medical orientation that stresses postural alignment, mobility and symmetry as goals of equestrian activity.

In the United States the adapted sports model and the treatment model have been modified and expanded into the current classification system that recognizes four areas: sport, therapy, education and recreation/leisure. Each area encompasses specific goals and techniques, is appropriate for certain individuals and requires different professional personnel as instructors or therapists. Yet all four areas overlap, complement and support each other (Figure 1) so that while riding for sport and recreation, a student also receives valuable physical and psychological benefits. For example, a young child riding in a program with educational goals is also participating in an enjoyable, exciting sport that contributes to self-esteem. The more than six hundred therapeutic riding programs in the United States vary widely in the populations of people with disabilities they serve, the goals they set for their riders, and in how they deliver their services. Most programs place a high degree of emphasis on the combination of learning a rewarding activity while attaining the best physical and functional levels possible. Within the United States, programs are encouraged to join the North American Riding for the Handicapped Association (NARHA) which sets accreditation standards for therapeutic riding programs and certification standards for instructors. NARHA makes liability and accident insurance available for riders, volunteers, and staff, holds seminars and conferences, promotes education and publishes data on therapeutic riding throughout North America.

It is easy to comprehend the social, recreational, and sport aspects of riding. This is one of the world's oldest and most popular leisure activities. Horseback riding is practiced in nearly every culture by men and women enjoying the close association with an animal. In therapeutic riding, children and adults with disabilities come together with a professional instructor, horse leader, sidewalkers and their special mount to experience a pleasurable activity. They learn the rules of a sport, the techniques of horsemanship, and methods of controlling their bodies to make the human-to-horse interaction meaningful. Students can enjoy practicing skills in indoor and outdoor rings, trail riding, or progressing on to drill team participation, dressage, and equestrian competition. Opportunities to participate in organized equestrian sports events continue to increase throughout the world as is evidenced by local, national, and international Special Olympic events, equestrian competition at the Para-Olympic Games, and at Pony Club Shows open to all qualified riders. When asking students why they ride, the most often heard response is "because I enjoy horseback riding," not because it is therapeutic. The recent shift in America to recognize the quality of life issues facing the person with disabilities is helping make a broader range of adapted sport opportunities available. Therapeutic riding is a leader in demonstrating how an adapted sport can become a meaningful recreation alternative for people with varying disabilities.

Less obvious to the observer but of equal importance in therapeutic riding, are psychotherapeutic and educational goals such as sequencing, teamwork, right-left discrimination, and following directions--goals that can be addressed as a horse and rider maneuver through an obstacle course. A relay race on horseback can be highly motivating while demanding attention to other riders in the ring and cooperation among teammates to achieve success. Hurrying, becoming verbally or physically abusive, or quitting has immediate negative results in the horse withholding the desired behavior or with the student's removal from the highly motivating opportunity to ride. Students develop a rapport with their teammate, and the horse, and they must concentrate to achieve the goals of their individual lesson.

A wide range of equine related activities are used to address physical, psychological, cognitive, behavioral, and communication goals. An example of an integrated lesson plan for a Down Syndrome child could be the following:

A. In one session the child rides in a saddle with stirrups and works on the posting trot in preparation for competition in Special Olympics.
B. In another session, the same child rides on a sheepskin fleece, sitting erect without holding on, developing trust and staying centered while the horse trots on the lunge line.

It is this combination of interesting and challenging experiences that makes therapeutic riding so motivating for the rider and interesting for professionals and volunteers. NARHA has established three organizational sections within the association's overall structure to address clients' special needs. The three sections of NARHA are the:

American Hippotherapy Association (AHA)
Competition Association of NARHA (CAN)
Equine Facilitated Mental Health Association (EFMHA)

In therapeutic riding the use of the horse by health care specialists to treat specific movement dysfunctions is called hippotherapy — laterally "treatment with the help of the horse." Hippotherapy is carried out by physical, occupational and speech therapists working with a horse expert and a specially trained horse. The client's role is not to influence or control the horse, but to actively respond by posturally adapting to the horse's guided movement. The rider's center of gravity is continually displaced with each step the horse takes, causing the rider to accommodate these changes with muscular activity and control to remain centered on his or her mount. Movement exploration including reaching and touching the moving horse, varying sitting postures, and performing graded exercises all accomplish goals of postural control and sensory integration. Arousal level, attending, body positions in space plus integration of sight, sound and motion all come into play as the multiple systems of the human-horse team act and react.

Equine assisted psychotherapy, another area of specialization within therapeutic riding, integrates the treatment protocols of the psychologist, psychiatrist and behavior specialist into equine activities. This form of treatment demonstrates the capability of the horse to assist the individual in realizing behavioral and emotional goals. In equine assisted psychotherapy, both on the ground and off the ground, equine activities are used to develop a sense of self, increase levels of trust, establish boundaries, and create awareness of the needs of living creatures through responsible care of the horse.

Every rider presents a unique set of abilities. Therapeutic riding develops lesson plans that build on and modify present abilities enabling clients better to meet the challenges of daily living. Meaningful lesson plans can often be formed by combining goals from all areas of therapeutic riding. An integrated lesson focuses on treatment goals from many perspectives while at the same time addressing quality of life issues. However, there are times where a client needs to effect a change or achieve a goal in a more proscribed area. In these instances professionally designed treatment plans carried out by medically licensed personnel use the unique attributes of the horse in specific treatments. All therapeutic riding sessions require teamwork, and whatever the goals are for a particular lesson and whatever the orientation is of the particular therapeutic riding team, the ultimate goal is to maximize each client's functional potential. As is true in any activity, the participant's perception of accomplishment and joy in achievement remain paramount.

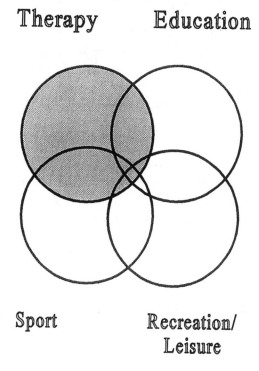

Therapeutic Riding Classifications
North American Riding for the Handicapped

Figure 1.

The Horse

Oh horse you are a wondrous thing,
No buttons to push, no engine that pings.
You start yourself, no clutch to slip,
No dead battery, no gears to strip.
No license buying every year,
With plates to screw on front and rear.
No gas fumes polluting each day,
Taking the joys of nature away.
No speed cops dashing into view,
Writing a ticket out to you.

Your super-treads all seem OK,
And hoofpick in hand, they should stay that way.
Your spark plugs never miss and fuss,
Your motor never makes us cuss,
Your frame is good for many a mile,
Your body never outdates its style.
Your needs are few, and happily met,
We honor you, we're in your debt!
You serve us well, as our riders you carry,
Making instructors, volunteers - the whole team merry.

Yes, Horse, you are a wondrous thing,
Teacher--Therapist--Friend,
your praises we sing!

Jean M. Tebay

WHEN IS THERAPEUTIC RIDING HIPPOTHERAPY?

Barbara Heine, P.T.

By it's very nature, **therapeutic riding** influences the whole person and the effect on all the body's systems can be profound. With an ever increasing number of people today seeking alternatives to traditional methods of treatment, it comes as no surprise that therapeutic riding or equine related therapies are as popular as they are effective. It was, therefore, a natural progression for therapeutic riding in North America to branch into the medical application of the horse - hippotherapy. Unfortunately, the use of this overall term has led to many misconceptions among therapeutic riding professionals.

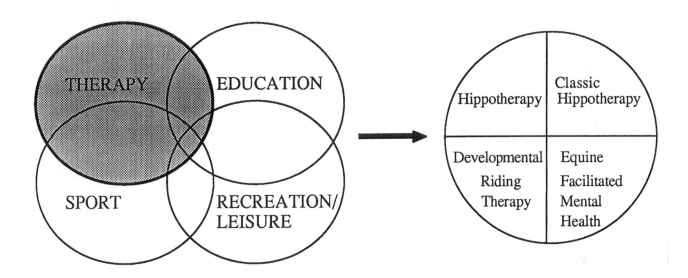

Figure 1.   Figure 2.

To delineate the four major areas relevant to therapeutic riding, North American Riding for the Handicapped Association [NARHA] has defined a model of four equal circles intersecting with the horse as the central focus (figure 1.) This article will address the therapy circle (figure 2), in an effort to dispel the confusion surrounding hippotherapy.

Any riding program using horse related activities for clients with physical, mental, cognitive, social or behavioral problems is a therapeutic riding program. When, therefore, does therapeutic riding become **hippotherapy** or **classic hippotherapy,** and what exactly is **developmental riding therapy**? Following are some examples of frequently asked questions.

A physical therapist (PT) volunteers in a consulting capacity once a month. Does this mean that your program offers hippotherapy?

An occupational therapist (OT) with a solid horse background consults for your program once a week and works one on one with selected clients to address specific areas of motor planning and sensory integration. The horse for these clients has been selected carefully for its movement and behavioral qualities. You notice that the therapist chooses to use a vaulting surcingle for these sessions and in each session the client assumes different positions on the horse such as kneeling and quadruped (on all fours). Is this hippotherapy, developmental riding therapy, or therapeutic riding?

Your program has a physical therapist who leases your facility and horses to provide hippotherapy treatment for several clients each week. The therapist bills each client directly. The clients sit astride the horse facing forward and backward, and occasionally are placed prone over the barrel. The therapist directs the treatment by advising the horse handler when changes in tempo and direction are required. Is this classic hippotherapy or hippotherapy?

Your therapeutic riding program has recently received a grant to purchase a trained vaulting horse. You plan to select several clients whom you feel would benefit enormously from this type of activity. One of your volunteers has had previous vaulting experience and is willing to work closely with your therapeutic riding instructor to develop this group activity. Will this be hippotherapy, developmental riding therapy, or therapeutic riding in the area of recreation and leisure?

Your therapeutic riding program would like to expand its services to include hippotherapy because there are several clients that you believe would benefit from a more specific one-on-one approach. A PT in a local sports medicine practice is very keen to become involved and he or she has ridden as a recreational sport as a child. What additional qualifications would this therapist need to provide direct hippotherapy treatment for these clients?

Questions like these highlight the often subtle differences between these various applications of the horse in a therapeutic setting. In today's litigious society, it is essential that people involved with therapeutic riding programs are informed not only about the role that a therapist can play, but also the requirements, qualifications and training necessary if that therapist is providing a direct service. It is the aim of this article to clarify these issues.

Hippotherapy literally means treatment with the help of a horse, from the Greek work "hippos", meaning horse. More specifically it is the 3-dimensional movement of the horse's hips and pelvis as the hind legs move forward at the walk that provides a movement challenge to the client.

Classic hippotherapy is so called because it reflects the German model of hippotherapy practiced widely throughout Europe since the 1960's. Since it is purely the horse's movement and the client's responses that constitute the treatment, classic hippotherapy should only be carried out by a physical, occupational therapist, or a speech and language pathologist with a certificate of clinical competence (SLP/CCC) who has focused his or her training in the following areas:

1. Development of body systems and interaction with the development of movement.
2. Effect of neuromuscular, musculoskeletal, cardiovascular, and a pulmonary dysfunction on growth and development, motor development and function.

In classic hippotherapy it is purely the horse's movement that influences the client. The client may be positioned astride the horse facing forward, backward, prone, or supine. The client interacts with, and responds to, the horse's movement. The therapist's responsibility is constantly to analyze the client's responses and adjust accordingly, the manner in which the horse is moving. This assumes that the therapist has sufficient understanding of the movement of the horse to direct the experienced horse handler/therapeutic riding instructor to alter the tempo and direction of the horse as indicated by the client's responses.

The primary focus of classic hippotherapy is the rider's posture and movement responses. However, other effects can and do occur in areas such as respiration, cognition and speech production. For example, if the treating therapist is a PT and his or her primary focus is to strengthen the trunk muscles and positively affect the client's posture, respiration and speech will improve as a consequence of the increases in trunk strength. That is the beauty of the horse as a treatment tool; these "other" changes occur although one is not focusing on them.

Hippotherapy, on the other hand, is a treatment approach that uses the movement of the horse based on the methodology of classic hippotherapy with the addition of the treatment principles that apply to the particular profession of the therapist providing the service. Hippotherapy can be applied by a physical therapist, an occupational therapist, a speech pathologist, a psychologist, or a psychotherapist.

It is a treatment approach that uses activities on the horse that are meaningful to the client and specifically address the particular goals established for that client. Hippotherapy provides a controlled environment and graded sensory input designed to elicit appropriate adaptive responses from the client. It does not teach specific skills associated with being on a horse, but it provides a foundation of improved neuromotor function and sensory processing that can be generalized to a wide variety of activities outside treatment. In other words, the client's adaptive responses to the environment and the horse's movement ultimately cause improvements in function.

Although hippotherapy is frequently used to achieve purely physical goals, it also affects psychological, cognitive, social, behavioral, and communication outcomes. The unique combination of the horse, the horse's movement and an environment that is not clinical gives hippotherapy a multidisciplinary nature making it an ideal co-treatment tool. In this extraordinary environment, all systems of the body are affected and co-treatments with, for instance, a physical/occupational therapist or occupational/speech therapist are particularly effective. An example of the way in which multiple systems of the body are affected is in the use of developmental positions. A young client may be asked to move from facing forwards to facing backwards and then to a quadruped (on all fours). In this position he or she may be asked to reach one hand down to pat the horse. This one activity (the transition, the quadruped position and the reaching activity), is overlaid on the constant rhythmical three-dimensional movement of the horse. Therefore, in addition to the facilitation of automatic postural responses and stimulation of trunk muscles, there are increases in sensory stimulation to the following systems of the body:
- vestibular - because the client is facing backwards while the horse is moving forwards
- proprioceptive - heavy touch pressure through the hips, knees, wrists, elbows and shoulder joints in the quadruped position
- tactile touching the soft warm coat of the horse.

This is a meaningful activity for any client who exhibits trunk weakness, poor pelvic control, decreased gross motor skills, poor motor planning and a diminished ability to process sensory information.

Developmental riding therapy is distinguished from either **classic hippotherapy** or **hippotherapy** by its broader professional participation, more diverse client population, and equine skills/training specific to the areas of dressage, horse-handling, and vaulting. Jan Spink, M.A., developed this technique in the late 1980's to address a growing need for a more specific philosophy and methodology that focused on a multidisciplinary approach to therapeutic riding. This approach incorporates the treatment techniques and expertise of six health or education professions: physical therapy, occupational therapist, speech therapy, rehabilitation or psychomotricity, special education, and psychology.

Some fundamental and distinctive elements of developmental riding therapy are:
1. Individual sessions with active therapist input, a client-centered focus, and graded control of sensory stimuli during mounted and non-mounted activities.

2. Use of developmental positions on the horse that directly correlate with specifically controlled movement challenges from the horse.

3. Development of interrelationships among the client, therapist, and horse.

4. Selected components of riding and vaulting skills.

5. Use of a horse that has been carefully screened for movement and behavioral qualities.

Developmental riding therapy involves the use of therapists or specialists who are thoroughly trained in horsemanship and in the philosophy and methods of equine-assisted therapy and the specific features of the system of developmental riding therapy (Spink 1987, 1990.) Developmental riding therapy can serve as an entry point for clients whose skills are not yet well enough developed for therapeutic group riding or vaulting. For the hippotherapy client who has met all long term goals, developmental riding therapy is an ideal transition to another program. The client is able to continue therapy in the highly motivating and pleasurable environment of the horse, but is provided with greater challenges through the use of specific riding or vaulting skills.

The Therapist's Role in Therapeutic Riding
If you are currently involved in the operation of a therapeutic riding program and are considering expanding your services to include hippotherapy here are some guidelines as to the qualifications, responsibilities and training requirements of therapists wishing to practice hippotherapy. Keep in mind, the use of the horse as a treatment tool does not mean that a therapist is a "hippotherapist" any more than an occupational therapist, using the principles of sensory integration, is a sensory integrationist, or a physical therapist using a pool is a hydrotherapist.

Any therapist providing direct treatment services in a classic hippotherapy or hippotherapy program must meet the following qualifications:

1. Is licensed or registered to practice a nationally recognized health care profession.

2. Maintains current professional liability insurance.

3. Has received training in the principles of classic hippotherapy, equine movement, and equine psychology through attendance at a minimum of one American Hippotherapy Association (AHA) approved 3-4 day course, "Introduction to Classic Hippotherapy." The completion of this course is one of the requirements of any therapist wishing to be registered with the AHA.

4. Is an NARHA registered instructor (minimum level) and if not, has an NARHA registered instructor assisting with all treatment sessions.

Legally, a therapist must be in direct attendance to the client at all times during a session. If a therapist, operating within the scope of their professional practices act, is conducting a group session, they will be actively engaged in the treatment of the whole group and focusing on each client, as and when appropriate. In such a case, treatment progress notes must be kept on each client in the group.

To practice hippotherapy, the treatment principles of a particular health profession are integrated into the hippotherapy setting. The actual treatment on the horse is only one part of a comprehensive treatment program that begins with an initial evaluation. A crucial part of this initial evaluation is the establishment of a treatment plan that incorporates both long and short term goals. Long term goals must be functional and relevant to each client's family/school/work situation; therefore, consultation with the client's family is necessary.

The treatment plan is developed based on the professional training and constraints of the professional practice act of the particular health professional providing the service. Choosing the horse whose movement best addresses the client's needs and appropriate equipment to facilitate the desired responses is an integral part of the treatment plan. Regular documentation is provided through progress notes recorded after each treatment.

Re-evaluation of each client should be carried out at 3-6 month intervals (or less, depending on the reimbursement source) to ensure that the treatment plan and treatment goals remain appropriate for the client. There will be occasions when re-evaluation confirms that a client has met/or not met all the long term goals and in the therapist's professional opinion, hippotherapy can no longer address the needs of that client. In this case, the client should be discharged from hippotherapy. It is the responsibility of the treating therapist to write a discharge summary and to communicate directly with the client and/or client's family to recommend further treatment such as physical therapy, occupational therapy or speech therapy, or a transition into another program. In the case of a client meeting all long term goals, an ideal opportunity is presented to transition that client to a therapeutic riding program where the learning of "real" riding (or vaulting) skills can add a new and exciting dimension to their lives. If the client's functional abilities and motivation are high it is quite likely that they can make the transition to able-bodied riding or vaulting classes or competitive equine sports.

Additional Roles For Therapists:
Therapists have much to offer any therapeutic riding program and may become involved in roles other than direct client service. These can include:

1. Consultation

2. Staff and volunteer training in body mechanics, physical and cognitive impairments, basic handling/transfer skills, precautions and contraindications

3. Community education

4. Liaison with the medical community

5. Recruitment of additional health care professionals

6. Referral of clients

By helping in this way, a therapist has an opportunity to observe the innumerable qualities of the horse as a treatment tool. This can often be such an enlightening experience that the therapist will be motivated to gain the additional skills and training necessary to provide direct service to some of your clients. Therapeutic riding instructors should remember that very few therapists come equipped with horse knowledge and riding skills. You can therefore help each other grow and learn.

The hippotherapy team of horse, client, sidewalkers, therapist, and therapeutic riding instructor are a wonderful example of a symbiotic relationship. No one part can operate without the other and the greater the harmony that exists among all members of the team, the greater the benefit to the client. The client's safety, progress and happiness after all, is the reason all of us love what we do and continue to strive to be better at it.

Author's note (1997):
At this time, a process does not exist for certification in hippotherapy in the US. Therapists wishing to practice hippotherapy must meet certain qualifications that include being registered with the AHA or working under the supervision of a therapist registered *with* the AHA.

It is not within the scope of this article to extrapolate these qualifications. For readers wanting more information, please contact the NARHA office.

REFERENCES:
1. Spink, J. (1993). *Developmental Riding Therapy - A Team Approach To Assessment and Treatment*; Therapy Skill Builders, a division of Communication Skill Builders.
2 *Hippotherapy Standards. 1995.* Draft 3/95; Approved by the AHA, March 4, 1995.

AMERICAN HIPPOTHERAPY ASSOCIATION POSITION PAPER ON THE PRESENT USE OF HIPPOTHERAPY IN THE UNITED STATES

American Hippotherapy Association
April 1996

Hippotherapy treatment using the multidimensional movement of the horse, has become a tool of choice for health professionals working with clients with a wide variety of problems especially those with movement dysfunctions. Hippotherapy is the overall term used to include a variety of applications of the use of the horse in treatment provided by physical therapists, occupational therapists and speech therapists. In hippotherapy a number of theoretical bases are used as a rationale of how to vary the use of the horse for specific client populations and functional outcomes. It is presently assumed that the success of hippotherapy can be explained by a number of existing theoretical models of treatment including but not limited to: sensory integration, motor learning, motor control, dynamical systems and psycholinguistic theories.

Hippotherapy as a tool has been used in treatments to achieve functional outcomes in therapy in the United States since the late 1970's. It has been used internationally for over 30 years. Hippotherapy is presently recognized as a treatment modality by 24 countries. In order to provide a forum for education, communication and research among health professionals using hippotherapy, the American Hippotherapy Association (AHA) was formed in 1992. It became an official Section of the North American Riding for the Handicapped Association (NARHA) in 1993. The AHA is composed primarily of physical therapists, occupational therapists, speech and language pathologists and others interested in utilizing the horse in treatment.

Hippotherapy is one part of a comprehensive treatment program. Treatment is based on an initial evaluation with the establishment of functional goals and a treatment plan. Regular documentation is provided through progress notes. A treatment plan is developed based on the professional training and constraints of the professional practice act of the particular health professional delivering the service (physical therapy, occupational therapist, speech/language pathologist). Treatment sessions are provided on an individual basis or in small groups directly by the licensed health care profession.

Therapists are encouraged to pursue specialized training in the use of the horse in treatment. AHA has developed a 3-4 day-standardized course "Introduction to Classic Hippotherapy - Principles and Applications" that provides a thorough overview. In 1997, the AHA was in the process of developing three intermediate level continuing education courses. Clinicians in the field have offered a number of other continuing education programs directly related to hippotherapy every year since 1984. AHA provides therapist registration that indicates that a therapist has met minimal educational and practice requirements in hippotherapy as determined by the AHA Registration and Standards Committee. AHA has developed hippotherapy program standards to be used in NARHA program accreditation where hippotherapy is offered as part of a treatment plan. Competencies focusing on the clinical and equine skills needed by health professionals using hippotherapy in their practice are currently being developed. Once the competencies are completed, it is projected that a certification process would be implemented within the following three to four years.

Since 1982, third party reimbursement has been commonly received for treatment that has included hippotherapy from a wide variety of insurance companies across the nation. Since hippotherapy is not presently considered one unique treatment, a variety of CPT-4 codes have been used to reflect the particular treatment application in which the horse is used and the particular profession of the therapist. The codes commonly used have included those for: therapeutic exercise, neuromuscular education, kinetic activities-therapeutic activities, sensory integrative activities, and individual speech therapy. Within the treatment session a variety of other treatment techniques other than the use of the horse are typically included such as soft tissue mobilization, joint mobilization, gait training, activities of daily living/self care, and others.

It is considered standard practice in professions that using experiential functional activities in natural environmental settings provides the client with one of the best opportunities to achieve functional outcomes. The horse can be considered a treatment tool used in a variety of ways just as a gymnastic ball, scooter board and suspended equipment can be used for a variety of purposes. The horse can also be used to provide select experiential activities in a natural environment just as a farm, a pumpkin canning activity, dance or a water environment can be used in different ways based on the treatment goals and the theoretical model being used by the therapist.

Horses used within hippotherapy need to meet criteria regarding movement quality, temperament and training. Even when an ideal horse is used, the treatment quality and results are based on the specialized hippotherapy training of the therapists, their clinical experience and expertise and how well they integrate the use of the horse into a comprehensive treatment program suitable for each client. Putting a client on a generic horse and having the horse move randomly is not considered hippotherapy and will not produce functional motor outcome in a consistent or efficient manner.

Hippotherapy as a tool is becoming widely accepted as a standard of practice by health care professionals. There are a number of universities including Springfield College, Columbia University, University of California at San Francisco, University of New Mexico, Colorado State University, and the University of Kentucky that specifically place their health professional students in affiliations that offer hippotherapy as a treatment option. A number of school districts pay for school-based therapy that includes hippotherapy in the treatment plan because it produces educationally relevant functional outcomes. In a number of states Medicare, Medicaid, and Medicaid waiver programs have paid for therapy services that include hippotherapy. Continuing education CEU's are routinely approved for courses approved by AHA and provided by clinicians with recognized expertise in hippotherapy. Articles on the use of the horse in treatment have been published in peer reviewed journals such as *Physical Therapy* and *Physical and Occupational Therapy in Pediatrics* as well as numerous articles in clinical publications. Presentations on hippotherapy have been given at regional, national and international professional conferences.

At this point in time, most health professionals in the United States are familiar with the concept of using the horse to achieve functional change in clients. For many health professionals, hippotherapy has become a tool of choice when working with clients with a wide variety of problems, especially those with a movement dysfunction.

May be reprinted by permission from the AHA.

CHAPTER 2

THE RIDER'S VIEW OF THEIR REHABILITATION

HOW THERAPEUTIC HORSEBACK RIDING WAS INSTRUMENTAL IN MY REHABILITATION

Sandy Dota

In 1980 while out trail riding, my horse was spooked by a dog, causing me to fall. The result of that fall was a spinal cord injury from a broken back. This injury left me a paraplegic. I have no use of my legs or control of my bodily functions from the waist down. When I came out of surgery, the doctor told me I would probably never walk again. I appreciated his honesty. Over the next few months, I would realize how my accident would create a major change in my life and that of my family. Not walking again would be only <u>one</u> of the many difficulties I'd have to learn to endure.

My main inconvenience has been loss of bowel and bladder control. Fear of incontinence or an embarrassing accident dictates where I can go and for how long. Usually, I didn't care to go anywhere at anytime. Being seen in public as a disabled person and in a wheelchair also made me extremely uncomfortable. During the first two years, I hardly left my house (except my excursions to the stable). Going to shopping malls was a horror because I felt everyone was staring at me. I no longer felt like a customer or typical shopper. I saw myself as this big clumsy obstacle in everyone's way. I got to the point where I just refused to go to stores which put an additional burden on my husband. I had lost all self-confidence and much self-esteem. This was not a good feeling.

I had a real need. I was not much good for myself or my family. Rehab and medical professionals were not much help. Their job was to constantly remind me of "reality" and the "real world" according to everyone else's point of view. I heard things like, "you've got to learn to adjust," or "you've got to learn to live with it." No encouragement was ever positive or upbeat. And you can just forget horseback riding, 'cause that doesn't fit into their reality at all; paraplegics CANNOT RIDE HORSES!

I was convinced of this until I came across an article in a newspaper about the Cheff Center for the Handicapped in Augusta, Michigan. The article focused on therapeutic horseback riding. From the information sent to me, I found out therapeutic riding is rehabilitative emotionally as well as physically, and at the same time it can be recreational. For me, just the thought of riding again was exciting and overwhelming. I was informed by the Cheff Center to contact Mrs. Octavia Brown at the Somerset Hills Handicapped Riding Club in Bedminster, N.J. After a "go ahead" from my surgeon, and a lot of "I hope you know what you are doing" from my family and friends, I was back in the saddle only ten months after my accident, this time on the back of a beautiful mare called Brandy. My own horse put me in the chair; Brandy took me out.

Animals have that innate ability to break through emotional barriers that drugs and the medical profession have difficulty accomplishing. Animals meet a human being's needs of honesty and affection, creating a valuable friendship. Most people would be astonished to think this is possible with a horse, but they have not met the horses and ponies in therapeutic riding programs.

My riding lessons had begun with a leader at Brandy's head and a side-walker on each side of me for balance and support. It took two years of lessons before I could be weaned of one side-walker, then the other, and finally the leader. I was now an independent rider again, just me and my horse, walking around the ring with an occasional bit of trotting. Although this was enough to make me happy, it was not enough for Brandy; she expected more of me. She taught me to trust her, and she would help me learn, by not always being consistent, to balance myself to increase my riding ability. Brandy was always totally tuned into my body and its needs. She ignored my distracting legs as they flopped and banged at her sides, all the while encouraging me to use my upper body for control and balance. She could transform the most timid personality into an assertive, self-confident individual. Although this horse may seem special or remarkable, almost every therapeutic riding program has a "Brandy." She is a representation of the personality and attitude required before a horse is accepted into a therapeutic riding program.

For me, Brandy represented a transition in my life, a kind of stepping stone. My weekly riding lessons with Brandy were all I looked forward to. She didn't care about my wheelchair or my disability; she responded only to my feelings for her. She made me feel worthwhile. Because she was so nurturing to me, I grew to trust her completely. In doing so, my riding improved dramatically. I was becoming more confident in myself and my capabilities, dwelling less and less on what I could <u>not</u> do. With Brandy, I began doing riding exhibitions and even started competing in horse shows. I couldn't imagine something like this was possible for any paraplegic, much less me. Through Brandy, I was allowed to find another reality, one I could learn to adjust to or live with; hers was not the reality of resignation and adjustment, but of "can do." Trust in her gave me the self-esteem I needed to progress and the self-confidence to follow through.

In 1985 I earned a position on the New Jersey Cerebral Palsy/Les Autres Equestrian Team and competed very successfully on the national level. We received the Governor's Trophy and New Jersey State Horse person of the Year award for 1985. This award had been given the previous year to the U.S. Olympic Equestrian Team. So as you can see, we were in pretty good company! Another rider from Somerset Hills and I were among fourteen top disabled riders in the U.S. who were invited to participate in Inspire '85, an event chaired by Nancy Reagan. We did three performances of a musical Pas de Deux on the Capitol Mall in Washington, D.C. My riding pursuits have since taken me and my family all over the U.S. and Canada. I have also taken an active interest in carriage driving and was reserve champion in 1988 at an ADS (American Driving Society) sanctioned show in New Jersey. When not competing in horse shows, I am working at them. I've been show secretary, scribe for dressage judges, and am also a judge myself (certified with the American Judging Association). I have also completed an instructors' training course to instruct horseback riding to people with disabilities and have been teaching since 1985. I have been on the faculty (in the instructor's position) of NARHA's[1] General Workshop and Instructor Workshop.

I currently have a horse that is being trained "in lightness" by Jean-Claude Racinet (a master of riding in lightness). This principle involves the absolute lightness of the horse to the hands, seat and legs of the rider. As the training progresses, the horse performs more and more in a self-maintained impulsion, carriage and collection, the rider practicing an almost permanent release of the aids. My personal goal is to perform higher level dressage exercises using the *lightness* approach, but the ultimate result will show how a horse trained in lightness can increase the abilities of disabled riders as well as able-bodied riders.

You are reading about the same person who several years ago could not handle being seen in public in a wheelchair, and at that time whose closest friend was a horse. True, even today when I go to shopping malls, people still stare. That's human nature. But, it's not my problem anymore. My chair is just a tool, something to make my life easier, just as eyeglasses are a tool to help someone see better. The point is, I go and I do. I now have the courage to at least try. My husband and my son are happy to have our household back to "normal" again. I've become very busy and totally committed to supporting and promoting therapeutic horseback riding and driving and their benefits.

"Who would have thought the same thing that put me in a wheelchair, namely horseback riding, would be the same thing to get me "back on my feet again" so to speak?

Sandy

[1] NARHA: North American Riding for the Handicapped Association, P.O. Box 33150, Denver, CO USA

A RIDER'S PERSPECTIVE

Arthur S. Hansen, DDS

Readers of this section should know that I am writing as a rider who is hemiplegic as a result of a right cerebral hemorrhage (CVA) in 1982 and subsequent brain surgery in 1983. Prior to the foregoing, I was an active dentist in a private practice and showed no signs of problems of the nature described. I also had no previous riding experience or contact with horses other than occasional "hack" rides as a teenager.

Since my surgery in 1983, I have attended rehabilitation sessions in which physical and occupational therapists used Bobath techniques. My riding began in 1984 during a particularly depressive period, more or less as a last resort. This last resort saved my life. The information I will share with you has been developed through a mentor/rider program, hippotherapy program and individual evaluation and experiment program. I ride for therapy; riding is secondary to therapy. **My riding has been** *"my therapy"* **whether it was hippotherapy, therapeutic riding or just riding on the Alaskan trails.**

The Horse

The horse is the most important element in therapy or therapeutic riding and the instructor must know and understand the horse. The ability of the horse will dictate the therapy that the rider will receive. In a controlled situation, the instructor must know how to engage the horse to gain the movement pattern that the therapist has requested for the rider. The instructor must know and understand the communications of the horse (i.e., tail swishing, head shaking) so as to develop the horse's potential for a rider. Not only must the instructor understand this aspect of the horse, but the horse's behavioral characteristics must be taught to the rider (if the rider is able to understand). This is an important aspect of rider improvement especially if sensory systems are impaired. The horse can replace these impairments to some degree if the rider and instructor are sensitive to the horse's actions. The higher the training level of the horse, the more this is true, due to the higher level of sensitivity of the horse to the rider's actions (i.e., leg pressure from high leg tone may cause the horse to do side passes or move sideways). The challenge in such a situation is for the rider to adjust the pressure or change position so as to stop or prevent unwanted movement of the horse. In this way the trained horse becomes the therapist by eliciting desirable activity from the rider. It cannot be over-emphasized how important the horse is to the rider.

The Horse Trainer

The trainer probably holds the key to the success of any therapeutic riding program or individual's therapy on horseback because it is the trainer who must be relied on to train the horse so it can be used to its fullest potential. The better the horse is trained, the greater it can be utilized in therapeutic riding. In order to do this, the trainer must understand how the horse is to be used by the rider and what must be done to draw the desired results out of the horse. In order to do this, the trainer must confer with the therapist, instructor and therapy team members.

The Therapist

The therapist must have determined a goal or several goals and a plan to attain them. The goals should be presented to the rider, instructor and the therapeutic riding team. Once this is done, the team can synergistically develop the best way to proceed. The therapist is the monitoring person for the rider to assure that the program progresses, is challenging, and that it is producing the desired results with the fewest side effects.

The Instructor

The instructor must instill confidence and enthusiasm for what the rider is doing. The primary goal of any therapeutic riding instructor should be to assist in integrating a medically, physically, or mentally compromised person into a society that considers itself "normal." It is to this end that all activities involving a client should be directed. In the process, the activities involved should in no way be demeaning or patronizing. Remember, riders are people too, and should be treated as such. They are not "problems" housed in a body, but people with a problem. In many cases they are extraordinary people who show courage, perseverance and drive beyond the norm. It also must be remembered that were it not for these people and their needs, there would be no need for the therapeutic riding programs. These riders need the instructors, but it must never be forgotten that the program is for the riders and the benefits they derive from it and not vice versa.

Challenge plays an important part in eliciting therapeutic progress. It is important for the instructors to challenge the riders, but at the same time they must monitor and minimize risks involved. Risk removal should not be carried to extremes, however, so as not to stifle the inner need for challenge. The risk-taking is very important in eliciting progress from the client. A rider's program also should be dynamic. Push the limits of the rider at each session. Vary activities for or during each session to keep the rider's interest. If the rider is able to talk, involve him in the activities and get feed-back on the results.

Find out what the rider likes or does not like, whether he has pain or not. Don't forget, however, that the rider's reactions will change as he progresses. Don't assume that things are static. If the program established for the rider is dynamic and progressive, noticeable changes can take place in a week or two, or even during a session, depending on the duration and frequency of the sessions. This will depend on the rider and the trainer's ability to accommodate him or her in the program. Once goals have been achieved, new goals should be developed, but the old goals should be incorporated in the process of attaining the new goals so progress is not lost, but reinforced.

The Volunteer It is the volunteer's job to assist the instructors and/or therapist to see that the sought-after goals are achieved by the rider. At the same time goals are being pursued, it must be remembered that progress is not always forward. Many things such as illness, depression or other outside distractions may impede progress. The volunteer must realize this and adjust to it. The rider may or may not realize ground has been lost and it is often only the urging and persistence of the volunteer that carries the rider through the rough times. A friendly smile means more than one could ever realize when the rider is in need.

Possibly the greatest improvement in riders will be in the areas of psychological well-being and self-esteem. The volunteer can play an important role in this area by praising the rider when it is earned and by keeping the rider interested and focused on the riding session.

Accomplishment is an important part of improving one's sense of well-being and renewing self-esteem. It is an important aspect of the volunteer's job to reinforce this sense of accomplishment as goals are attained. This can be done by direct observation and comment or indirectly by starting at higher levels of difficulty as goals are attained. BE DYNAMIC, but above all, BE PATIENT, because progress is often painstakingly slow. The words of my instructor to "hurry slowly" seem appropriate. He was speaking of training horses, but I believe it applies equally well to the therapeutic rider.

The Rider
The rider, next to the horse, has the most important job of all. If therapeutic riding is going to be successful, the rider must communicate in his or her own way with the therapeutic riding team and the horse. The rider must be consistent and persistent in his or her riding activities if established goals are going to be attained. My experience, with input from others, shows that progress is slow in a once-a-week program and all efforts should be made to ride at least three days a week, or seven days a week if possible. Progress is patterned and sequential and the more the patterns can be repeated on a regular basis, the greater the progress.

Children and adult riders should not be mixed--this can be embarrassing and demeaning for the adults and hinder progress; even grouping persons with different disabilities can cause problems, i.e., hypertonic and hypotonic in the same class (each of these requires different activities). Be careful not to tell the rider he or she can not do something if he or she really can. It may be your or someone else's perception that he or she can not in order to remove a risk. It could also inhibit challenge-taking and stop progress. Neither safety nor a rider's need for challenge need

be compromised, as long as thought is given to both for a progressive and dynamic therapeutic riding plan. This certainly requires a delicate balance at times, and all factors must be considered on a "value-to-the-rider" basis. For the rider, frequent and consistent therapeutic riding is an effective adjunct to clinic therapy. The therapy or therapeutic riding team (horse, trainer, instructor, therapist, and volunteers) must think in terms of progress and change in order to assist the rider to attain his full potential.

My riding has been "my therapy" whether it was hippotherapy, therapeutic riding or just hacking on the Alaskan trails. My horse is "my therapist" and facilitates my therapy with or without my own assistance or anyone elses."

CHAPTER 3

RESEARCH REVIEW

The Review of Research in Therapeutic Riding

Karen P. DePauw, Ph.D.

A comprehensive review of the research on therapeutic horseback riding was undertaken and reported by DePauw in 1986. Based upon a review of the literature, she wrote of the need to: "... (a) collect empirical evidence supporting the claimed benefits, (b) develop appropriate evaluation instruments/tools, (c) identify effective intervention techniques, (d) provide for accessibility of publications/information from Europe, and (e) develop printed materials and audiovisuals for the health professional community" (DePauw, 1986).

Less than ten years later, significant progress has been made in each of the five recommendations identified above. Instrumental to the progress made in the last two recommendations are the efforts of the editor (B. Engel[1]) and authors of this book, organizations such as the North American Riding for the Handicapped Association (NARHA) and the Delta Society, national and international conferences on Therapeutic Riding and their published abstracts and proceedings, and the efforts of numerous individuals (e.g., L. McCowan[2], J. Tebay[3], F. Joswick[4]) in disseminating information worldwide.

In addition, progress has been made in establishing the empirical bases for valid, accurate assessment and in effective therapeutic riding intervention programs. This progress is due to the efforts of such individuals as J. Copeland, R. Dismuke-Blakely, B. Glasow, J. Tebay, and V.M. Fox among others. The purpose of this section is to provide the reader with a brief synopsis of current research in North America on therapeutic riding and to offer a suggested framework for future research.

After reviewing published articles, conference presentations/proceedings and other materials on therapeutic riding available since 1986, it appears that a portion of the published information has expanded beyond reports of therapeutic riding intervention programs, training programs for instructors, certification programs, and curriculum innovations. Even though this information still comprises the overwhelming majority of available information, the pertinent literature now contains a variety of studies which support the positive changes or benefits of therapeutic riding programs and the application of such programs to different population groupings (e.g., persons with cerebral palsy, elderly, head injured, mentally retarded).

Relative to the three commonly identified aspects of therapeutic riding (medicine, education, sport), most of the research has been conducted on the medical or physical benefits (therapeutic, rehabilitative) especially as applied to those with physical impairments. The research conducted since 1986 has been reported primarily in

---

[1] Engel, B. (1992). *Therapeutic Riding Programs: Instruction and Rehabilitation*, Durango, CO. 81301
[2] McCowan, J. The Cheff Center, Augusta, MI 49012.
[3] Tebay, F. Therapeutic Riding Services, PO Box 41, Riderwood, MD 21139.
[4] Joswick, F. Fran Joswick Therapeutic Riding Center, 26282 Oso Road, San Juan Capistrano, CA 92675.

the following areas: balance, sensory-motor programming (SI--sensory integration, NDT--neurodevelopmental therapy, perceptual-motor training), strength, coordination, posture, and other physical benefits.

Included among the recent findings are the following: (a) improved posture of children with cerebral palsy (Bertoti, 1988), improved balance among children with mental retardation (Biery & Kaufman, 1989), improved arm and leg coordination (Brock, 1988), positive changes in balance, mobility, and posture of physically impaired persons (Copeland, 1986, 1989) and developmentally delayed persons (Walsh, 1989), and increased relaxation of spasticity found among persons with cerebral palsy (Glasow, 1986). In addition, research has brought to light contraindications for those with structural scoliosis of greater than 30-40 degrees and for those with atlantoaxial instability found primarily with Down Syndrome individuals (Tebay & Schlesinger, 1986). Use of sensory integration and NDT techniques have been reported to be effective, as well as "centered" riding (Donahue, 1986).

In addition to the studies identified above, a limited amount of research has been conducted in other areas. The means of assessing performance and measuring change have improved and have become increasingly more sophisticated (Bieber, 1986, Brock, 1987; Fox, 1986). Valid measuring devices remain critical to assessing change accurately.

Dismuke-Blakeley (1981, 1984, 1990) remains the sole pioneer in research on improvement in speech and language as a result of therapeutic riding programs. Increasing interest has been shown in an integrated therapy approach but to date (e.g., Johnson, Elitsky, & Bailey, 1990), very little research has been reported.

In addition, very few research reports were found about other educational or sport benefits of therapeutic riding. Only one author was found to have investigated aspects of therapeutic riding related to sport participation (Bieber, 1986) whereas two authors reported their findings on the psychosocial aspects of riding (Good, 1986) and psychosocial re-education of "problem children" (Jollinier, 1986).

Early proponents of therapeutic riding "knew" that therapeutic riding was beneficial to participants via their observations but had very little other objective or empirical data. Current therapeutic riding programs have been designed around, and research data collected on, the *a prior* determined categories of benefits (e.g., medical, educational, sport) reported by these early proponents. Although the research data seem increasingly to support the claims of the benefits of therapeutic riding, these findings must be published in scholarly journals in order to be more readily accessible to the academic community and other interested persons. Further, a meta-analysis of the existing research could reveal the overall effectiveness of the programs.

That which remains unstudied, or perhaps understudied:
- Are there reasons *why* therapeutic riding is beneficial?
- Although the "product" (benefits) is known, an understanding of the process remains relatively unknown.
- Why does therapeutic riding work?
- How does therapeutic riding effect change in riders?

Therapeutic riding research must now move from reliance upon descriptive and experimental (quasi-) research designs to more naturalistic inquiry using qualitative research paradigms. This type of research requires direct observation and analysis of the process. Perhaps the answer to why therapeutic riding works lies in understanding the interactions among the rider, the instructor, the horse, and the environment. Among the understanding the interactions among the rider, the instructor, the horse, and the environment. Among the questions to be posed is the role of the human-animal companion bond (physiological, psychological), the three dimensional movement of the horse, nature and extent of the sensory stimulation received during riding, and the environment (physical, learning, emotional) in a successful therapeutic riding program. Thus, the next phase of therapeutic riding research needs to examine the human-horse-environment interaction. Inasmuch as learning (or change) occurs as a result of the person-environment interaction, it follows that an examination of the role of the horse in this interaction is of paramount importance.

As suggested by Copeland, McGibbon, and Freeman (1990), "... a theoretical framework is imperative in therapeutic riding as we evolve from practicing technicians applying techniques, to professionals basing our programs on a foundation of testable hypotheses and research data." One such framework for future research on therapeutic riding should include an examination of the interaction among (a) the three-dimensional movement of the horse, (b) sensory stimulation and its integrative effects, and (c) the horse-human bond (human-animal companion bond) in the therapeutic riding setting.

REFERENCES:

Bertoti, (1988). *Effect of Therapeutic Horseback Riding on Posture in Children with Cerebral Palsy.* 6th International Congress of Therapeutic Riding. Toronto, Canada.

Bieber, N. (1986a). Characteristics of physically disabled riders participating in equestrian competition at the national level. In Sherrill, C. (Ed) *Sport and Disabled Athletes.* Champaign, IL: Human Kinetics.

Bieber, N. (1986b). Therapeutic riding: The special educator's perspective. Abstract of paper presented at the *Delta Society International Conference.* Boston, MA.

Brock, B. (1988). *Effect of Therapeutic Horseback Riding on Physically Disabled Adults.* Doctoral Dissertation: U of Indiana.

Copeland, J.C. (1986). A study of four physically disabled riders with twenty-five years of combined riding experience. Abstract of paper presented at the *Delta Society International Conference.* Boston, MA.

Copeland, J.C. (1989). Therapeutic riding as a treatment adjunct after selective posterior lumbar rhizotomy surgery. Abstract of paper presented at 5th *International Conference on the Relationship between Humans and Animals.* Monaco.

Copeland, J.C., McGibbon, N., & Freeman, G. (1990). Theoretical perspectives in therapeutic riding. Abstract of paper presented at *Delta Society Ninth Annual Conference,* October 11-13.

DePauw, K.P. (1986). Horseback riding for individuals with disabilities: Programs, philosophy, and research. *Adapted Physical Activity Quarterly,* 3, 217-226.

Dismuke, R.P.M. (1981). Therapeutic horsemanship. *The Quarter Horse Journal.* 34-37.

Dismuke, R.P.M. (1984). Rehabilitative horseback riding for children with language disorders. In C.K. Anderson, B.L. Hart, & L.A. Hart (Eds), *Pet Connection.* 131-140. Minneapolis: University of Minneapolis, Center to Study Human-Animal Relationships and Environment.

Dismuke-Blakely, R.P.M. (1990). Combined speech/language and occupational therapy through rehabilitative riding. Abstract of paper presented at *Delta Society Ninth Annual Conference.*

Donahue, K. (1986). Centered riding for the physically disabled rider. Abstract of paper presented at *Delta Society International Conference.* Boston MA.

Glasow, B. (1986). Hippotherapy: the horse as a therapeutic modality. *People-Animals-Environment.* 30-31.

Good. C.L. (1986). Psychosocial aspects of riding for adult disabled equestrians. Abstract of paper presented at *Delta Society International Conference.* Boston, MA.

Fox, V.M. (1986 Winter). Measurement device for therapeutic horseback riding. *People-Animals-Environment*. 33

Johnson, L.M., Elitsky, L., Bailey, D. (1990). A holistic approach to therapeutic riding. Abstract of paper presented at *Delta Society Ninth Annual Conference,* October 11-13, 1990.

Jollinier, M. (1989). Horse riding activity and psycho-social re-education in problem children. Abstract of paper presented at *5th International Conference on the Relationship between Humans and Animals.* Monaco

Joswick, F., Kittredge, M., McCowan, L. et al. (1986). *Aspects and Answers*. Michigan: Cheff Center.

Tebay, J. & Schlesinger, R. (1986 Spring). Riding therapy as a contraindication for Down syndrome individuals with atlantoaxial instability. *People-Animals-Environment*. 31-32.

Walsh, L. (1989). The therapeutic value of horseback riding and the developmental milestones accomplished through horseback riding. Abstract of paper presented at *5th International Conference on the Relationship between Humans and Animals*, Monaco.

HIPPOTHERAPY AS A SPECIFIC TREATMENT:
A REVIEW OF CURRENT LITERATURE

Amy Wheeler, PT

Hippos is the Greek word for horse. Hippotherapy literally means treatment with the help of a horse. Hippotherapy is a treatment approach that is gaining popularity with physical, occupational and speech therapists. Riding skills are not the focus of hippotherapy; rather; the movement of the horse is used to elicit change in the person. The person responds to the movements of the horse with automatic postural responses.

Movement of the Horse's Pelvis

The horse provides a repetitive rhythmical movement to the rider's pelvis and lower trunk. With each step the horse takes, the rider is moved through a similar pattern. As the horse pushes off and swings one of his hind legs forward, his pelvis drops on that side and his pelvis and trunk rotate. This produces lateral pelvic tilt in the rider. As the horse's leg swings forward, he laterally flexes his spine. This produces pelvic rotation in the rider. As the horse steps and shifts his center of gravity, lateral pelvic displacement occurs in the rider. While these three dimensional movements are occurring, the rider is carried forward through space. The three-dimensional movement of the horse allows the individual to experience movement patterns in a functional way. Similar to the techniques used by proprioceptive neuromuscular facilitation, the horse is able to move the person through diagonal movement sequences. The rhythmical motion of the horse also provides the rider with some rhythmic stabilization to the pelvis and trunk (Wham, 1992). This facilitation of the pelvis and trunk is important to the development of a stable base from which to perform functional activities.

The movement in the horse's pelvis at the walk is very similar to that of the human pelvis during gait. There have been several studies in recent years that attempt to measure and explain any differences between horse and human gait. Fleck, in a 1992 master's thesis at the University of Delaware, used 16 mm films to compare the pelvic movements of 24 normal children while walking on a treadmill and while riding a horse walking on an equine treadmill. She found that linear displacements of the children's pelvises during walking and riding differed in magnitude but not in timing or sequence. That is, the timing and frequency of the horse and the human's movement are similar but the magnitude is not, in part because a horse is so much larger. Freeman (1992) used quantitative kinematic analysis to measure the movement of the horse's pelvis at a walk. Her measurements revealed the following information. The horse's pelvis moves 3.92 degrees in the sagittal plane, 6.98 degrees in the coronal plane, and 9.08 degrees in the transverse plane. These measurements of equine pelvic movement are similar to adult pelvic movement parameters found by Perry and Sutherland. Perry reported five degrees in the sagittal plane, seven degrees in the coronal plane, and ten degrees in the transverse plane. Sutherland (1980), in a study of 186 normal children, found that there were two to three degrees of pelvic motion in the sagittal plane, ten degrees in the frontal plane (five degrees during weight assumption and five degrees during terminal stance and toe-off) and approximately 20 degrees in the transverse plane (ten degrees on either side of the frontal plane).

Skill Acquisition during Hippotherapy

The horse's cadence in steps/minute is also similar to an adult's cadence. The average adult walks at approximately 110-120 steps/minute and a large horse walks at a speed of 100-120 steps/minute (Barnes, 1993, Hippotherapy DACUM Committee, 1990, Rosenzweig, 1992). Most hippotherapy sessions in the United States last approximately one half-hour (Glasow, personal communication, 1994). During a half-hour

Hippotherapy DACUM Committee, 1990, Rosenzweig, 1992). Most hippotherapy sessions in the United States last approximately one half-hour (Glasow, personal communication, 1994). During a half-hour session, the rider is exposed to and has the opportunity to practice a skill often. A horse that walks at 100 steps/minutes will take more than 3000 steps during a session. This will give the rider literally thousands of opportunities to practice specific skills such as a weight shift and maintaining the midline position (Wham, 1992).

According to motor learning theory, repetition in a variety of settings is important to help a person learn a task. During a hippotherapy session, the rider has that chance. In the beginning, the horse's movements will be closely monitored. The movement of the horse can be directed to elicit certain responses in the rider. For example, upward transitions will cause a flexor response. As the horse moves forward from a halt, the person is moved backward and must use flexor muscles to maintain an upright position. During a downward transition, an extensor response is elicited.

Riede (1988) reported that the overall treatment goal of hippotherapy is automatic postural stability in alignment with the center of gravity. When the horse begins to move, the person's pelvis moves into a posterior pelvic tilt, there is realignment of the trunk on the pelvis, the head moves into slight flexion, and the eyes are horizontal (Citterio, 1985). This is a functional position that allows the rider to respond to the movement of the horse and interact with the environment.

Movement of the horse in long straight lines is the initial focus of treatment (Citterio, 1985, Glasow, 1985 and 1988, Rosenzweig, 1992, Spink, 1993). This will emphasize flexion and extension in the rider. As the person gains trunk control and the pelvis is able to move both in the anterior and posterior directions to follow the movement of the horse, transitions from low to high impulsion and lengthening and shortening of the stride at the walk can be done. A transition from a halt to a walk or vice versa is the biggest challenge to an individual's flexion/extension control. As the person is able to respond and react to these activities with appropriate righting responses and trunk control, movements in other planes can be addressed.

Frontal plane movements that emphasize lateral flexion are the next steps in the progression. This is the ability of the person to elongate and shorten trunk musculature. This automatic reciprocal lengthening and shortening is an important component of weight shifting. Lengthening and shortening in the rider is encouraged when the horse is asked to bend. As the horse bends and moves through curves there is increased rotation in his pelvis. The increased pelvic rotation in the horse facilitates lateral flexion in the pelvis and trunk of the rider (Rosenzweig, 1992). As the horse moves around a circle, the subject falls toward the outside of the curve because of centrifugal force (Citterio, 1985). The person experiences a weight shift to the outside and elongation of the trunk on that side. There is a shortening on the inside. The person has moved their center of gravity over their new base of support to prevent falling. A weight shift also happens each time the horse takes a step. There is elevation of the rider's pelvis on the same side as the horse's hind leg that is in a stance phase. This is the same as in a human gait (Wham, 1992).

Long shallow curves can be combined with changes in direction to encourage a weight shift across the midline and encourage lateral flexion from one side to the other. Many schooling figures (circles, serpentine, figure eights and changes of direction) have curves in them. The smaller and tighter the curves the more challenging they are to the rider because the rotational component of the horse's movement becomes larger.

Rotational movement in the trunk and pelvis of the rider can be emphasized by having the horse perform lateral movements. The horse moves with a distinct diagonal component when doing movements like the rein back (walking backwards) and two track movements (the horse is not moving straight ahead but diagonally). It has also been documented that having the horse increase his length of stride at the walk will encourage rotation in the rider (Spink, 1993; Author-personal experience). As the horse walks forward, there is increased lateral trunk flexion because of his increased length of stride. This lateral trunk flexion in the horse is perceived as rotation to the rider because the horse and rider's pelvises are at ninety degree angles to each other.

As with the developmental sequence off the horse, movements and skills are not practiced in isolation. For instance, as a rider is working on weight shifting and medial/lateral control, the horse can be asked to lengthen or shorten his stride or the speed of the transitions can be changed. This will challenge the rider's anterior/posterior control. Different movements can be performed by the horse to facilitate other responses in the rider.

Postural Control During Hippotherapy Sessions

As mentioned earlier, during a hippotherapy session the rider does not control the horse and is not taught riding skills. Instead, the rider reacts to the movement of the horse. In the beginning, these reactions are a consequence of automatic postural responses and reflexes with no cortical input (Citterio, 1985). The person is actively involved but that does not mean that the person has to be cognitively or volitionally reacting to the movement. The rider is actively involved at a subconscious level when automatic responses are elicited (Glasow, 1985. Schmidt, 1988).

As the horse continues to walk, the person experiences a repetitive rhythmical movement. It is an open task; it does not have a discrete beginning and end (Carr & Shepherd, 1987; Schmidt, 1988). The repetitiveness of this task helps generate a positive expectation for the rider. He or she knows what to expect and when, as the movement of the horse becomes more familiar. This allows the person to anticipate, prepare, and respond appropriately. The rider is able to anticipate an action that is already familiar (DeLubersac, 1985). Later, the rider can be challenged to respond and adapt to variations of this familiar action, for example a lengthening of the horse's stride or a change of direction. The person begins to use both feedback and feed forward mechanisms for postural control (Carr & Shepherd, 1987; Schmidt, 1988).

Effects of Hippotherapy on Balance

Throughout the therapeutic riding literature there are claims to the benefits of using the horse as a therapeutic modality. Unfortunately, most of the studies are hampered by small sample size, poor control, and limited repeatability. Only a few studies have attempted to look specifically at hippotherapy and its effects. Standing balance is one area that is often purported to change after participation in a therapeutic riding or hippotherapy program.

Biery and Kauffman (1989) examined the effects of therapeutic horseback riding on balance in eight children with mental retardation. They reported an improvement in balance as indicated by significant changes in standing and quadruped balance test scores after involvement in a twenty-four-week program of riding. Subjects rode once per week for twenty minute sessions that included a five minute warm-up, ten minutes of intense exercise, and five minutes of cool-down.

Bertoti reported an improvement in the posture of children with cerebral palsy after participation in a therapeutic riding program. She developed an objective measure of posture, The Posture Assessment Scale, for the study (Bertoti, 1988). The families of these children also reported improvements in balance and functional activities (Bertoti, 1988). Wingate (1982) examined therapeutic riding as an integrative program for children with cerebral palsy. She had seven children in her study. They rode for one hour, twice a week for five weeks. The families of four of the participants reported improved posture, less falling when walking, improved sitting posture, independence in functional skills, such as taking a shower, improved head control, a decrease in lower extremity hypertonicity, improved gait, and improved self image. Mackay-Lyons et al (1988) reported on ten patients with multiple sclerosis who participated in a nine-week trial of hippotherapy sessions conducted twice per week. Their attendance rate was 92.1%. They reported no significant change in postural sway measurements and functional mobility ratings after the hippotherapy. However, four patients reported increased standing balance during activities of daily living (ADL's.)

Riede (1988) reported in his book, *Physiotherapy on the Horse*, on several European studies that have examined the effects of hippotherapy. Brauer, in a 1971 study, evaluated children before and after participation in twenty-five riding sessions. He reported improved relaxation, improved coordination and balance, and improved range of motion. Meier (1976) reported improved coordination of movement sequences and increased stimulation of back extensors. Von Bausenwein (1989) measured a decrease in reflex activity in eleven children with cerebral palsy after participation in hippotherapy. Hardt, in a 1980 study, studied nine subjects with cerebral palsy walking on a treadmill before and after each session of hippotherapy. He reported a decrease in adductor spasticity and improvements in postural components during gait which were evaluated subjectively.

Validity of Hippotherapy

Hippotherapy has face validity especially if looked at from the motor control/motor learning point of view. The repetitive rhythmical motion of the horse allows the rider to learn to adapt, anticipate, and react to a moving object. During hippotherapy sessions, the participants are able to practice functional tasks (weight shifting, balance reactions, and equilibrium responses) in a variety of settings.

Hippotherapy uses principles from the traditional therapeutic exercise techniques and puts them into a novel situation. The person is able to feel the motion of the horse as they are moved through space. This affects the motor control and motor learning of the rider. The sensory input provided by the horse is able to be used as an adjunct to the therapist's hands.

Despite its growing use as a therapeutic modality, little has been done in the area of research. Most of the studies in the literature are hampered by small sample size, poor design, and decreased reproducibility. If hippotherapy is to become an accepted adjunct to therapy, it must have research to quantify what is happening on the horse.

REFERENCES:
Barnes, T. 1993. Hippotherapy DACUM Committee (1990). J. Tebay, Riderwood, MD.
Bertoti, DB. 1988. **Effect of therapeutic horseback riding on posture in children with cerebral palsy.** *Physical Therapy*, 68(10) 1505-1512.

Biery, M., Kauffman, M. 1989. **The effect of therapeutic horseback riding on balance**. Adapted Physical Activity Quarterly,6(3) 221-229.

Bauer, (1988). In D. Reide Physiotherapy in the horse. Delta Society, Renton WA.

Carr, Sheperd, 1987. *Movement Science: Foundation for Physical Therapy in Rehabilitation*, Aspen Publishers, Rockville, MD.

Citterio, DN. 1985. **The influence of the horse in neuromotorial evolution**. In the *Proceedings of 5th International Congress on Therapeutic Riding*. ANIRE Association, Milan, Italy.

DeLubersac, R. 1985. **The psychomotor mechanism, riding and the horse** in the *Proceedings of 5th International Congress of Therapeutic Riding*, ANIRE, Milan, Italy.

Fleck, CA. 1997. **Hippotherapy: Mechanics of human walking and horseback riding**. In *Rehabilitation with the aid of a horse: A collection of studies*.(Ed). B. Engel. Barbara Engel Therapy Services, Durango, CO.

Freeman, G. `1992. **Assessment of the client in hippotherapy** in *Therapeutic Riding Programs: Instruction and Rehabilitation*. (Ed). B. Engel. Barbara Engel Therapy Services, Durango CO.

Glasow, B. 1985. in the *Proceedings of 5th International Congress of Therapeutic Riding*, ANIRE, Milan, Italy.

Mackay-Lyons, M., et el. (1988). **Effect of therapeutic riding on patients with multiple sclerosis, a preliminary trial**. *Physiotherapy*, 40(2) 104-109.

Meier, 1988. In D Reide *Physiotherapy in the horse*. Delta Society, Renton WA.

Perry, J. 1975. **Cerebral palsy gait** in *Orthopedic Aspects of Cerebral Palsy*. R.L. Amilson (ed) Philadelphia: J.B. Lippincott Co. 71-88.

Riede, D. 1988. *Physiotherapy on the horse*. Delta Society, Renten WA.

Rosenzweig, M. (1992). **The value of the horse to the rider** in *Therapeutic Riding Programs: Instruction and Rehabilitation*, (Ed) B. Engel, Barbara Engel Therapy Services, Durango, CO.

Schmidt, R.A. 1988. *Motor Control and Learning*. Champaign, Homer Kinetics Publishers, Inc.

Spink, J. 1993. *Developmental Riding Therapy*. Therapy Skill Builders, Tucson AZ.

Sutherland, D.H., Olshen, R., Cooper, L., Woo, S.LT. 1980. **The Development of motor gait**. *Journal of Bone and Joint Surgery*.

Wingate, 1982. **Feasibility of horseback riding as a therapeutic and integrative program for handicapped children**. *Physical Therapy* 62(2) 184-186

Wham, (1992). **Rhythmic facilitation: A method of treatment neuromotor disorders using the rhythm & movement of the horse** in *Therapeutic Riding Programs: Instruction and Rehabilitation*, ed B. Engel, Barbara Engel Therapy Services, Durango, CO.

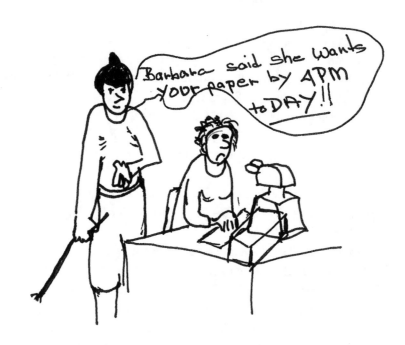

CHAPTER 4

INDICATIONS AND CONTRAINDICATIONS TO HIPPOTHERAPY WITH CLIENTS WITH PHYSICAL DYSFUNCTIONS

TO RIDE OR NOT TO RIDE: IS THAT REALLY THE QUESTION?

Linda Mitchell, MS, PT

CASE HISTORY--PART 1

It was Matthew's first time on a horse or even near enough to the horse to feel its breath on his hand as he cautiously reached out to pet its nose. The smiling, freckle-faced five year old had been referred to the equine-assisted therapy program by his physical therapist. The therapist was concerned with Matthew's low muscle tone, fear of heights, and decreased postural control. The therapist had obtained a physician's referral for the consulting riding therapist, and shared as much information as possible about her perception of this child and how he might be helped by using the horse in therapy. Based on this information an evaluation on the horse was scheduled and planned.

A short, sturdy horse was selected on the basis of Matthew's fear of heights. Because it was anticipated that he might need a feeling of security, yet should be given an opportunity to feel and respond to as much of the horse's movement as possible, the equipment selected was a bareback pad and anti-cast surcingle. A brief "off horse" assessment was conducted to verify prior information and to establish rapport between Matthew and this new therapist. Matthew was introduced to his horse "Yoda," and was assisted in mounting. He was in an excited, anticipatory state.

It was immediately apparent that Matthew did not include `midline' in his repertoire of strategies for balance. As Yoda stood quietly and Matthew was encouraged to relax and adjust, he remained tense, gripping the surcingle handle, first with both hands, then one, then the other, in an attempt to find a secure enough posture to request the horse to walk. Matthew's trunk was pulled into collapsed flexion. He was tightly gripping with his legs and moving his pelvis, searching for stability between anterior and posterior tilt, and between right and left weight bearing, but just not able to center and organize.

After a few minutes, it was decided to go ahead and depart at a walk to see if a rhythmical gait in long straight lines would assist Matthew or further disorganize him. The side helpers were instructed to give firm tactile support and to reassure him as needed. And, with much encouragement, Matthew finally took a deep breath and shouted out the words "Walk on, Wo Ha!"

The ride lasted twelve minutes. The results were disastrous. Throughout the ride Matthew struggled, without success, to feel secure enough to enjoy what he knew was **supposed** to be fun! With every stride he changed his strategy. With every defeat, he lost a little more control, until he could no longer count on any of his sensory systems to give him a clear message of where he was, let alone what to do about it. He began to attempt a dismount from the moving horse, only he could not find a way, and could not express that he wanted off. The surcingle handle became an obstacle, an intrusion on his space, a distraction from his ability to focus.

His chatter increased, but was scattered and full of questions unrelated to his ride. Matthew was asked if he wanted the horse to "whoa," and he immediately shouted "Whoa" to whomever would hear it. He was then assisted to the ground, where he displayed difficulty finding his base of support, and organizing enough balance to walk through the gate to his Mom. He had no desire to further interact with Yoda, and when asked if he'd enjoyed his ride, he responded, "That was fun! Are we going home now?"

DISCUSSION

Matthew is a classic example of a five year-old child who should be an excellent candidate for equine-assisted therapy. First of all, he does not demonstrate any of the listed "contraindications," has no significant medical or orthopedic problems, and exhibits sensorimotor dysfunction that could be changed through the rhythmical, symmetrical input of the moving horse. A logical "recipe" was followed in the planning and execution of his riding evaluation. Yet Matthew's first ride portrayed a very different picture from the expected outcome, thus illustrating the premise of this paper: the importance of regular, ongoing, individualized assessment of each rider by knowledgeable and skilled professionals in each therapeutic riding program.

INDICATIONS, CONTRAINDICATIONS AND PRECAUTIONS

Lists are available through NARHA[1] and CanTRA[2] publications and in the training manuals of the Hippotherapy Curriculum Committee[3] that present a summary of the collaborative research efforts, clinical findings, and professional opinions of experts in the field. They are meant to serve as guidelines for decision making, particularly with respect to the medical aspects of various disabilities and their diagnosis. But, without backup knowledge and understanding, no list can serve as a bible or a cookbook. The author is working with populations served by therapeutic riding programs, running the gamut from recreational to medically-oriented, and **every decision is essentially a judgement call based on skilled observation** and problem solving. The ability to break down the total picture of a client into variable components is the best answer to the questions of accountability, liability, and quality of service.

And so the issue expands from a question of whether or not a person should ride at all to the real "why" or "why not," as well as the "how," "when," "where," and "with whom" should they ride, if at all. The use of the horse in therapy encompasses a rationale which can be as simple or as complex as the level of understanding one has, as well as the scope of the perspective of the whole person with individual needs and abilities. Combine this premise with a sound working knowledge of the tool (the horse) and its potential, and a firm foundation is established for quality practice.

RATIONALE

Above all, the preliminary assessment must rule out the fact that damage or physical harm may be done to the client. This is the basis of any list of contraindications and precautions, compiled in accordance with the actual physical effect of the moving horse on its rider. Prior to the placement of a client in a program, as well as throughout treatment, these questions must be asked:

- What is moving, what is not moving, and WHY?
- Is the effect, or projected effect, a desirable one?
- Is there any reason this interaction of horse and rider should not be allowed to occur?
- And are there any changes that can be made to obtain or improve a desirable result?

Once the absence of contraindications is verified, a reason should be clear for using the horse in some way to uniquely affect an area of dysfunction, and to assist in accomplishing a therapeutic goal. Again, an

Once the absence of contraindications is verified, a reason should be clear for using the horse in some way to uniquely affect an area of dysfunction, and to assist in accomplishing a therapeutic goal. Again, an understanding of the sensorimotor impact in the exchange between horse and rider is critical to the safe, purposeful and appropriate use of the horse in treatment.

VARIABLE
The impact of the horse is strong and powerful; the changes effected are subtle and intense. Fragile, sensitive nervous systems are constantly asked to gather and integrate sensory information and to design a strategy for response. The most minute change in sensory input has immense potential for realizing a desirable difference in the response of the client. Thus, it is the responsibility and ability of the **trained clinician** to assess and adapt, in both the planning and the treatment stages of every program, utilizing a working knowledge of the changeable components: namely, the horse, the equipment, the position or activities, and, finally, the movement used in order to accomplish change in the rider's response.

CASE HISTORY--PART 2
Matthew returned to the stable with his Mom on the day following his on-horse assessment. He sported a "shiner" on his left eye that Rocky would have been proud of! When asked about it, his Mom reported that he had fallen off the couch the night before, and just seemed to have been "off-balance." This finding was definitely in keeping with the therapist's assessment that some changes needed to be made if Matthew were to ride again. Yesterday's short ride had indeed had devastating results. The new plan had already been formulated. In view of the fact that Yoda's movement had served only to further disorganize a child who apparently struggled with severe inability to organize his posture, a different horse was selected for Matthew to try. Although "Donnie" was taller than Yoda, he was also broader, and had a much shorter, slower stride, thus providing minimal movement input and a larger base of support. The idea was to maximize the ways of addressing Matthew's need for stability and provide it to him in a very different way.

The surcingle had interfered and disoriented Matthew, as it required more motor planning and ability to weight-shift into his arms and hands than Matthew was able to manage on the horse. So the surcingle was eliminated from his visual and tactile field, thus allowing him options for interacting with only one dependable surface, Donnie's back. Matthew was mounted on Donnie on a thick bareback pad, and reminded that he had the power to control Donnie through voice commands of "walk" and "whoa". The side helpers were instructed to engage in minimal verbal interaction with Matthew and to give guarding rather than tactile assistance, with the idea of providing him a structured, safe environment, focused and distraction-free, within the boundaries of which he could problem-solve his responses. Using the organization offered by Donnie's movement, Matthew began to find his own strategies for dynamic stability. He demonstrated awareness of being off-center, attempts to correct to mid-line, visual attention to his task of staying on this moving horse, a minimum of conversation, and repeated appropriate use of the command to "Whoa" when he needed to reorganize. In addition, Matthew began on his own tactile exploration of Donnie through changing his own position, hugging Donnie's neck, reaching for his tail, and even stopping the horse so he could lie back and touch the horse's rump and "belly". This time, the ride lasted 15 minutes, with Matthew asking if he could stop Donnie and dismount. At the end of the ride, he turned and faced the horse, patted and thanked him, and fed him a carrot, before returning to his mother's side, proud and much more "together" than the day before.

COMMENTARY

For all of us in therapeutic riding, Matthew's experience holds a twofold message: one of caution, flavored with creative encouragement. The instructor's insightful perspective, based on skilled observation, and conclusions based on experience allowed the boy not only to continue the ride but to maximize his potential for a positive and worthwhile learning experience. **Without the benefit of such expertise, despite the best intentions, a child like Matthew would, at best, be prevented from entering a program. Or, in an even more damaging scenario, he might be allowed to continue without recognition of the harm being repeatedly allowed to occur.** It is simply not possible to assure quality and safety through the use of a checklist or a "cookbook" method of client selection and screening. Horses are not generically beneficial to everyone with a disability or even with certain disabilities. But, with the right understanding and the required, trained professional judgement, even the strictest rules can be revised, resulting in a uniquely powerful effect on the quality of the lives that are touched by this unique treatment.

[1] North American Riding for the Handicapped, Box 33150, Denver, CO 80233 USA

[2] Canadian Therapeutic Riding Association (CanTRA), P.O. Box 1055, Guelph, Ont, N1H 6J6, Canada.

[3] Hippotherapy Curriculum Committee, Therapeutic Riding Services, PO Box 41, Riderwood, MD 21139

INDICATIONS AND CONTRAINDICATIONS FOR HIPPOTHERAPY AND EQUINE-ASSISTED OCCUPATIONAL, PHYSICAL or SPEECH THERAPY

Barbara T. Engel, M.Ed, OTR

Anytime a therapist decides to add a new procedure to his or her treatment methods, the therapist must examine the advisability of this new procedure. Will the procedure be effective with my client? Is the procedure appropriate for the client's age, disability, and functional status? Is the procedure safe for this client and will the benefits of this procedure outweigh the risk? Will the therapist achieve his or her goals with the client in an optimum amount of time in a cost-effective way? Precautions are necessary with any method of treatment that are being considered. This is especially true in selecting the horse as a tool. This article will discuss many aspects of using the horse in therapy.

In selecting the horse as a treatment tool for a client, there are many factors to be considered. Contraindications can arise due to a horse with poor movement qualities, lack of trained staff, lack of equipment or lack of adequate and safe facilities. Just as in traditional treatment, one must have a facility that provides the space necessary to accomplish the type of treatment one wishes to practice. Certain equipment is necessary for specific clients. When using a horse, we must have a horse that will provide the type of movement necessary for a specific client. The availability of necessary transfer devices such as a ramp or lift must be at the facility. We must have a team of trained people. The therapist must have a good understanding in the etiology and treatment methods for a specific dysfunction that is present in the client he or she plans to treat with a horse. Equestrian skills are also necessary so horse suitability can be determined for a client and how the horse's movement and stimulation will confront the goals to be met. The therapist must be able to do an extensive evaluation since one is dealing with two moving bodies, the client and the horse, who will interact with and influence each other. The therapist must have extensive knowledge of known data in the field of therapeutic riding to decide which diagnoses and syndromes are appropriate or which could cause harm to a client.

Contraindications can occur for any of the reasons mentioned in addition to diagnostic considerations.

STAFF SUITABILITY

A physical therapist becomes interested in hippotherapy. She has worked for six years after graduation, in an orthopedic-sports medicine practice with adults. Your center's population consists of children with neurological-based problems. She took the introduction course to hippotherapy and states she went on many trail rides as a child. Is she qualified to practice hippotherapy with your center's clients?

An occupational therapist with twelve years experiences in inpatient psychiatric rehabilitation and head of their recreation program wishes to change her focus. She had a back yard pony as a child but never had any training. She read about hippotherapy and took the beginner hippotherapy course. Would she be qualified to provide hippotherapy for your clients with cerebral palsy, sensory integrative dysfunction, and developmentally delayed kids?

A speech pathologist has worked in the school system for 20 years. Her work station was a six feet by six feet room where she sat facing a child across the table. She had no experience with movement effects on the vocal

35

system. One day she heard a lecture about hippotherapy and its use in speech-pathology. She always loved horses though had never ridden one. She decided the change of that environment would be good for her. She found a center that needed a speech-pathologist. Would you hire her?

None of these therapists are qualified to do hippotherapy nor to do physical therapy, occupational therapy, or speech therapy with the horse. Suitability to work with a particular diagnosis is dependent on the training and experience a therapist has had. Using the horse as a tool adds another dimension and requires additional training. One cannot practice neurodevelopment technique (NDT), sensory integration (SI) or cranial sacral therapy without extensive training nor can one use a horse as a tool without the knowledge of the horse's biomechanics, behavior and communication system or how to manipulate his movements by applying aids to facilitate the client. Why is all this important in equine-assisted therapy? Because the apparatus one is using is mobile, large, fast, and can be unpredictable. The therapist is working with two living bodies who must interact with each other. One must know their clients's problems to understand the client's reaction to the horse and the outcome of treatment. The equestrian setting is more dynamic, complicated and distractable than settings occupational therapists, physical therapists, and speech pathologists are used to. The presence or lack of qualification will greatly determine indications and contraindications for treatment. The level of riding skill, horsemanship knowledge and treatment experience with the horse will further qualify a therapist for the more complex client.

THE HORSE SUITABILITY
It is the three-dimensional movement of the horse that is historically attributed with the therapeutic value to the client. If a client cannot accommodate the movement of a specific horse (the horse's movement is too much or too little for the client) then the therapeutic value has been lost. Horses' movements vary depending on breed, size, stride length, balance, rhythm, willingness, attitude, conditioning, and training. A horse that meets all these criteria can become stiff with two days in a stall. Without the conditioning prior to the therapy session, his value has been lost. A horse with flawed movement may transfer that movement to the client. The wrong horse may be a contraindication for one client and just right for another.

EQUIPMENT
If the therapist is planning to work with clients who use wheelchairs or those who have moderate degrees of instability, a ramp or ramps will be needed. If a ramp is not available, it will limit the type of client one can treat. Not only is a mount from the ground hard and unbalancing on a horse with a well conditioned rider, it is much harder on the horse with a person with a disability and an equine massage therapist would not recommend it. There are mechanical lifts that can allows some clients to transfer independently or to assist a difficult [heavy or poor mobility] client to transfer. Some clients can transfer from a mounting block, and a few agile ones may be able to mount from the ground. Tack is another consideration one must take into account when placing a client on a horse. The wrong tack (saddle, surcingle, pad, reins) can make riding unsafe, the horse sore, and/or make the client uncomfortable, or provide the wrong results.

FACILITY
Safety is a prime consideration in the equestrian environment for anyone involved with horses. The facility can be one that considers all safety factors or one that has accidents waiting to happen. Arenas must have good footing and secure fences. Anywhere that a client will go must be safe for his/her level of function. The lack of a proper riding facility is a contraindication to treatment with the horse as a modality.

To consider using the horse as a treatment tool, some features we need to examine:

1. How will the movement of a specific horse address the goals we have established?
2. Will this horse cause more spasticity?
3. Will the mounting and dismounting procedure make the client's problem worse?
4. Could unpredictable movements by the horse cause the rider harm? (physically or mentally)
5. What size horse, gait and pace is necessary to improve the client's problem?
6. Has there been documentation that the horse as a tool is an appropriate treatment technique to treat your client's dysfunction?
7. Does the riding center have the special equipment and a clean safe facility to meet your client's needs?
8. Do you know how to transfer one moving body (client) to another moving body (horse)?
9. Can the client safely accommodate the movement of the horse to be used?
10. Which horse will you choose for the five year-old child with spastic cerebral palsy? The fourteen hand Arab with her short-quick gait, the 12 hands pony with her stiff-choppy gait or the 15^3 hand Quarter Horse with his smooth rhythmic gait, or the thirteen hand Haflinger with her broad back and smooth easy movements?
11. Is riding appropriate for all persons with multiple sclerosis? with spastic cerebral palsy? With Down Syndrome?

> *Sensory Integration's Jane Ayres once said, "If you do not know--don't do it." This may be very true for this equestrian activity*

THE CLIENT

How does one determine which client can best be treated by hippotherapy, or by equine-assisted therapy by an occupational therapy, physical therapy, or speech therapy? The following discussion will consider the specific disabilities and some of the considerations that each therapist must make. One must always remember that each client is different. We do not go by disability alone. Twenty-five years ago there were 'Strokes,' 'CPs,' 'Retards' and so on. Now we consider each person with his or her disability - one child with CP will differ from another with CP. It is no longer true, as stated in many articles, that riding is good for (all) those with cerebral palsy, spina bifida, multiple sclerosis. Under particular circumstances and with certain complications, riding may not be appropriate.

The following are therefore guidelines. If one is not sure, seek help and do not experiment with your client without the expertise to do so. It must also be mentioned that countries have different standards due to insurance or government regulations. Indications, contraindications and precautions may vary.

INDICATIONS FOR HIPPOTHERAPY AND EQUINE ASSISTED OCCUPATIONAL, PHYSICAL OR SPEECH THERAPIES INCLUDE:

- Neurological movement dysfunctions of diverse etiology
- Developmental disabilities
- Sensory integrative dysfunctions
- Perceptual motor and coordination dysfunctions
- Arousal and reactive responses
- Speech and language delay
- Bone and joint dysfunction

PRECAUTIONS TO HIPPOTHERAPY OR RIDING WITH ALL TYPES OF DISABILITIES INCLUDE:

- ▸ Poor endurance - watching for signs of fatigue
- ▸ Any medical condition that puts the client at risk without physician's approval
- ▸ Diabetes
- ▸ Severe sensory loss -at risk for skin breakdown
- ▸ Behavior problems which may cause a safety problem to horse, staff or client
- ▸ Any medically unstable condition
- ▸ Allergies/asthma agitated by the horse or its environment
- ▸ Anti-clotting therapy and/or prone to an embolism
- ▸ Fear of the horse or its movements

CONTRAINDICATIONS TO TREATMENT WITH THE USE OF THE HORSE WITH ALL TYPES OF DISABILITIES INCLUDE:

- ▸ Lack of progress to meet therapy goals within a reasonable time
- ▸ Conditions that produce negative results, aggravates a condition or cause pain
- ▸ More weight than a horse can comfortably carry without disturbance of his gait, balance, rhythm and muscling.

  A sound horse with good conformation who is well muscled, supple, balanced and in excellent condition may carry a well conditioned -supple and balanced rider who weighs 250 lbs. but can only carry a normal stiff, unbalanced rider weighing 140 pounds [S. Harris & J. Harman DMV]. With this in mind, our horses would be able to carry less weight with our riders with disabilities.

- ▸ Heart and circulatory conditions that would prevent strenuous activity or are aggravated by riding. Also, uncontrolled hypertension and or stress.
- ▸ Uncontrolled bleeding disorders
- ▸ A person with high blood pressure who might react to stress with increased blood pressure and hypertension.
- ▸ Severe allergies to the horse or it's environment, also noted sun reactions due to medications. Sun reactions may require an indoor arena if available.
- ▸ Uncontrollable behavior problems that could cause injury to the horse or staff
- ▸ Indwelling catheter for females
- ▸ Some medically unstable conditions

THE SPINAL COLUMN:
Contraindications to riding therapy or hippotherapy include:
- ▸ Post spinal surgery - before eight to 12 months after surgery or when the physician says a solid bony fusion has occurred and riding can continue. Also post surgeries until stabilized.
- ▸ Inflammation of the spine and/or its disc that worsen while riding
- ▸ Pain or sensory loss that increases when riding
- ▸ Degeneration of moderate to severe degrees of the spine
- ▸ Pathological fractures of the spine

- Osteoporosis of moderate to severe degree
- Osteogenesis imperfecta
- Bechterew's disease
- Scheuermann's disease with inflammation
- Scoliosis, structural lordosis, and kyphosis of moderate to severe degrees
- Spondylolisthesis
- A body jacket with a chin support
- Atlantoaxial instability
- Regression

Precautions to hippotherapy or riding therapy include:

- Spinal fusion of small areas of the spine that allow adequate mobility in the spine to accommodate the movement from the horse
- When spinal fusion causes limited mobility of the spine
- Mild degenerative disease with a physician's approval and monitoring, and no negative results from riding
- All spinal curves - structural and functional must be carefully monitored - contraindicated if the curve gets worse
- Spinal curves that do not respond to therapy
- A client with any type of body jacket - must provide stability and balance in upright posture without pain or tension. Clients need to be monitored carefully
- Plates, wiring, Luque sublaminae and Harrington Rods must be approved by a physician and precautions must be known by client and family.

THE HIPS:
When sitting astride a horse, one balances on the three points of the pelvis. The condition and mobility of the pelvis and hips are, therefore, of prime concern. Riding requires a degree of movement of the hips.

Precautions to hippotherapy or riding include:

- Limited hip mobility
- Artificial hip
- Degeneration of the hip joint.

Contraindications to hippotherapy or riding include:

- Lack of range of motion to straddle the horse if manipulation of the spine, the pelvis and legs cannot accommodate appropriate posture to sit astride
- Ossification of the hip joint(s)

- Severe degeneration of the hip joint
- Pain of the hip joint while riding which does not subside

NEUROLOGICAL CONDITIONS:

The spinal column is directly affected by the movement stimulations from the horse through the seat of the rider. Special attention must be paid to the spinal column's reaction to the movement and stimulation from the horse. According to Strauss, the righting reaction of the spine for walking is a major goal of hippotherapy (not necessarily equine-assisted therapy.) If this cannot be obtained then goals need to be re-evaluated.

Contraindications to hippotherapy and riding include:

- A very large head which cannot be fitted with a helmet or which places the spine at risk due to lack of support
- Open area in the skull without a shunt - and a helmet cannot be fitted exactly
- Lack of head/neck stability that cannot be controlled
- Spina Bifida with pain
- Spina Bifida without pain but cannot gain sitting balance
- Spina Bifida with increased neurological signs
- Spina Bifida with skin irritation that can not be corrected
- Spina Bifida with increased spinal curve while riding
- Spina Bifida with a tethered spinal cord that becomes a greater risk with low level involvement
- Chiari II malformation symptoms.
- Seizures that cause reactions that can frighten or injure the team (horse and staff)
- Seizures with a convulsive nature, loss of postural control - either flaccid or spastic
- Vestibular hypersensitivity that cause severe fear
- The inability to be controlled on the horse.

Precautions to hippotherapy or riding include:

- Open area to skull with a well fitted helmet - specific to this client to prevent infection Shunt
- Low tone or spasticity that could lead to a dislocated hip
- Any subluxation or dislocation must be carefully monitored by the therapist and physician.
- Poor head control of a child
- Spinal cord involvement (complete) above the T-6 level
- Hydrocephalus with a shunt
- Spina Bifida
- Skin breakdown must be monitored on surfaces affected by riding
- All spinal cord injury involvement
- Lack of sitting balance in an adult despite cause
- Down Syndrome with low tone (absent Atlantoaxial instability) must be carefully observed for negative signs and must be clinically reviewed by their physician
- All low toned clients must be carefully monitored for any negative signs such as decreased balance while riding

- ▸ Hypertonus needs to be monitored for changes in function
- ▸ Lack of potential of righting and strengthening the spine
- ▸ Seizure disorders are mild (little change of awareness and minor motor reactions) with a trained team
- ▸ Seizure disorders that cause lack of awareness with no improvement due to riding with a trained team

References:

Strauss, I. (1995). *Hippotherapy*. Ontario Therapeutic Riding Association, Canada.
NARHA. (1997). NARHA Operating Center Standards & Accreditation Manual, Denver CO.

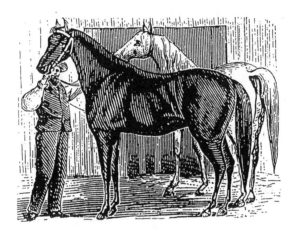

CHAPTER 5

DEFINITION OF TERMS IN HIPPOTHERAPY, THERAPEUTIC RIDING, AND DRESSAGE

GLOSSARY OF TERMS USED IN THERAPEUTIC RIDING

Barbara T Engel, M.Ed., OTR

ADA

American with Disabilities Act is the civil rights law passed in 1990 for people with disabilities in USA.

ADAPTIVE EQUIPMENT

1) Riding equipment changed in structure or form to allow a person with a disability to ride.

2) Equipment that has been specially developed to allow a physically disabled person to ride a horse.

3) Equipment used to elicit specific responses.

ADAPTIVE PHYSICAL EDUCATION

Physical education modified for a special population who cannot take part in regular physical education activities.

ADAPTIVE RIDING

Horseback riding adapted for a special population.

AIDS (HORSE)

Methods used to communicate with the horse - leg aids, seat and weight aids, hand aids, spurs, whip and voice aids.

ANIMAL ASSISTED ACTIVITIES (AAA)

A person who provides AAA possesses specialized knowledge of animals and the populations with which they interact in delivering motivational, educational, recreational and/or therapeutic animal-oriented activities. Volunteers are often involved in AAA. Individuals may work independently when they have specialized training. This group may include but is not limited to such individuals.

ANIMAL-ASSISTED THERAPY (AAT)

is a goal-directed intervention in which an animal that meets specific criteria is an integral part of the treatment process. AAT is directed and/or delivered by health/human service professionals with specialized expertise. It is used within the scope of practice of their profession. AAT is designed to promote improvement in human physical, social, emotional, and/or cognitive functioning. AAT is provided in a variety of settings, and may be group or individual in nature. This process is documented and evaluated. An alternate term to identify such action is "pet-facilitated therapy." A less acceptable term is "pet therapy."

ARENA

A place set aside for the performance of riding activities on the flat. The arena is enclosed by solid walls in an indoor arenas or a safe fence or rail outdoors.

AROUSAL

Level of being alert in order to attend, to learn or to behave appropriately to a given situation. A state of arousal that is to high may cause over activity, or fight-flight reaction; under arousal may cause doziness, day dreaming, or being spaced out.

ASSISTANT RIDING INSTRUCTOR

A person who is qualified to teach people with disabilities in a therapeutic riding center and who has passed current tests and standards; in the U.S.A. established by NARHA - see NARHA.

BARN MANAGER

A person who is in charge of the daily operation of barn activities and supervision or care of the horses.

BEAT

A footfall within a gait. A hoof, or pair of hooves virtually simultaneously, strike the ground together.

BEDDING

Used in a stall, such as straw, peat, or wood shavings.

BONDING

The establishment of an attachment/union between two or more persons, person and animal, or among animals.

BRIDLE

A harness composed of leather of webbing that provides a means of communicating with the horse.

CAST

A horse is said to be cast when he is lying in such a way that he can not stand up without assistance - such as rolling over toward a wall with the legs against the stall wall and unable to roll back over.

CENTER - therapeutic riding

The location of an organization involved in any aspect of therapeutic riding.

CENTERED RIDING

A teaching technique developed by Sally Swift based on the classic art of equitation stressing the rider's sense of natural balance by a process of building blocks or processes.

CERTIFIED OCCUPATIONAL THERAPIST ASSISTANT (COTA™)(COTA™/ L)

A person with credentials as an occupational therapy assistant who works under the supervision of an occupational therapist registered and who treats diseases and injuries by use of activities with the emphasis on adaption.

CLASSIC ART OF EQUITATION

Training of a horse and rider in the art of riding developed during the 16th through 17th centuries - now called dressage. It is the harmony between horse and rider.

CLASSIC HIPPOTHERAPY

Hippotherapy following the German methods based on classic dressage as it applies to rehabilitation.

CONDITIONING

Gymnastic exercises performed with the horse to condition his muscles, supple him, and increase cardiovascular activity and general health

CONFIDENTIAL RECORDS

Any records related to personal or medical information of clients, riders or staff

CONFORMATION

The physical structure of a horse. Horses of different breeds vary in structure just as humans of different backgrounds vary in structure. The conformation of a cold blooded horse is different from a thoroughbred or a warm blood or a Quarter Horse, or an Arabian. Each is bred to perform give tasks. The way a horse is built. Good conformation is functional for the work that the horse will do. Deficits can be a problem for a horse working in one area but not in another

DELTA SOCIETY

An organization headquartered in Renton, WA, that supports research studies and educates people on how companion animals benefit human physical and emotional well-being; establishes community programs to build a partnership between animals and people; operates the national information center and library for field of human-animal interactions.

DEVELOPMENTAL EQUINE-ASSISTED THERAPY

A specific treatment method, using NDT and/or SI treatment technique, carried out by a specially trained physical or occupational therapist during a treatment session with a client with neuromuscular dysfunctions.

DISABILITY

Restriction or lack (resulting from impairment) of ability to perform an activity in the manner or within the range considered normal for a human being (World Health Organization, 1980). A person with a disability may not have a handicap in certain situations.

DOCUMENTATION

Specific records which state factual information. Documentation can be for employee records (job descriptions, disciplinary actions, etc); client evaluation and progress reports; operating procedures. All documentation is a legal record. They should be written so that they will stand up in any legal action.. With this is mind the person doing the documentation will write them factually and precisely.

DRESSAGE

Means training of the horse (in any discipline) to improve movement, develop muscles, supple, develop balance, develop submission and responsiveness to the aids in a systematic way based on the muscular development of the horse.

DYSFUNCTION

Abnormal or impaired function.

EQUINE-ASSISTIVE THERAPY

Treatment with the use of the horse in an equine setting by a qualified health care professional.

EQUINE-FACILITATED PSYCHOTHERAPY

Treatment by a psychologist, behavioralist, or psychiatrist in the treatment of social or emotional disorders.

EQUINE FIRST-AID KIT

A kit that contains items for emergency purposes and for the regular medical care of horses. The kit should include any tack or other equipment needed while dealing with an emergency.

EQUITATION

The art of riding.

FACILITY

The location of a therapeutic riding center where riding or management activities are held.

FARRIER

A person who cares for, trims or shoes the feet of the horse.

FLEXIBILITY

The ability to move the joints freely.

FOREHAND

The head, neck, shoulders and forelegs of the horse.

FORWARD

To or toward the direction tin which the horse should be going.

FOOTING

The ground cover of an arena.

FRIGHT, FLIGHT, FIGHT REACTION

A reaction seen in horse and people. The reaction is set off when the person or horse senses danger, stress or something unfamiliar. The initial reaction is fright, with increased stimuli results in flight. If the horse or person cannot escape, fight is initiated

GAIT

The horse has several natural gaits including walk, trot, canter, gallop.

GUIDELINE

Directions, instructions and/or regulations developed for implementation by a government, an organization, a Center, a supervisor which are to be followed without question [unless modification is requested].

HAND (horse term)

A horse is measured by the linear measurement equals to 4 inches or one hand. A fourteen hand horse equals 56 inches at the withes.

HANDICAP (human)

Disadvantage for a given individual, resulting from an impairment or a disability, that limits or prevents the fulfillment of a role that is normal (depending on age, sex, and social and cultural factors) for that individual (World Health Organization, 1980).

A handicap may not indicate a physical or mental disability.

HEADER

Also caller a horse leader. A person who stands at the head of a horse while the rider is mounting to keep the horse relaxed and still.

HEAD INSTRUCTOR

Persons who have the training and meet the qualification to be in charge of riding instruction at a therapeutic riding center. A head instructor must pass the current required certification course (within his or her country) to be eligible to instruct persons with disabilities. A head riding instructor is in charge of all other riding instructors at the center, consultants and volunteers.

HEALTH CARE PROFESSIONAL

A person with qualifications who is licensed in a nationally recognized health profession; is qualified to bill a third-party payee. See licensed/credentialed health professional

HELMET

A helmet is a piece of equipment that covers the head of **any** rider while mounted in a NARHA program. The **riding helmet** must be a currently approved riding helmet tested for safety for horseback riding activities with a secure full harness and approved by NARHA, in the USA, for the current year. The use of light weight helmets must meet the current NARHA's guidelines, in the USA, for light weight helmets. All helmets MUST fit the head according to guidelines. A helmet that is too large or too small is dangerous.

HIPPOTHERAPIST

Does not exist. To be a hippotherapist would indicate a profession in hippotherapy. **There is no such profession in the US.** Sorry therapists - you have to get your business cards reprinted? Hippotherapy is a specialized method of treatment very much like neuromuscular developmental techniques (NDT) or sensory integration (SI). Hippotherapy is practiced by specially trained occupational, physical or speech therapist in the practice of their professions. To use this form of treatment one must be an occupational, or physical or speech therapists. The therapist must have training in the theory of classic hippotherapy, (a minimum of a three- day course) and in the use of equine movements in the treatment of neurological disorders; can apply this knowledge to augment his or her professional skills in physical therapy /or occupational or speech therapy to treat clients with mild to severe movement disorders (Hippotherapy Curriculum Development Project 1988/Hippotherapy Section of NARHA 1991). The individual who practices hippotherapy must meet the current standards for this modality according to their national organization within their country. In 1997 there were no international standards.

HIPPOTHERAPY

"Hippos" means horse in Greek. "Treatment with the help of the horse." A treatment for clients with movement dysfunctions and/or neurological disorders used by physical or occupational therapists trained as hippotherapists. In classic hippotherapy, the horse influences the client rather than the client controlling the horse (Hippotherapy Curriculum Development Project, 1991). The therapist may use exercises or activities to achieve specific treatment goals.

HORSE

Any equine animal such as a pony, horse, donkey or mule used in a therapeutic riding program.

HORSE HEADER

A person, normally the horse handler, who stands at the head of a horse while a rider mounts the horse.

HORSE HANDLER

A person who has had training in horsemanship skills and knows the psychological and physical needs of a horse. This person maybe the horse leader.

HORSE LEADER

A person who has had training in horsemanship skills and knows the psychological and physical needs of a horse. In addition, he or she knows how to handle a horse with specific needs for the disabled rider.

HUMAN-ANIMAL BONDING

The attachment that develops between humans and animals involving strong feelings and psychological ties. Studies have supported that the love and attentiveness given by people to animals is reciprocal and both animals and people benefit (Anderson, 1983).

IMPAIRMENT

Loss or abnormality of psychological, physiological, or anatomical structure or function.

INSIDE

The direction toward which the horse should be laterally positioned or bent. The side that is toward the center of the ring.

IRREGULAR

Impure, unlevel or uneven gait. Does not mean unsteady in tempo.

LEADER

One who leads a project or a group. The person in charge. A leader is a person who can attract followers. Without followers one can direct (or oder) but cannot lead.

LICENSED/CREDENTIALED HEALTH PROFESSIONALS

A health professional who has completed a course in a recognized filed and is licensed and/or certified by federal, state and national organization to practice in a specific field and is approved to bill third part agents such as medicare, medi-aid, or insurance carriers.

LONG REINING

A technique used in hippotherapy and training. The horse is "driven" from the ground by using reins that reach from the bit to one stride or more behind the horse. The client sits on the horse while the handler controls and reins from behind the horse.

LONGEING

Moving a horse around on a circle with the longer in the middle having the horse on a **longeline**. The purpose is to control the horse in his gaits, to bend and supple him. Longeing can be used to train a rider in developing a seat and balance. A horse should never be raced around the circle for pure exercise since this does not develop balance or development of appropriate muscles.

LONGER OR LONGEUR

A person who has been trained in the techniques of longeing as a method of training or as the longeur for a vaulting group.

METER

A unit of measurement in the metric system. A riding ring, such as a dressage arena, is measured by the metric system. 1 meter = 39.37 inches.

MODALITY

A form of treatment.

MOUNTING BLOCK

A device used for mounting a rider to the horse.

MOUNTING RAMP

A ramp designed for mounting a person onto the horse from a wheelchair. It is also used by ambulatory riders since it is kinder to the horse's back than ground mounting.

NORTH AMERICAN RIDING FOR THE HANDICAPPED ASSOCIATION (NARHA)

NARHA is the service organization in the U.S.A. created to promote the well-being of individuals with disabilities through equine activities.

NARHA REGISTERED INSTRUCTOR CERTIFICATION (CRTRI)

A person who has passed the requirements set by NARHA necessary to qualify for the title of a registered riding instructor.

NARHA ADVANCED REGISTERED INSTRUCTOR CERTIFICATION (CATRI)

A person who has passed the requirements set by NARHA necessary to qualify for the title of an advanced riding instructor.

NARHA MASTERS INSTRUCTOR CERTIFICATION (CMTRI)

A person who has taken a written examination and has passed the qualification that NARHA has set for the master's level certification for riding instructors in the U.S.A.

NDT

Neuro-developmental technique - a treatment method used by occupational and physical therapists and speech pathologists with persons who have deficits in their neurological systems.

NEAR-SIDE

The left side of the horse.

OCCUPATIONAL THERAPIST REGISTERED (OTR ™) /or licensed-OTR ™/L

A person with a credential in occupational therapy who treats disease and injury by using activities with emphasis on adaptation (Clark & Allen, 1985). Occupational therapists are licenced in some states but not all. They are certified nationally.

OFF-SIDE

The right side of the horse.

OPERATING CENTER

An organization that provides therapeutic riding activities to persons with and without disabilities.

OPERATING STANDARDS FOR HIPPOTHERAPY (NARHA)

If hippotherapy is used at a center that is requesting or being accredited, these standards must be in place.

PARTICIPANTS OF THERAPEUTIC RIDING CENTERS

Any person who receives services from a therapeutic riding program.

PHYSICAL THERAPIST--PT.

A person with a degree in physical therapy who treats disease and injury by physical means, such as light, heat, cold, water, ultrasound, massage and exercise with emphasis on mobility (Clark & Allen 1985). Physical therapists are licensed by each state - not nationally.

PRAXIS

The ability to organize, plan and execute skills. The sequential component of praxis are imitation, ideation, initiation, construction, feedback, feed-forward, grading, timing, sequencing, and motor planning.

PROBLEM SOLVING

The mental process by which one sequentially identifies a problem, interprets aspects of the situation, and selects a method to alleviate the problem (Fleming, 1991).

PROFESSIONAL

A person professing or declaring to have an occupation that requires advanced training. Having much experience and great skill in a specific role. Claiming to be a professional (in a specific field) can take on the legal responsibility of the status so claimed.

RECREATION SPECIALIST

A person with a degree in recreation who is skilled to work in the field of recreation but does not have the additional medical skills necessary to be a recreational therapist and work with persons with disabilities.

RECREATIONAL THERAPIST--RTR

A person with a degree in recreational therapy who works with persons with disabilities, using recreational and leisure activities to help the individual to re-enter a social life and community living.

REMEDIAL RIDING

Riding activities adapted to help the client gain educational and psychological goals under the direction of a specially trained educator or therapist.

REGULARITY

Correctness of the gait to include purity, evenness, and levelness.

REMEDIAL VAULTING

Vaulting which is adapted to help the client to gain educational and psychological goals under the direction of a specially trained educator or therapist.

RIDING ON THE FLAT

Riding in an arena or arena type area - working on gymnastic type exercises.

RIDING THERAPY

The integration by therapists of neurophysical or psychosocial treatment procedures with exercises and horsemanship to gain specific medical goals. Riding therapy is a part of equine-assisted therapy.

RHYTHM

The characteristic sequence of footfalls and phases of a given gait.

SCHOOLING FIGURES.

Circles, figure eights, straight lines, curves, and other patterns used in riding training to develop precise control of a horse through one's aids or actions.

SENSORY INTEGRATION (SI)

The ability of the brain to organize and coordinate sensation and behavior, which leads to adaptive responses that permit a higher level of function. Sensory integration procedures are initiated by the client with the therapist manipulating the environment to gain specific therapeutic results. The sensory integration procedure is a part of the occupational therapy practice and can also be carried out by SI trained physical therapists. Sensory Integration is a specific treatment technique developed by A. Jean Ayres and her associates for children who have been identified by specific test measures to have deficits in sensory integration.

SENSORIMOTOR INTEGRATION

This term refers to a group of techniques used by therapists to treat neurological disorders. It may incorporate sensory integration methods along with other techniques to increase a person's function. Vestibular or tactile stimulation by themselves are included here since this is not sensory integration.

SEQUENCING

The step by step procedure required to plan a step, to accomplish an activity, to develop a skill.

SHEEPSKIN

A pad made out of real or artificial sheepskin secured with a surcingle. The pad is used with clients during exercises with a therapist or with riders who are more comfortable with the softness of sheepskin. It can be used with a standard surcingle or with a **vaulting** surcingle.

SHOEING

Having shoes put on the horse's feet.

SIDE-AID or AID, SIDEWALKER.

A person who has been trained to help a rider. This person walks next to the horse at the rider's side (so he or she can place his or her arm across the rider's thigh when necessary), may help the rider with balance, provides necessary security, and/or may help the rider carry through with a lesson. "Side-aid" is more often use by therapists since the term is more descriptive to the task.

SPECIAL EDUCATION

Educational programs which are adapted to meet learning needs for a population with special needs (and problems).

SPECIAL NEEDS POPULATION

Persons with special needs--these can be physical, psychological, psych-social, or a combination of these.

SPEECH AND LANGUAGE PATHOLOGIST

A person with a degree in speech and language pathology who treats persons with deficits in speech and language, both visual and verbal.

SPEECH TEACHER

A speech teacher trained to develop normal speech and communication. May be a BS degree. This person does not have a medical background to work with those who have pathological problems.

SPORTS VAULTING

The same as vaulting. Gymnastics on horseback. Vaulting is carried out according to the primary six vaulting exercises and additional creative exercises called "kur." Vaulting is an equine sport.

SUPPLING THE HORSE

Riding exercises to increase the lateral flexibility and balance of the horse.

SURCINGLE

A girth placed around the horse's barrel just behind the withers - used for training or to hold on a blanket. In therapeutic riding it can be uses with a sheep skin during therapy.

TACK

That which is placed on the horse to train or to ride a horse, such as a bridle, surcingle, and saddle.

TACKING-UP

To prepare a horse for riding by 'tacking-up' by putting on the bridle, pad, saddle, etc.

TACTILE DEFENSIVE

Inability to tolerate or process touch - over sensitive.

TEAM

A team is a group that works closely together to purse a single objective. A therapeutic riding team consists of a minimum of a horse, a rider or client, and an instructor or therapist. The team may consist of a horse, a rider or client, an instructor, a therapist, a leader, and one or two sidewalkers or helpers.

THERAPEUTIC RIDING

Therapeutic riding uses equine activities to promote physical, cognitive, emotional and social vitality in persons with disabilities. Therapeutic riding includes activities in sport, leisure and recreation, education and in therapy. The emphasis in sport is the acquisition of skills for recreation and/or competition directed by therapeutic riding instructors. Sport may include riding, driving and vaulting. Recreation and leisure equine activities are carried out by instructors or recreational specialists or recreational therapists. Therapy is a specific goal directed treatment using equine activities carried out by licensed/credentialed health care professional (able to bill third party payors).

THERAPEUTIC VAULTING

Standard vaulting exercises performed at the level of the special vaulter. Sports vaulting for special needs vaulters.

THERAPY

The method employed in effecting the cure or management of disease. Implies diagnosis using special criteria (or diagnostic and procedural coding systems used in medicine for billing purposes); involves prescribed treatment by a health care professional who is liable for his or her actions according to the standards of his or her specialty, and is billable to third-party payers (i.e., insurance carriers). Hippotherapy and equine-assisted therapy are recognized treatment procedures when used by especially trained physical, occupational, or speech therapists in a treatment situation by the American Physical Therapy Association, by the American Occupational Therapy Association, or by the Speech and Language Association.

TOPLINE

The horse's outline from the ears along the top of its neck and back to its tail.

TRACKING UP

The hind feet step into the tracks of the forefeet.

TT.E.A.M.

The Tellington-Jones Equine Awareness Method, a unique training protocol developed by Linda Tellington-Jones for the horse to make him safer, more attentive to the handler, less distracted by the environment, more pleasurable, less stressful to the ride and a better performer. The training method involves a detailed step by step procedure (taught during a series of courses) which produces a friendly horse who is eager to learn (Tellington-Jones, Bruns 1988).

VAULTING

The gymnastics on a moving back. Vaulting is carried out according to the primary vaulting exercises and additional creative exercises called kur. Vaulting is an equine sport.

VAULTING SURCINGLE

A surcingle with handles. A vaulting surcingle used with a bareback pad or sheepskin, mainly for holding on, can be constructed of leather or webbing with two handles (internally secured to a metal plate) and can flex at the center. A vaulting girth used in gymnastic vaulting, must be constructed with a solid plate (internally) from well below the handle on one side, across the top to well below the handle on the other side. The construction of this vaulting girth is much stronger than the one required for "therapeutic riding."

VAULTING THERAPY

The integration by therapists of neurophysical or psychosocial treatment procedures with exercises and vaulting to gain specific medical goals. Vaulting therapy is a part of equine-assisted therapy.

VETERINARIAN

A doctor of veterinarian medicine who treats animals.

VOLUNTEER

Any person who is not paid for their service who is involved in any activities of a therapeutic riding center.

WARMUP

Exercising the horse from the ground on a longe or riding the horse to warm up his muscles, supple him and prepare his body for the work ahead. Warm-up exercises may take from ten minutes at a walk, then trot and canter to twenty minutes for an older horse.

ADDITIONAL TERMS?

_____

_____

_____

_____

_____

_____

_____

_____

_____

_____

_____

_____

_____

DRESSAGE and RIDING TERMS AND INTERPRETATIONS

DRESSAGE - WHAT IS IT?

Obedience is necessary for suppleness---without suppleness the horse cannot bend, flex, or engage. If he cannot bend, he cannot go straight. " Dressage is a basis for training horses of all types. When basic dressage training is completed, a horse should be not only a pleasure to ride but also prepared for specialized training in any discipline," (S.E, Harris, 1996). " Dressage is based on classical principles and methods proven over several centuries," (S.E. Harris,1996). The harmony between horse and rider permits the horse to carry out all movements with mental and physical enjoyment and being supple, rhythmic, and forward is what reflects the beauty and grace. Dressage is the gymnastic training of the horse on a developmental basis to develop his muscles and coordination to perform the horse's normal way of going.

Basic training provides one with a horse that is responsive and pleasant to ride. *"To confirm that the horse's muscles are supple, and loose, and that it moves forward in clear and steady rhythm, accepting contact with the bit." (AHSA training level definition).*

"To confirm that the horse in addition to the requirements of Training level, has developed thrust (pushing power from the hindquareters) and achieved a degree of balance and throughness (AHSA first level definition). A therapy horse should have all these qualities to provide a client with quality movement therapy. In addition, lateral movements are frequently mentioned to facilitate lateral trunk flexion and extension in the client. Without the training and first level skills in a horse, lateral movements will not be balanced, rhythmic and fluid.

1	A X	ENTER WORKING TROT SITTING HALT. SALUTE.PROCEED WORKING TROT SITTING
2	C E X	TRACK LEFT. TURN LEFT CIRCLE LEFT 20 M
3	X B	CIRCLE RIGHT 20 M
4	C	HALT 5 SECONDS. PROCEED WORKING TROT
5	HZF F	FREE WALK ON LONG REIN WORKING WALK
6	A E-B	WORKING TROT SITTING HALF CIRCLE RIGHT 20 M
7	B	WORKING CANTER RIGHT LEAD AND IMMEDIATELY
8	B B	CIRCLE RIGHT 20 M STRAIGHT AHEAD
9	F KXM	WORKING TROT SITTING CHANGE REIN
10	M E-B	WORKING TROT SITTING HALF CIRCLE LEFT 20 M
11	B	WORKING CANTER LEFT LEAD AND IMMEDIATELY
12	B B	CIRCLE LEFT 20 M STRAIGHT AHEAD
13	M HXF	WORKING TROT SITTING CHANGE REIN
14	A X	DOWN CENTER LINE HALT. SALUTE.

TRAINING LEVEL-TEST 4 (when a horse is balanced enough to canter on a 20 M circle)

1	A X	ENTER WORKING TROT HALT. SALUTE. PROCEED WORKING TROT
2	C S-L	TRACK LEFT LEG YIELD LEFT
3	L L A	CIRCLE RIGHT 10 M STRAIGHT AHEAD TRACK RIGHT
4	V-I	LEG YIELD RIGHT
5	I I C	CIRCLE LEFT 10 M STRAIGHT AHEAD TRACK LEFT
6	HXF F	LENGTHEN STRIDE IN TROT RISING WORKING TROT
7	A	HALT 5 SECONDS. PROCEED WORKING WALK
8	KXH H	FREE WALK ON LONG REIN WORKING WALK
9	C M	WORKING TROT WORKING CANTER RIGHT LEAD
10	B	CIRCLE RIGHT 10 M
11	K-H H	LENGTHEN STRIDE IN CANTER WORKING CANTER
12	MXK	CHANGE REIN. AT X CHANGE OF LEAD THROUGH TROT
13	B	CIRCLE LEFT 10 M
14	H-K K	LENGTHEN STRIDE IN CANTER WORKING CANTER
15	A FXH H	WORKING TROT LENGTHEN STRIDE IN TROT WORKING TROT
16	B X G	TURN RIGHT TURN RIGHT HALT. SALUTE.

FIRST LEVEL-TEST 4 (end of first year of training)

DRESSAGE TESTS

Tests are established to determine if the horse has accomplished a level of competency at a sequential level. The purpose of the tests are not to train to accomplish **a test** but to train to accomplish coordination and muscling in order to accomplish skills. Each test level addresses a horse with a year or more of training. In competition one competes against oneself, in that one tries to improve on one's scores at progressively higher levels. Ribbon placement only shows how your test score places you with in that group of riders who may not be that skilled to start. It may not show improvement in skills for the years you and or your horse have worked.

ABOVE-THE-BIT

- The head and nose are too high or forward.
- There is no effect "through" the horse with the movement coming from the hindquarters, through the back and to the bit.
- The reins do not have contact with the mouth. The rider has little or poor control of the horse. Muscles of the hindquarters, back and neck are tense.
- Being behind the vertical does not necessarily mean the horse is behind the bit.
- Develop the wrong neck muscles (develops the lower neck muscles rather then the upper neck muscles.)

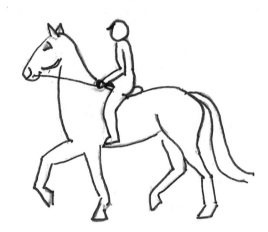

ACCEPTANCE

The lack of evasion, resistance or protest. The horse shows an unresistant willingness to allow the maintenance of a steady contact.

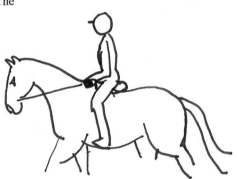

AIDS

The communication with the horse. A continuous exchange of information from the rider to the horse and the horse to the rider. Communication to the horse must be clear and exact in order for the horse to understand. The horse must be kept attentive to the rider's communication so he is always ready for change.

Horse's method of communication is body attitude, lack of alertness and resistance to aids either because of being unwilling or not being in condition to do what is asked of him.

Rider's method of communication is through the seat, torso, legs, hands, balance, weight shift, flexion and relaxation of muscles, and rein and voice aids.

ARM AIDS (not a true aid but an influence)

The arms follow the movement of the horse's head/neck while the hands remain still but can be used to restrain the horse by momentarily bracing with the back.

ALIGNMENT

The alignment of the horse's body parts from tail to poll.

ASTRIDE
   A person sitting on a horse with one leg on each side.

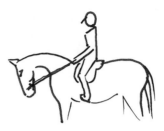

BACK AID
   Tensing, extending or restricting the back muscles aids in the communication in halting the horse, collection and lateral work.

BALANCE - horse
The horse needs to learn a new way of balancing himself when a rider is astride. **The weight of a rider threatens the natural sense of balance of a horse.** Training is required for the horse to learn longitudinal flexion (around the rider's leg) and to develop the hindquarter to shift his center of gravity toward his haunches. Balance in the horse with a rider astride is cultivated first at the walk, then trot and later canter. In each gait and with each exercise flexion is developed. The horse's balance is also influenced by the rider's balance since any weight shift off the center of gravity or involuntary hand action will imbalance the horse. The correct seat is a question of balance, and it places the rider in balance with the horse. The horse's balance is important since the rider re-organizes his or her balance with every step of the horse's action. Longitudinal balance prevents sluggishness and running while lateral balance prevents drifting sideways and uneven strides.

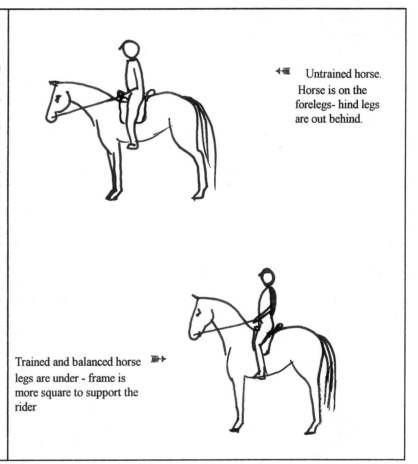

Untrained horse. Horse is on the forelegs- hind legs are out behind.

Trained and balanced horse legs are under - frame is more square to support the rider

BALANCE-human
   Riding requires the balance of the upper body, the neck and the head. The upper torso is free to move separately from the pelvis. Centered Riding - the centering process - relaxes and softens the rider, deepens the seat, drops the center of gravity, and balances the body.

BEAT
   A footfall within a gait. A hoof or pair of hooves striking the ground at the same time. By this definition the walk has four beats, the trot has two, the canter has three.

BEHIND-THE-BIT

The horse has no contact with the bit. The rider has no contact with the horse. The horse cannot lengthen (stretch) the neck that helps stretch the back.

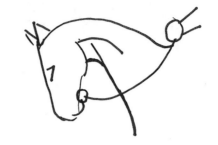

BENDING

Going forward with the total body bent to the bend, in which the horse is going without the shoulders or haunches falling in or breaking the flow of the curve. The horse's body is adjusted to the bend of the curve. The power flows through the body of the horse from the hindquarter to the head.

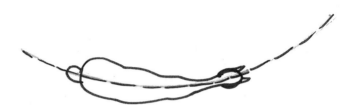

BRIDLE

Includes the headstall, bit and reins. The total head harness.

CADENCE

Cadence requires rhythm, acceptance of the bit, impulsion, self-carriage in connection with collection and extension to give the pace an energetic lift of the feet from the ground as though the horse was bouncing through the air .

CARRIAGE

The posture of the horse.

COLLECTION:

Collection is a combination of engagement and flexion of the haunches. It causes the shortening of the horse's frame by bringing the hindquarters under him to carry more of the weight of the rider. The forehand becomes lighter, the horse appears to go uphill as he elevates his withers and neck. The frame shortens in stages as the horse's training progresses. Collection begins from self-carriage, to a rectangular frame, to a square frame at the higher levels. In dressage tests each level of testing requires increased collection from a triangular frame to a square frame with the horse carrying increasingly , more of the rider's weight on his hindquarters.

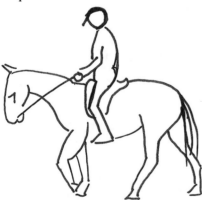

**SELF-CARRIAGE
WITHOUT COLLECTION**
Horse's weight is forward

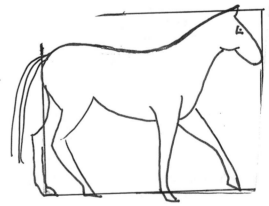

BEGINNING COLLECTION
Neck is raised allowing the hind to drop

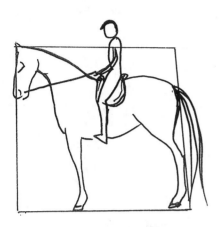

**COLLECTION WITH THE HORSE
IS A NEAR SQUARE FRAME**
The legs are under the horse carrying
the rider's weight

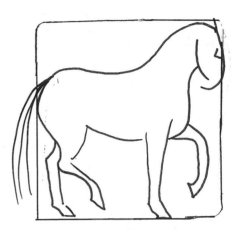

**ADVANCED COLLECTION
NECK IS RAISED, RUMP TUCKED UNDER**
The horse appears to go uphill

CONFORMATION
   The bone structural formation of the horse.
CONFORMATION FAULTS
   Faults are errors in conformation that may produce negative movements, lameness, or other problems. See *Therapeutic Riding I Strategies for Instructors* for detailed faults.
CONNECTION
   State in which there is no blockage, break or slack in the association that joins the horse and rider into a single unit. Unrestricted flow of energy and influence from and through the rider to and through the horse.

CONTACT
   The connection of bringing suppleness, regularity in tempo and engagement from the haunches over the back and connecting into the hands - and accepting the bit with the leg aid contact. The tipping under of the haunches will shorten the line from the shoulder to the buttocks. Contact engages the hind legs under the horse's body to accommodate the additional weight of the rider. Contact is the acceptance of the bit that comes from the hocks through the body moving the horse forward with leg aids to the bit.

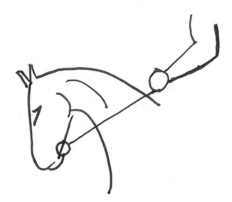

THE HORSE COMES FROM BEHIND INTO THE BIT
The horse maintains contact with the bit without pulling on the reins-
the contact on the reins remains light. The horse holds his head with the upper
neck muscles rather then holding it up by leaning on the bit.

DEEP SEAT

Allowing the seat muscles to relax and the legs and thighs to spread and drop as in figure A. The rider's weight sits on the pelvic bones and crotch. A deep seat takes the tension off the horse's back (hollow back) and allows it to round the top line. A deep seat allows full contact with the horse through the seat and thighs.

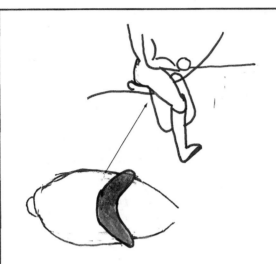

Figure A. DEEP SEAT shows the buttocks and thigh from below -bottom-left.
- allows full contact through seat & thighs to the spinal column and balance through the seat-thigh area.

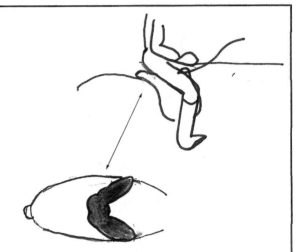

Figure B. - FORKED SEAT
on the bottom-left - shows the buttocks from below -buttocks not down and soft -more weigh on knees - increased tension on horse's back but less contact with the horse.

ELASTIC

The ability to stretch and contract the musculature smoothly.

ENGAGEMENT

Engagement is developed through training and progresses at different levels. Initial engagement refers to the horse's response to the rider's demand to increase performance. Engagement is developed through, lateral -total body- flexion to develop the engagement of the hind legs (engagement & disengagement - the pushes off). It is the degree that a horse reaches with his hind legs forward under his body. Engagement of the pelvis is the tilt under of the pelvic bone.

FOOTING

The ground cover of an arena. The quality of the footing is important to preserve the horse's legs and to make a ride comfortable

FLEXION

Articulation of the joint so that the angle between the bones is decreased.

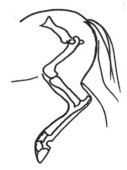

FREEDOM

The horse carrying the rider's weight without tension before asking for contact should be free of restrictions to the natural way of going.

GAITS

Is the manner of movement on foot. Good movement is healthy for the horse, easy to ride to and attractive to look at. The quality of the therapy is dependent on the quality of gait:

The quality of gait is dependent on:

1) **rhythm,**
2) **suppleness,**
3) **straightness,**
4) **acceptance of the bit,**

5) **impulsion,**
6) **collection,**
7) **cadence,**
8) **lightness.**

Walk - a four-beat gait with the left hind foot leading, following the left fore, right hind and the right fore.

Trot -.is a two-beat diagonal gait with the right hind and left fore, followed by suspension, left hind and right fore and suspension

Canter - a three-beat gait with suspension. The right hind, the left hind and right fore, left fore followed by suspension.

Gallop - is a four-beat gait with suspension.

Working walk -A regular, energetic, unconstrained walk used in the early stages of training. The horse maintains a light contact.

Collected walk - on the bit, moves energetically forward with the neck arched and raised to the degree of training. The pace has a marching rhythm forward but is not fast.

Working trot - properly balanced, supple poll, remains on the bit, goes forward with even and elastic steps and has good hock actions.

Collected trot - On the bit, moves forward with the neck raised and some arch. Hocks are well engaged (flex). He remains energetic with impulsion. Engagement of the hindquarters allows the shoulders to move with greater ease. Horse's steps are shorter then on the working trot.

Working canter - Good balance, on the bit, forward, light, cadenced, stride with good hock action-not ready for a collected canter

Collected canter - On the bit, he moves forward with an arched and raised neck, lightness in the front.

HALF-HALT

Used for re-balancing and gaining the attention of the horse. It can be brought into action by re-balancing the rider, engagement of the hind legs to bring the horse into the hands, bringing the center back and making the forehand light (S. Swift 1985). The half halt is used before any transition or change in direction.

HAND AIDS

Hands remain still and soft. They are used to communicate with the mouth through the bit by momentary flexing of fingers, squeezing.

HEADSTALL

That which goes over the head of the horse to hold the bit and the reins.

HORSE'S MOVEMENTS

The horse's movement will be balanced, free of restrictions, forward and flowing.

IMPULSION

The power thrust from the haunches propels the horse forward through the swing back and a relaxed neck. The horse's desire to move forward with an elastic step, supple back and engagement and thrust of the hindquarters. The hindquarters are energetically lifted - the feet from the ground by flexion of the joints. The increased activity of the hind joints causes flexion and rotation of these joints. This allows slow, graceful effortless movements. The willingness to go forward is the lower level requirement of impulsion that requires suppleness. **Impulsion enables the horse to carry the rider softly since it reduces the jarring effect of the legs hitting the ground. It requires less energy of the horse since he has become more balanced and the joints are stronger.** The perfection of impulsion requires good rhythm, cadence in the horse's natural gaits.

LEG-YIELDING

When the horse moves away from the pressure of the rider's leg pressure but remains forward and straight.

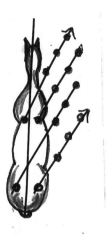

LIGHT CONTACT or LIGHTNESS

Light contact indicates the horse's willingness to remain on the bit without leaning on the bit (this means that one can hold his hand still and not feel the weight of the horse's head in the reins.) He holds his head and neck within the requested frame - he holds and maintains an arched neck (to the degree of training). The horse must develop neck muscles along the top of his neck to hold his head in this way. A horse with weight on the forehand cannot maintain light contact on the bit for very long if at all. The horse moves with agility and grace. A horse trained to lightness allows the rider to use subtle commands, a big advantage for persons with disabilities or in directing a horse in hippotherapy.

OBEDIENCE

When a horse responds without resistance to the command of the aids.

"ON THE AIDS"

The horse has learned to respond to the rider's seat, legs, and hands.

ON THE BIT"

Acceptance of the bit is the lower level of "on the bit." "On the bit" involves the total frame of the horse. The neck is slightly raised with the face vertical (depending on the level of training). There is no resistance. This provides the connection between the hand and the leg (hands -bit - leg). "On the bit" indicates the horse accepts and reaches for the bit. He does not avoid it by pulling his head in (behind the bit) or putting his nose too high or stretching forward (above the bit). The amount of contact of a trained horse is no more then a gentle soft pull on the fingers.

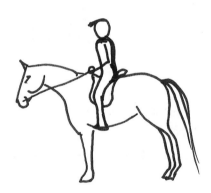

PACES

The pace refers to the horse's rhythm, speed and length of the stride. It should be energetic, regular, straight and free with the shoulders swinging forward and backward with ease.

PURITY

Correctness of the order and timing of the footfalls of the gait.

REGULARITY

The correctness of gait - evenness, levelness and purity.

RHYTHM

Regularity and correctness of the horse's footfall, the beat of his gaits. The rhythm should not change as the horse moves through circles, straight lines, curves or changes gaits.

DEFINITION OF TERMS IN HIPPOTHERAPY, THERAPEUTIC RIDING, AND DRESSAGE

RELAXATION

The lack of physical tension and mental calmness of the horse while he performs as requested by his rider (submission). Relaxation is a prerequisite of all work, in both mind (trusting the rider) and body. Relaxation is reflected in longitudinal flexion of the horse that produces more energy and rounding out his top line. Longitudinal flexion allows the horse to lower his haunches and step further under himself. It is the foundation of all suppling. A horse who is **not** relaxed - strung out, tenses and above the bit, usually with a depressed back will vibrate the tension throughout his body. The stiff legs will traumatize his impact on the ground. This impact will be transmitted to the rider further transmitting tension from the horse to the rider. Yielding of the jaw indicates a total state of relaxation. Yielding of the jaw is accomplished by a pressure of the fist on the reins without any movement from the arms causing a feeling of melting reins.

RESISTANCE

The horse shows resistance by:

Putting the tongue out,
Grinding the teeth,
Taking hold of the bit with his teeth,
Swinging the tail
Being above or behind the bit
Throwing his head

SCHOOLING FIGURES

The riding of patterns such as circles, straight lines, turns or any combination. These exercises train the horse to bend, go straight, respond to transition and to respond to the rider's aids willingly. In hippotherapy they can be used to cause postural adjustments and vestibular stimulation. They can also decrease boredom and fading out in the horse by causing the horse to stay attentive.

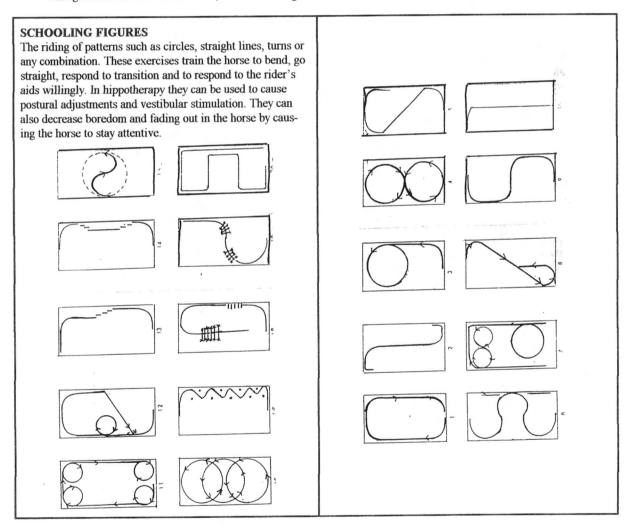

"SCHWUNG"

The transmission of the energy from the hind legs " dynamics and spring."

59

SEAT

The seat is important because a correct seat influence correct movement. It maintains the rider's center of gravity with the center of gravity of the horse. It provides good communication with the horse and allows the horse to move freely without restriction from the rider (even in hippotherapy the passenger can restrict the movement of the horse). The seat is related to balance and relaxation that allows the rider to go with the horse's motion. Only with a balanced and secure seat will the rider's center of gravity follow the horse's center of gravity. In dressage the rider sits "in" or deep in the horse not on top of the horse. The points of balance are the two seat bones and the crotch forming a triangle. The influence of the rider on the horse originates from the triangle. The influence from the horse to the rider is transmitted through this triangle. The legs of the rider are in a walk phase position. If the knees are pulled up this causes the rider to be in a "chair position" and the contact through the buttocks is greatly decreased and the communication lost. In jumping, the rider stays light in the saddle so as not to interfere with the withers and frees the horse to jump. The contact through the buttocks is lost and the influence to the spine is minimal.

SEAT AIDS

Driving seat, engaging aid. The seat is used by pushing the buttocks forward to move the horse forward (driving seat), bracing the seat to restrain the horse, weight shifting for turning, and balancing the seat as a half-halt. Seat aids are used in combination with other aids.

SECURE OR INDEPENDENT SEAT

Places one in balance with the horse and provides the rider security. The seat moves with the horse - the torso becomes independent and flexes, extends and straightens above the hips. This allows the horse to move in rhythm and forward without interference. Without a secure seat a rider cannot use his or her hands, arms, and legs independent of each other. The secure seat allows one to work toward lightness (sensitivity and quick response) in the use of aids. The secure seat is obtained by holding the legs with the inside thigh muscles allowing the legs to hang straight; the knees are forward with the weight in the heels and the chest is up and out with the shoulders back.

SELF-CARRIAGE

The relationship of the hooves of the horse to the mass of its body providing the horse with stability (Swift, 1985). Placing a rider on the horse's back requires the horse to change his method of balance. As the horse is gymnastically trained, he will progress from carrying major weight on the forehand to balancing weight over his four feet, to carrying weight over the hind quarters. A state in which the horse carries itself without taking support of balancing on the rider's hand/reins.

SHOULDER-IN

An exercise that promotes flexion or bending which in turn strengthens the hindquarters. Shoulder-in at the walk and trot will make the horse bend and use the joints in his hind legs while causing him to raise in the forehand. The horse's legs must cross with clearly defined flexion of all joints. This not only helps the horse to balance but also helps to strengthen the joints of the legs.

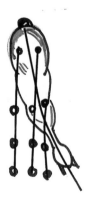

STRAIGHTNESS

To work the energy through the horse and forward. The hind feet work on the same track as the fore feet. The horse is symmetrical and balanced. Straightness requires the rider to sit straight - with the horse's hind feet placed in the step of the fore feet. Straightness cannot be obtained without the horse's ability to bend and to be supple.

STRIDES

The amount of ground covered in each step. A lengthened stride requires more power from the hind legs. The horse does not go faster but covers more ground. A shortened stride requires the horse to shorten his steps but maintain his rhythm and timing.

SUBMISSION

Obedience is displayed by always being focused, being willing to accept the aids with light contact and with no resistance. The horse shows his confidence in his behavior, in the ease of execution in his movements. Submission is displayed by the horse for example, by moving away from light pressure while be tacked-up or lowering the head for bridling.

SUPPLENESS

Is caused by thrust. A supple horse can bend laterally, shorten or lengthen in his frame without loss of balance. Through correct gymnastic exercises the horse will become balanced and in turn supple (S. Swift 1985). Suppleness increases with the degree of training. Lateral movements which lead to suppleness require of the horse a great deal of work to develop the muscles necessary for such movements.

SUSPENSION

The action of the legs when they momentarily are suspended in the air.

TEMPO

Speed measured in meter per minutes. Speed of the horse's rhythm.

TENSION

Tension prevents the horse from using his body well. The back becomes stiff and he is uncomfortable to ride. His back muscles contract. His walk becomes shorter in stride and stiffer because the joints do not bend as much. The horse is not happy. The rider becomes stiffer from the stiff horse.

TRANSITION

Changes from the halt or one gait to another, from one speed to another within a gait.

THROUGHNESS

The supple, elastic, unblocked, connected state of the horse's musculature that permits an unrestricted flow of energy from back to front allowing the reins to make a connection with the hind legs; or the push of the hind legs to drive through to the bit. The rider can feel this as a force flowing through the horse rather then the force from the hind legs ending at the buttocks of the rider.

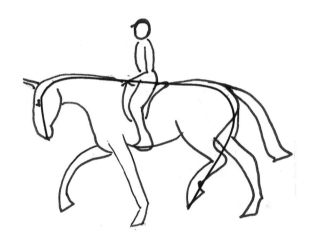

WEIGHT AIDS

The rider uses his weight to adjust to the horse's center of gravity or to change the horse's center of gravity. The rider can shift his or her weight to shift the horse's center of gravity. If a rider wants to turn right, he or she turns the spine and faces the direction of the turn. The rider's weight is shifted from equal weight on both buttocks to more weight on the right buttocks causing the horse to respond to the shift and to turn right. The **seat** always remains the same - only the weight distribution changes and/or the leg or hips change. The rider does not lean forward, or collapse the hips or shoulders. The rider's hips and shoulders must always remain parallel to those of the horse.

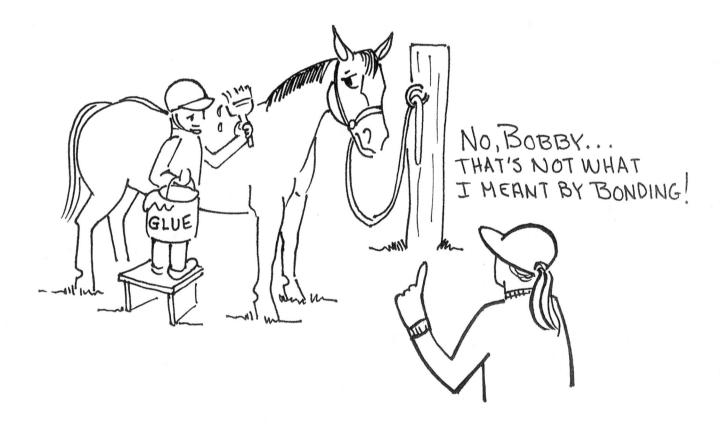

HIPPOTHERAPY and EQUINE-ASSISTED THERAPY TERMS

ACTIVITY ANALYSIS
To breake down an activity so that it can be examined and taught in sequential parts.

AMERICAN HIPPOTHERAPY ASSOCIATION (AHA)
The American Association of occupational, physical, and speech pathologists involved in treating clients with the use of the horse.
The Association is a section under the North American Riding for the Handicapped (NARHA) and can be contacted through NARHA.

BACKRIDING
When two people ride on a horse together. In therapeutic horseback riding, backriding is used in therapy to develop posture in the front rider, the client, by the backrider, a therapist. A trained instructor may backride a child under the direct supervision of the therapist. Backriding is considered a treatment with the therapist using NDT or CranioSacral techniques. To a limited degree, an instructor may backride a child who has normal or near normal gross motor skills until that child feels secure, for one to three sessions.

CLASSIC HIPPOTHERAPY
The client sits astride a specially trained therapy horse. The horse influences the client through its movements controlled by the instructor. The client is a passenger on the horse and does not control the horse. The client is positioned on and actively responds to the movement of the horse. The therapist directs the movement of the horse and analyzes the client's responses and adjusts the movement according to the treatment goals. (Adapted from the Definition of Classic Hippotherapy, American Hippotherapy Association)

CO-THERAPY
The treatment of a client by two disciplines in joint treatments such as occupational and physical therapy or occupational and speech therapy.

DEVELOPMENTAL RIDING THERAPY
Described as a specific systems approach for intervention based on psychomotricity techniques which is carried out by a treatment team. This technique was developed by Jan Spink, MA

DEVELOPMENTAL VAULTING
Vaulting (gymnastic activities on the back of a horse) for persons with special needs, supervised by a vaulting instructor.

DEVELOPMENTAL EQUINE-ASSISTED THERAPY
A specific treatment method, using NDT treatment techniques, which are carried out by a specially trained physical or occupational therapist during a treatment session with a client with a neuromuscular dysfunction.

EQUINE-ASSISTED THERAPY
This can include any treatments performed by a recognized health care professional that involves treatment other than hippotherapy. Therapy may include any horsemanship activities on or off the horse. An example may be grooming the horse to gain range of motion, balance and gross and fine motor coordination.

EQUINE FACILITATED PSYCHOTHERAPY
Treatment of social and behavioral disorders by a licenced professional in the field of psychology or psychiatry using the horse as a tool for intervention.

EQUIPMENT USED IN HIPPOTHERAPY
The horse wears a bridle with a snaffle bit, a pad and vaulting surcingle and side-reins; or a saddle and saddle pad with or without side reins. If the horse is long-reined side-reins are normally used.

FEEDBACK
Information about what has actually happened that is given to an individual.

FEED FORWARD
The anticipation of what is to happen by an individual.

HIPPOTHERAPIST
There is no such person since there is to field of hippotherapy.

HIPPOTHERAPY

"Hippos" means horse in Greek. "Treatment with the help of the horse." A treatment for clients with movement dysfunctions and/or neurological disorders used by physical or occupational therapists or speech pathologists with special training to use this medium as a tools. Hippotherapy is based on Classic Hippotherapy. Hippotherapy may include meaningful activities while on the horse that enhance the client's level of function. The therapist may use exercises or activities to achieve specific treatment goals.

HOLISTIC

An approach that deals with the multi-dimensional aspect of human functions.

KINETICS

The science of the effects of motion on matter in relation to the forces acting on them. Only when the kinetics of the horse's motion is as clearly understood as the movement responses of the rider, can the therapist accurately assess the effects of the riding on the patient. Only then can the therapist correctly apply riding therapy - the appropriate amount and understand the contraindications.

LONG REINING

Driving the horse from the ground from behind the horse with long reins while a client is astride, allows the instructor to collect the horse and to perform lateral movements to which the client must develop the coordination to remained balance and to flow with the horse's movements.

MATCHING THE HORSE TO THE RIDER

Consider and match the rhythm, stride, sensitivity, activity level, height, width of the back of the horse to that of the client.

MOTOR PLANNING

The ability to create, to use and combine various motor skills to perform new complex tasks.

MOVEMENT

Movement is the change of place or position. A horse does not move the same with a rider astride as he does when he walks, trots, canters freely. A horse is trained with gymnastic exercises to strengthen and engage his hindquarters, strengthen and round his back, to move in a relaxed way with regularity, freedom of movement where his muscle groups work well together. (S. Harris 1996.)

MOVEMENT INFLUENCE ON THE CLIENT - THREE-DIMENSIONAL MOVEMENT OF THE HORSE

The influence of the horse is the swinging movement of the horse's gait causing a forward and backward movement of the client as the horse increases and decreases the movement caused by the pushing off and putting down a foot. The client also moves up and down as the horse steps under himself and then stretches the leg out. As the horse alternates his stride from right to left the client receives a side to side motion. The side to side - forward and backward produce a rotational movement to the client's spine since the influence from the horse is transmitted through the triangular base of the seat (seat bones and crotch). It is this three-dimensional movement from the horse that simulates the human gait. During the horse's complete four step walk the client's shoulders and pelvis perform a circular movement in the spine that combines rotation, compression, decompression and lateral tilt (Riede, 1988, Strauss 1995). The harmony of movement between horse and client is developed. The client learns to move to the preferred movement of the horse. The horse must therefore have the quality of movement that is to be transferred to the client. If the movement is flawed, the client will receive that flawed movement (Strauss, 1995.) The horse's movement influences all major human systems including respiration and oral, cardiovascular, digestive, arousal and attention, auditory, visual, vestibular/proprioceptive, tactile - sensory processing, postural, cortical organization, limbic, muscle tone and equilibrium and movement.

MOUNTING

The process of getting onto the horse. For persons who can walk and lift their legs, a step-up stair-platform with a handrail can be used. For clients with more severe disabilities a ramp is used. The ramp places the client at the level where a chair transfer requires a stand and pivot turn, and side sitting on the pad or saddle. The client's right leg is then helped over the neck of the horse. A well-trained horse will lower his head for this process. Dismounting is done in the reverse pattern.

PRAXIS

The ability to organize, plan and execute a skill in a refined and efficient manner.

RIDING THERAPY

The integration by therapists of neurophysical or psychosocial treatment procedures with exercises and horsemanship to gain specific medical goals. Riding therapy is a part of equine-assisted therapy.

SEAT

In order for the three-dimensional movements of the horse to influence the client, the client must obtain the balanced deep seat used in classic dressage. Without the contact of the pelvic and pubic bones the transmission through the spine is not obtained (Strauss 1995, von Dietz, 1994). A good seat is a natural seat. A soft and supple seat is created by having the client or rider relax and stretch. Such a rider/client then softly follows all the movements of the horse in order to balance. Balance is of course the basis for a good and secure seat. The soft, relaxed, and balanced seat develops in the rider the fine feel for the horse.

SENSORY MODULATION DYSFUNCTION

The inability to inhibit or process sensory stimulation -includes tactile defensiveness which may cause a flight, fright or fight reaction.

SENSORY INTEGRATION (SI International)

The ability of normal individuals to take in sensory information derived from the environment and from the movement of their bodies, to process and integrate these sensory inputs within the central nervous system, and to use this information to plan and organize behavior.

THEORETICAL MODELS FOR HIPPOTHERAPY

Sensory Integration Theory, Motor Learning Theory, Motor Control Theory, Dynamical Systems Theory and Psycholinguistic Theory (American Hippotherapy Position Paper 1996)

THERAPY HORSE

Considerations: Conformation, soundness, biomechanics, temperament, people oriented, submissive and wants to please, is physically and mentally broke. The therapy horse transmits to the rider its good or bad movements. The horse must be trained, conditioned and exercised to provide the client the maximum movement quality.

TEAM TREATMENT

Interdisciplinary - A variety of professionals working together as a team but using the skills of their own professions. They may work with a client together or separately but maintain clear communication and interaction with the total team. The team may consist of a nurse, occupational, physical, physician, psychological, recreational therapist, social worker and speech therapist. Or it could be just a speech therapist, occupational therapist, and a physical therapist and of course the client/family.

VESTIBULAR SYSTEM

The system which give a sense of movement. All sensations are processed in connection with the vestibular system. Dysfunctions in this system can causes problems in visual tracking, sequencing and timing, auditory and language skills. If damage has occurred to either the right side or to the left side, deficits may be more pronounced to that area that it affects.

ADDITIONAL TERMS.

_____

_____

_____

_____

_____

_____

_____

_____

_____

CHAPTER 6

THE USE OF THE HORSE AS A THERAPY TOOL

THERAPEUTIC USE OF THE HORSE IN HEALTH CARE SETTINGS

Barbara T. Engel, M.Ed, OTR

"The rhythmic movement of the horse's back, together with the physical contact and the motivation created through use of a living exercise apparatus, meets all the requirements of modern kinesitherapy techniques: increased flow of impulses from the periphery through proprioceptive, tactile, and vestibular stimulation; and improved activation of the voluntary motor control loop (periphery-cerebellum-parietal lobe-frontal lobe-periphery" (Riede, 1988, ie.). As early as the 1500's, physicians found that riding was beneficial to health. The Greeks used horseback riding with people who were found to have incurable problems in order to improve their spirits (Mayberry, 1978). In 1750 Francisco Fuller, in the first sports medicine text, mentioned equitation and its implications for maintenance of physical exercise and the effects it has on the mind and body.

Benefits which have been attributed to riding during the 1600-1800's are: stimulation of the digestive system, alleviating gout, relieving tuberculosis, influencing body metabolism, increasing strength in weak bodies, helping psychological problems, and improving general wellness of body and soul (De Pauw, 1986). Riders who were seriously injured were reported as making remarkable recoveries after they began to ride again as well as helping to relieve their psychological stress (Riede, 1988). The movement of the horse at a walking gait and the resulting swinging motions of its back are transferred to the rider; these actions closely approximate the same movement impulses or sequences that occur when a person walks normally (Heipertz, 1981).

The current use of the horse in medical care has developed since the late 1950's, mainly by German physicians and therapists. In 1965 Joseph J. Bauer and Dr. R.E. Renaud began using riding to rehabilitate patients. Clients involved in rehabilitation have included those with such disorders as multiple sclerosis, closed head injuries, orthopedic disorders, cerebral palsy, behavioral disorders and developmental disabilities. In the late 1970's, a few therapists, including physical therapist Barbara Glasow, who studied hippotherapy in Germany, began to spearhead the development of hippotherapy in the United States. International Congresses for Therapeutic Riding began in 1964 in Paris, France; 1976 in Basle, Switzerland; 1979 in Warwick, England; 1982 in Hamburg, Germany; 1985 in Milan, Italy; 1988 in Toronto, Canada; and 1991 in Aarhus, Denmark. These Congresses have been especially helpful in the exchange of information leading toward the development of the treatment applications of the horse.

Heipertz (1981) points out that the type, degree and quality of the horse's movement are important since these movements provide the therapeutic effects sought for the rider. If the horse's gait is blemished it will transmit flawed movement responses in the client (Strauss 1995). In addition, the facilities where activities occur must be appropriate for treatment purposes. A third essential element is a therapy team of qualified specialists. The treatment team consists of a therapist who is well trained in *equine-assisted therapeutic methods, in the theory of Hippotherapy and Riding theory*, a specially selected and trained horse that can produce 1st and 2nd level dressage movements (lengthening, leg yield, travers, shoulder-in), a skilled riding instructor who can produce and influence the horse's movements, and trained support assistants or helpers. The use of the horse for therapeutic purposes combines the ability to produce specific movement in the horse along with traditional therapy techniques used by physical therapists, occupational therapists, speech pathologists, and other health care practitioners.

References

Bauer, J.J. (1972). *Riding for Rehabilitation*. Toronto: Canadian Stage and Arts Publications Ltd.

DePauw, K.P. Horseback riding for Individual with Disabilities: Program, Philosophy and Research. *Adaptive Physical Activity Quarterly*. 3,3, 217-226.

Heipertz, W. (1981). *Therapeutic Riding*. English Ed. Ottawa: National Printers Inc..

Mayberry, R. (1978). The mystique of the horse is strong medicine: Riding as therapeutic recreation. *Rehabilitation Literature*.

Riede, D. (1988). *Physiotherapy on the Horse*. Renton: The Delta Society.

Strauss, I. (1995). *Hippotherapy: Neurophysiological Therapy on the Horse*. Ontario, Canada. Ontario Therapeutic Riding Association

THE VALUE OF THE HORSE'S MOTION TO THE RIDER

Marcee Rosenzweig, PT

For several decades it has been observed that the movement of the horse's pelvis at the walk is similar to the movement of the human pelvis at the walk. A rider sitting astride a horse experiences unimpeded repetitive pelvic motion similar to the pelvic motion of normal human gait.

The well-trained therapy horse which has a symmetrical and rhythmic gait will impart this motion to the rider's pelvis. Therefore, the horse's movement provides an invaluable method of training or re-training pelvic and trunk control.

An understanding of the effects of the three separate components of movement at the walk is the key to comprehending the value of the horse's motion to the rider. First, the acceleration/deceleration of the horse's movement influences the anterior/posterior tilt of the rider's pelvis. As the horse's hind leg pushes off and passes through the swing phase of gait (acceleration) the rider's pelvis moves into a posterior tilt. As the hind leg strikes the ground (deceleration) the pelvis becomes anteriorly tilted. The rider's pelvis is at a ninety degree angle to the horse's pelvis. Therefore, as the horse pushes off with his hind leg and thus rotates his pelvis, the second component, lateral flexion of the rider's pelvis, occurs. The third component of the movement occurs as the horse swings his hind leg forward, which laterally flexes his trunk. This motion produces rotation in the rider's trunk and pelvis. All three components of movement are at their peak, i.e., anterior pelvic tilt, forward rotation, and lateral flexion, when the horse's hind leg is directly underneath him.

One other valuable aspect of the horse's movement is the stride length. The stride length of the average horse (14.3 to 15.2 hands) is very similar to the stride length of the human adult. In the re-education of human gait, a horse is invaluable in producing this feeling of a proper stride length. The horse walks at a rate of 100 - 120 beats per minute, whereas the adult walks at 110-120 beats per minute (Reide, 1988). This provides a rate of movement at which the trunk and pelvis of the rider can learn to accommodate the motion. A pony which has a choppier gait because of its shorter stride is never appropriate as a hippotherapy horse. (The pony's acceleration along the vertical is too high [Reide, 1988]). The motion of the horse's back and pelvis at the walk is the valuable tool which is essential for the development of trunk control in therapeutic riding and hippotherapy. To date, no apparatus has been developed which can replicate this movement.

Summary

- ◘ A horse 14.3 to 15.2 hands:
    - • has a stride length similar to the stride length of the human adult
    - • walks at a rate of 100-120 beats per minute
- ◘ An adult human walks at 110-120 beats per minute.
- ◘ The rhythm of the forward movement (swing phase of the walking gait) of the horse must synchronize with the rhythm (swing phase of the walking gait) of the human to provide therapeutic motion to the trunk and pelvis of the human.
- ◘ A pony cannot approximate the rhythm of an adult's walking gait

References

Glasow, B. (1984), *Hippotherapy: The Horse as a Therapeutic Modality*. New York: Warwick.

Heipertz, W., Heipertz-Hengst, C., Kroger, A, & Kuprian W. (1977). *Therapeutisches Reiten* [Therapeutic Riding]. Stuttgart, Germany: Franckh'che Verlagshandlung.

Hippotherapy Curriculum Development Committee. (1991). *Introduction to Hippotherapy - Module C. Instructor Resource Book.*

Maryland: Riderwood.

Reide, D. (1988). *Physiotherapy on the Horse*. Therapeutic Riding Service: MDn.

ACUPUNCTURE-MANDARIN: A THEORETICAL APPROACH TO THERAPEUTIC HORSEBACK RIDING

Ho Ming Hsia, BA., DC

Based on my observation and knowledge - combining these two together, I have come to the conclusion that therapeutic riding causes the production of a Human Growth Hormone. Another name for this growth hormone is Myotropin, which helps muscles growth and maintains muscle masses.

There is one very important point in acupuncture/meridian therapy, called Gate of Life (Ming Meng, Mandarin pronunciation) , that is located at the L5/S1 vertebrae. During the riding, these two segments are moved in opposite directions; S1 segment moves forward, L5 segment moves backward and vise versa. As the beautiful and faithful animal walks creating a rhythmical movement between L5/S1, resembles rubbing, better yet, massaging the point. The stimulation to this point induces Myotropin production and the passive muscle movements resemble exercise, which force the muscles to contract and relax. This process will re-start the circulation in the involved areas, and in turn, the nutritional supplies, including the Myptropin, will pour in. Thus the involved areas will begin the repair process and muscle masses will increase also.

I believe therapeutic riding is for anyone suffering from pain and decreased range of motion regardless of etiology.

Ho Ming Hsia, BA, DC
Arlington, Texas

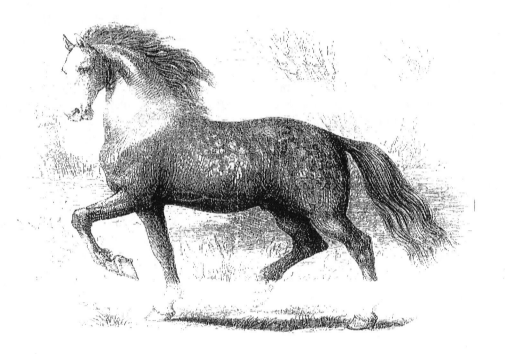

EQUINE-ASSISTED THERAPIES

Barbara T. Engel, M.Ed, OTR

Equine-assisted therapy is an umbrella term that includes methods of treatment used by physicians, psychiatrists and paramedical personnel. It includes: hippotherapy, occupational, physical therapy, speech and language pathology and equine-facilitated mental health. Treatment with the use of a horse differs from therapeutic riding in general in that treatment deals with specific problems and therapeutic riding deals with global motor abilities. Treatments are carried out by licensed health care professional and general therapeutic riding sessions are carried out by instructors-teachers

As programs in therapeutic riding have grown since 1952, an increasing focus has been directed toward the use of the horse as a modality by health care professionals for the treatment of specific disorders resulting from a variety of disabilities. The health care practitioner can make use of "therapeutic" elements that have advanced the therapeutic sports riding field. As professionals involved in the enhancement of human movement and function, and knowledgeable in the subject of human biomechanics, they now will study the biomechanics of the horse. A therapist can manipulate the horse so that the biomechanics of the horse are used to increase the biomechanics of the client. Through their special knowledge and training in a multitude of therapy techniques, therapists can manipulate the horse and its environment to meet therapy goals of their clients. In addition they can stimulate the client using more traditional hippotherapy treatment methods in order to gain exceptional results.

In order for the field to advance, several processes must occur:
● **Information must be disbursed** to health care professionals and physicians; to professional horse trainers interested in the field of hippotherapy riding, to the general community interested in the medical use of the horse, and to the population it serves. This goal is slowly being met as more therapists are trained and the field is becoming more well-known.

● **Advancement of trained hippotherapy and equine-facilitated psychotherapy teams**. Equine-facilitated therapy is a **team undertaking** involving:
   1. Therapists are specifically trained in the use of a horse as a modality.
   2. An instructor who has been trained in at least first, and preferably second level dressage skills.
   3. A horse who is sound, trained to be submissive and maintained to first/second level dressage and who meets the conformation and qualities necessary in a therapy horse.
   4. A sound understanding of classic dressage riding skills (riding theory).
   5. A reasonable ability to understand basic dressage riding without which one cannot fully understand the value of the horse to the rider.

● **Sharing of information** by all those who are involved in the field of hippotherapy and equine-facilitated psychotherapy.

● **Continued education** available to practitioner of hippotherapy and equine-facilitated psychotherapy. This is available through national and international organizations such as the Federation for Riding for the

Disabled and the American Hippotherapy Association. There are practitioner-specialists in the field of equine-assisted therapy who have gained the special knowledge in their own professional field - in addition to specific knowledge on equine-assisted therapy - necessary to further train others in the field. Education is available from a well trained and experienced 2nd level dressage instructor or therapists who ride at novice level horse trials or at least 1st level dressage.

- **Literature** is limited, but there are important books and conference papers that are a must to read for professional advancements.

- Pursuit of individual and group **research projects** and the publication of the results of these projects. Hippotherapy and equine-assisted therapies cannot endure without documentation showing the values and improvements of clients with this form of therapy. In a world where health-care monies are limited, the practitioners must demonstrate and document superior results over more traditional and less costly therapies. In the German-speaking countries, researching and presenting papers is a requirement for reimbursement and most are written by physicians. There is a wealth of manuscripts, but, sadly to say, most of us do not read German to make use of them.

This section includes the disciplines of medicine, occupational and physical therapy, speech/language pathology, equine-facilitated psychotherapy and recreational therapy. The text includes different treatment approaches used by knowledgeable practitioners in the field. The section is not intended to provide the reader with an in-depth knowledge of the equine-assisted therapies but to present the contributing author's points of view, to provide the reader with a concept of treatment approaches, and to stimulate interest in this dynamic field of rehabilitation. It will provide the reader with the basic parameters necessary for using the horse as a treatment tool. To become knowledgeable in this field, one must read extensively, study in courses, seminars, and with the experts in the field. Not only does one need to ride well under the instruction of a highly-trained dressage instructor, but one also needs to understand riding theory from the old masters (their theories are still true) to provide a true understanding of how movements of the horse are transposed to the rider and can be utilized for the benefit of the client.

Therapists may find a degrees of success without a horse with appropriate qualifications, either in English or Western type riding, or the theory base of riding. But they will never become the skilled clinician to truly modulate their clients' disability to the fullest extent. If one experiences burn-out there must be a problem - either a lack of skill, a lack of theory based knowledge, a lack of attachment to the horse as this marvelous instrument, or the inability to create dramatic changes. The author for one could never become burned out through this wonderful medium. If you do not love what you do and cannot cause change - burnout can come quickly!

AN INTRODUCTION TO TREATMENT
WITH THE USE OF THE HORSE

Kyle Hamilton, MS, PT

The traditional treatment setting in hospitals has no modality to match the versatility of the horse. This alive and moving "apparatus" provides a multitude of stimuli to treat a variety of diagnoses. The horse can assist the client in attaining motor skills that would be difficult or slow in coming in the clinic.

Any therapist trained in movement dysfunctions can design a workable treatment plan using the horse as the primary modality, but the therapist should be well-versed in horse handling skills. It takes many months of working with horses to be able to "read" them, just as it takes many months of hands-on treatment to properly evaluate and treat clients. Programs that use a therapist to draw up lesson plans yet not participate in the treatment of the rider, miss a vital ingredient in their approach. Only by instantaneous feedback will the therapist realize the benefits or short-comings of the exercise.

The therapist working as a "hippotherapist" or equine-assisted therapist should have at least attended a hands-on clinic taught by a reputable specialist in the field. In 1991, there was no certification for "hippotherapists" except in Germany, Switzerland, Austria and Italy. Other countries have developed courses to certify their therapists. A group of therapists in the United States under the direction of Jean Tebay[1] began working toward this end. The American Hippotherapy Association presently registers physical and occupational therapists that meet their basic requirements to practice as a "hippotherapist".

To work as a hippotherapist, the therapist must be a competent rider. To make this more objective, the therapist should at least be able to ride a horse in all training level dressage tests (accurately but not necessarily in competition). Germany is more specific, requiring more of a second level riding test which includes lateral movements. Many programs would not be in existence if this level of riding ability were a requirement. The horse must be well-chosen and properly cared for, both mentally and physically. Ideally, a variety of horses to choose from for different diagnoses would be wonderful. A horse of 14 to 15.3 hands high seems to be a good height to provide that lovely, swinging gait so necessary for proper client treatment.

The horse and therapist must be a team.
One cannot stress this too strongly. Hacking out in the fields/mountains will develop a strong bond between the horse and the rider, and ring work will make both responsive to subtle cues. A good working knowledge of dressage school figures will help add variety to your program, while maintaining an objective measurement (i.e., three 20 meter circles to the left at "A", followed by a three loop serpentine the length of the dressage arena).

The evaluation of the client should determine the treatment plan. This simple statement is often neglected and the treatment team goes around and around like a pony ride, leading to boredom and insubordination on the part

---

[1] Jean Tebay, Therapeutic Riding Services, Riderwood, MD 21139, USA

A horse must be a "happy camper" to fully participate in any program. He does not understand that he must provide an even, rhythmic pace to best benefit his or her rider. A sour horse is a dangerous horse. Critically evaluate the client's weaknesses, choose the mount to address those weaknesses, and provide proper school figures to challenge the client to strengthen those weak areas. Keeping the treatment focused on the objective can make documentation easier.

To avoid a sour horse, provide lots of turnout time, trail riding and short treatment sessions. Horses enjoy routines, but not drudgery. Do not overwork the poor beast!

More and more good articles are being written about therapeutic riding; take the time to read these to add to your repertoire. Be sure you understand the difference between riding for sport, therapeutic riding, and equine-assisted therapy/hippotherapy so that you can represent your program properly.

Enjoy working with clients, your staff, and your horse - an amazing living "apparatus."

CHAPTER 7

THE THERAPIST

THOUGHTS FOR THERAPISTS

Nancy H. McGibbon, PT

The rider's smiling face, proud look of achievement, new-found freedom of mobility, and renewed energy and purpose are enough to pique your interest if you are a therapist who is considering a new treatment approach. Perhaps you have been working in the field for a number of years and are looking for new motivational treatment options or you are fresh out of school and see hippotherapy as a natural integration of the techniques and theory learned in class. On the surface, hippotherapy looks like the ideal holistic treatment as it incorporates psychological and motivational as well as sensorimotor goals. It's hard to think of many clients who would not benefit from it. Is it too good to be true? Not really, but the therapeutic use of the horse, which looks deceptively easy, requires a great deal of knowledge, experience, and good sound judgement.

Extensive horse knowledge is a prerequisite for any therapist considering equine-assisted therapy. The steady, kind, patient and obedient therapy horse is in reality a complex and variable creature, that you understand better than any modality used in the clinic. Unlike the ultrasound machine or a piece of exercise equipment, no two horses are alike, and even a seasoned "therapy horse" is not necessarily safe or appropriate for all clients. If you do not have extensive horse experience, an introductory hippotherapy workshop provides as excellent overview, but it will not give you the depth and range of knowledge necessary to immediately use this treatment as part of a client's therapeutic program. The use of the horse presents a greater safety risk to the client than traditional clinical treatment. Thus, it is your obligation to become thoroughly familiar with the horse's temperament, basic instincts, body language, and movement characteristics before even considering incorporating equine activities into a treatment plan. Lectures and workshops are no substitute for experience: regular riding, handling, grooming, and "hanging out" with all sizes, types, and breeds of horses is necessary to gain this experience. The more hours spent with horses, the better the judgement the therapist will use in enhancing treatment safety and efficacy.

The work environment in hippotherapy is ideal for a therapist who enjoys the outdoors, who likes working with animals as well as people, and who enjoys creative, non-traditional treatment approaches. However, there are some drawbacks. One-on-one therapy requires much walking on soft and sometimes uneven ground, and you must be willing to tolerate dust, horse hair, and outdoor temperature variations. It is physically impossible to treat, hands-on, the same number of clients per week that one would see in the clinic, and a single therapist-client session requires a minimum of one to two additional trained staff. In order to proceed with a safe, effective therapy session, many factors must be coordinated: the horse, horse and rider equipment, team members, facility, and weather. Clearly, the logistics are more complicated than in the clinic.

A horse professional, in addition to you, and in whom you have complete confidence, is an essential member of the treatment team. As the therapist, you cannot handle simultaneously both the horse and the client and you will need to rely on the expertise of a horse handler to produce the desired equine movement and behavior. In spite of this, you are still ultimately responsible for the entire treatment team, for monitoring both client and horse, and for making key decisions regarding horse-client interaction.

Considering backriding? What could be more fun than riding a horse and treating a client at the same time! Well, you may want to reconsider unless you are a very experienced rider. Backriding is not the same as hippotherapy; it is strictly a technique for client handling. It allows you to be at the same level as the client and to be able to provide bilateral facilitation or support. However, before proceeding with this technique, ask yourself the following questions: *If the horse should spook or buck, can I maintain an independent seat?* i.e. can I maintain my balance and security on the horse without falling off? *Is my horse's back strong enough to carry the combined weight of myself and my client? Is backriding truly necessary, or could I effectively assist this client from the ground?* You must be aware that backriding presents an increased risk to the client. Consider carefully before utilizing this particular technique.

Insurance and liability issues that arise in any treatment situation are even more critical when a horse is involved. What is one's personal liability? Will your malpractice insurance cover this particular activity since it is somewhat out of the ordinary? Does your state practice act acknowledge the use of hippotherapy for client treatment? Will these therapy sessions be adequately reimbursed or can one afford to donate these services? Do not automatically assume that by volunteering your services your liability is reduced.

Professionalism must be maintained in spite of the outdoor, non-medical, recreational atmosphere. If you are considering affiliation with an established therapeutic riding center, check its credentials. Is it accredited by a national organization? Does it operate under the strictest safety guidelines? One needs to critique it in the same way one would any facility which offers professional services. Do the staff and volunteers dress professionally and appropriately? Are they mature and responsible? Will they inspire confidence in the clients and client families? Do they work well together as a team? Is the facility maintained well with regard to both horses and equipment? Can one carry out the treatment in a quiet, controlled environment without concern for unexpected trail riders, neighborhood dogs, or motorized bikes paying a surprise visit?

Getting started in hippotherapy is best done by volunteering to be a therapeutic riding consultant a few hours per week at an established program. As a consultant, you would advise the therapeutic riding instructor on rider posture and positioning, appropriate exercises, and special equipment and, at the same time, gain knowledge and experience in assessing horse-rider interaction. Assisting a rider as a side-walker will gives you helpful information on tone and postural response changes due to equine movement. In addition, working in close proximity to the horse will improve your confidence and provide experience in reading the horse's language.

Hippotherapy workshops in combination with increasing hands-on experience provide the groundwork for an exciting and rewarding therapeutic experience.

TRAINING REQUIREMENTS OF THE THERAPIST PRACTICING HIPPOTHERAPY

Barbara T. Engel, M.Ed, OTR

Hippotherapy is a treatment procedure used in increasingly more countries. The training of therapists, and the professional qualifications of these therapists, varies from country to country. Courses vary in length and in intensity. They may last a few days to many months to the inclusion in curricula of university. There are many reasons this variation occurs. For instance, the field of practice is comparatively new. Though there are more than twenty-five years of experience in the use of hippotherapy. This is a short history of a field of rehabilitation and medicine. Literature dating back to 460 BC, the 1500's, the 1600's, the 1700's briefly mentions the value of riding the horse for medical purposes.

The Austrians, Germans and Swiss were the pioneers of hippotherapy (a physiotherapy modality) in the 1960's. A medical model was developed in Canada in the late 1960's. In the late 1970's, the therapists in the US, lead by Barbara Glasow, began to develop a therapy model. Many lectures and courses were held that included leaders in the field from European countries.

In the US, the formal development of hippotherapy practice began with the formation of the National Hippotherapy Curriculum Development Committee in 1986. This group was spearheaded by Jean Tebay and Barbara Glasow. A core group of eighteen occupational and physical therapists took part in a ten day hippotherapy course in Germany. Following this course, several intense workshops and meetings were held. The outcome of these meetings was the formation of the AMERICAN HIPPOTHERAPY ASSOCIATION. In 1993 this group was accepted as a 'section' of the North American Riding for the Handicapped (NARHA.)

Hippotherapy, though always a treatment, means different things in different countries. This can be easily explained. In many European countries, the emphasis of physical therapy and occupational therapy is different from those in the U.S. The professions may differ from country to country. For example, Germany requires explicit supervision by a physician and only physiotherapists are involved in hippotherapy. Their insurance companies place specific limits on the way treatments are done. Many physicians are considerably involved in the treatment process. In the US, depending on the state, agency, and insurance carrier, therapists are more in control of and responsible for the treatment situation. Agencies or schools may request therapy where the physician may only receive reports. Therapists (occupational therapists, physical therapists and speech therapists) may also treat clients on a private basis and may not require the physician's approval. This freedom encourages continued education in a field of choice and allows a therapist the ability for exploration and the development of progressive techniques that will bring about the best results for their clients. This concept carries over into the practice of hippotherapy.

The therapist uses the horse as a treatment modality within his or her own orientation of practice. Hippotherapy is a neurological-based treatment and requires a solid foundation in neurology. It is generally accepted that comprehensive training in NDT (neurodevelopmental techniques) is necessary to practice hippotherapy. Most occupational and physical therapists working with clients who have neurological dysfunctions have training in NDT. Most pediatric occupational therapists have been trained in sensory integration techniques, a major occupational therapy-neurological treatment method. Some physical therapists have also been trained in sensory integration. Occupational therapists and speech-pathologists in the U.S. have traditionally had a strong neurological base since they are involved in cognitive function oriented rehabilitation. Besides these major treatment techniques, myofascial release, craniosacral therapy, PNF, Feldenkrais techniques and many other methods are incorporated in both physical therapy and occupational therapy treatments. Therapists using hippotherapy incorporate these techniques within their philosophy of treatment. These techniques are applied to the new dimension of using the horse as an instrument upon which treatment is based.

For example, hand rehabilitation is mainly a speciality within occupational therapy. A hand therapist could use hippotherapy to redevelop sensory processing. The movement and sensation carried from the horse through the client's body would be used to stimulate the arm after stabilization of major wrist surgery. As sensation increases this could be followed by functional activities such as manipulation of the reins and grooming the horse requiring a varied finger and wrist manipulation. The therapy session would vary greatly from that of a physical therapist working on balance reaction with a person following a stroke. The general hippotherapy process may be the same, but the techniques injected are different.

Any new technique requires extensive study and this is true of hippotherapy. Since hippotherapy involves another living being, it requires a wide range of training and knowledge. The horse at a walking gait, the movement of four steps, creates in the rider a circular movement. The rider's shoulders follow the horse's shoulders and the rider's seat follows the horse's hindquarters creating the rotational movement. The rotational movement of the spine, a three-dimensional movement with rotation, compression, decompression and lateral tilt are stated as a major therapeutic effect to the client. A therapist must understand how this occurs and what is required to have this occur. The rider's or client's seat is the base for the transmission of the rotational sensation. In classic riding terms what does this mean?

The horse's walk transfers to the rider's trunk the same movement pattern that the rider experiences while walking with his or her two legs. The trunk muscles are stimulated in a generally normal way of a person with a physical dysfunction (Reide, Strauss.) This may be true with a horse who has been trained to a level that produces a soft and relaxed gait, acceptance of the bit, impulsion, collection, suppleness and obedience. These are the requirements that Dr. Reide states in his book as a requirement in 1st and 2nd level dressage. If the horse has a flawed gait, or that is stiff and out of shape, has poor conformation or the wrong movement pattern for a specific client this will transfer to the rider, and will not provide "the same movement pattern that the rider experiences while walking." How can a therapist determine this? Reliance on the instructor may be the answer. But how does the therapist know that the instructor is knowledgeable enough to decide this? I asked an instructor what her training was - she said "I have competed for ten years - what more do you want?" Her knowledge was limited to intermediate stadium jumping with no flat work or teaching training. Without the knowledge one cannot gauge the knowledge of another.

Biomechanics are "the mechanics of the living organism, especially of the levers and arches of the skeleton, and the forces applied to them by the muscles and gravity." (Gold Medical Dictionary.) The biokinetics of the horse's motion must be understood since these are the movements to which the client responds. Can the therapist assess the effects of this motion for the client?

Next the therapist must be able to decide who is appropriate for therapy on a horse. Strauss (1995) stresses that certain movement abilities must be present in order for the client to accommodate the influences the horse provides to the client. After one has determined a client is appropriate, the therapist must analyze the biomechanics of the client to decide what moves need to be facilitated. How is this done? Placing a four year-old cerebral palsy boy on a horse with a therapist walking next to him does not justify a therapist charging for a therapy session. This is little more than a pony ride. Though hippotherapy can be fun for both client and therapist, it is a highly sophisticated treatment technique and requires detailed knowledge. The more we are involved with the procedure, the more we realize its complexity.

A therapist who plans to use the horse in treatment needs to learn many things about the horse
- His orientation and reactions to his world and environment
- His natural sensory perception and reactions to horses, persons, and things
- His basic physical, mental and social needs
- His conformation qualities
- The horse's biomechanics
- His needs for exercise, development and maintenance "to be a therapy horse"
- How his balance is affected by the rider's weight.

A therapist can only guess the following if he or she does not possess good riding skills:
- The therapist needs to learn beginning riding skills using a deep classic seat, and to learn what the "seat" is
- Why one uses a classic seat in hippotherapy
- Be familiar with the horse's sensitive reaction to the rider's communication
- Understand the movement of the horse and how the person astride can upset the balance of the horse or the horse upsets the balance of the rider
- Be familiar with horse characteristics and their meanings. The therapy horse must have the following characteristics: a soft and relaxed gait, acceptance of the bit, impulsion, collection, suppleness, and obedience

The therapist must know:
- How to stimulate trunk and neck extension and head balance
- How to move the horse to manipulate the spine, the pelvis or the shoulder girdle
- How to develop arousal and attention
- How to increase or decrease stimulation from the horse
- How to increase sensory processing
- How to encourage a good gait and t is a good gait
- How the horse should or should not be lead
- How to perform NDT on the horse
- How SI can performed on the horse?

This lists include only a fraction of what one must learn, but they give the reader a beginning. Most of us learn well when we are involved in the treatment process. Apprenticing in this field with a knowledgeable therapist is the best start. Nevertheless, one must be sure that we have the foundation upon which we can claim we are qualified to use hippotherapy as a treatment.

The American Hippotherapy Association has developed baseline criteria. In 1993, it established a registration of therapists that met the basic knowledge by taking required courses to practice hippotherapy and to advise others in hippotherapy. In 1996-97, the association was developing a theoretical base for hippotherapy practiced in the U.S. Further development includes a certification process, guidelines for the practice of hippotherapy at a NARHA Center and guidelines for backriding. Indications and contraindication are presently in place but will need continual revision as knowledge increases. Riding is NOT GOOD for everyone.

There are therapists with in-depth neurological knowledge who have not acquired the recommended riding skills yet have produced good results with their clients. Their excellent skills would be greatly improved with the additional riding skills. Hippotherapy is based on the riding seat. If one has not developed a good riding seat, one cannot understand its complexity or how to develop it in others. This is not a living therapy ball. The movements are much too complex.

After you have acquired all this knowledge, will you become a **hippotherapist**? The answer is **NO**. The profession of hippotherapy does not exist. There are no certified hippotherapists in the U.S. but a test to become certified in the practice of hippotherapy is now available. There are physical therapists, occupational therapists, and speech pathologists using hippotherapy within their practice. In the same sense, one does not become a sensory integrationalist or a neurodevelopmentalist. So those of us who did not think this process through must have our professional cards reprinted.

THE INSTRUCTOR/THERAPIST TREATMENT TEAM

Molly Lingua-Mundy, LPT

As *therapeutic riding* has grown into a highly developed form of therapy for persons with disabilities, professionals from many specialties are now involved with the client's/rider's program. These professionals include physical and occupational therapists, speech/language pathologists, and psychologists, each bringing their area of expertise to the therapeutic riding program. Each must work with the therapeutic riding instructor to ensure a safe and comprehensive program. It is important to examine and develop ways in which an instructor/therapist treatment team can be effective.

The cooperation required is not as difficult or as overwhelming as it may seem. One often overlooks the fact that, although the therapist and instructor may speak different languages, they see similar things. For example, a therapist talks about "postural alignment" while the instructor refers to "conformation." The instructor talks about a horse "being lame", and a therapist discusses its "gait deviations." Another key similarity is that both are interested in the good of the patient/rider (hereafter referred to as "client.") Both strive to uphold the credo *"Do No Harm!,"* which is so important in this litigation-happy world.

There are 5 basic ways the instructor and therapist can interact in the therapeutic riding setting:
1) **TOTALLY INTEGRATED**; 50/50
Here, both professionals are working with the client, either at the same time or separately. The therapist works on therapeutic goals while the instructor concentrates on riding skills. For example, after the therapist improves muscle tone and postural alignment--therapeutic goals, the instructor can work on steering (a riding goal.) As a team, the therapist works with the instructor to facilitate the success of the session, and vice versa. This type of collaboration must be carefully planned, practiced and executed so as not to bombard the client with too many, or worse, conflicting cues. In the session there may be little or no dialogue, or possibly just a pleasant exchange of ideas between the professionals. Whatever works for the two of them suffices.

2) **THERAPIST AS OCCASIONAL CONSULTANT**
This situation is called the "program's therapist." The therapist evaluates or screens the clients prior to their first session in order to determine whether the client is an appropriate referral based on his own therapeutic judgment or criteria and the program's guidelines. It is vital to recognize that therapeutic riding is not for everyone. The therapist then assists the instructor in selection of the horse, equipment and appropriate class for the client. During the first session, the therapist assists the instructor on proper mounting, "warm-up" exercises, activities, and dismounting to ensure a safe, FUN and therapeutic ride. Thereafter, the therapist is consulted as needed.

3) **CLIENT-SPECIFIC THERAPIST**
In this type of interaction, the therapist comes to the program with the client(s) from his or her institutional setting. He or she knows the client(s) well, and can often assist the instructor in the challenging behavioral and/or physical issues which may arise. The therapist may stand along-side the instructor, giving guidance and feedback as needed, or may assist in side-walking a client(s). This is a perfect opportunity for the team members to intertwine their goals--improving attention span, group skills, and upper extremity control. The session should be an opportunity for sharing and collaboration, rather than a chance for the therapist to retreat to the lounge for some rest and relaxation.

4) THERAPIST AS AN ADVISOR

In this situation, the therapist may be available for consultation over the telephone, sit on the program's advisory board, or consult only for particularly challenging clients. This type of interaction relies on excellent communication between the team members, even more than in other types of interactions. The therapist is usually not present at the program site. Therefore, the instructor and therapist must communicate outside of the session their needs and concerns clearly and succinctly without misunderstanding. This interaction is typically found at the well-established therapeutic riding centers, and is not recommended for less-experienced instructors and therapists.

5) INSTRUCTOR AS CONSULTANT TO THE THERAPIST

Equine-assisted therapy has grown tremendously in recent years. Examples such as hippotherapy and developmental equine-assisted therapy have proven to health care and medical professionals just how powerful the movement of the horse can be in the treatment of disabilities. As therapists are learning of this therapeutic technique through journals, seminars, and client case studies, they are becoming anxious to participate.

Despite their enthusiasm, the therapists may not have a good, clear understanding of therapeutic riding. To provide optimal treatment for the client, the therapist must work closely with the instructor. Even someone skilled and experienced in the use of equine movement needs an instructor's expertise to ensure the success of the treatment. After all, how can one person effectively treat the client, closely monitor the horse, and supervise the side-aides at the same time?

The therapist and instructor work together on horse selection, equipment, and school figures to be used to address the client's goals. During the session, the therapist concentrates mainly on the client while the instructor concentrates on the horse and the quality of its movement. The program should be approached as a medical treatment, with the team members working closely and effectively together to provide a safe, therapeutic and fun experience for the client.

For all of the possible types of therapist/instructor treatment teams, there are a few key points to remember:

How to Find a "Good" Therapist

As more and more therapists become interested in therapeutic riding, programs increasingly have the opportunity to involve a therapist to enhance or develop the program. However, not every "Polly P.T." or "Oliver O.T." is right for a program. The therapist must have clinical experience treating the particular client population for that program. For example, a physical therapist with several years of sports medicine experience is not a choice for cerebral palsy clients. An occupational therapist with experience in the geriatric acute hospital care setting does not have the knowledge required to work with developmentally-delayed children. If the clients are neurologically involved, the therapist should have strong neuro-developmental technique (NDT) background. Otherwise, it may be more work than it is worth to re-educate the orthopedic therapist in neurological disabilities.

Communication

Once the therapist has been selected or has found an appropriate therapeutic riding program, the two professionals must make sure they understand each other's terminology. Although in an optimal case, the therapist would have a strong equine background and the instructor would have a background in health care, this is not always possible. The professionals must teach each other, learn from each other, and in doing so, lay the groundwork for good communication, better understanding and TEAMWORK. This sharing of knowledge can be achieved by reading books, attending courses, and observing one another.

It is very important to agree on similar terminology. When two "experts" team up, they must ensure that they understand each other's professional terms and jargon to be effective, even when it varies from region to region in states and country. The instructor/therapist treatment team is an exciting and vital part of the success of a comprehensive therapeutic riding program. The teamwork may be intense, consultatory, or sporadic depending on the program's and team members' needs. The team members should not be afraid to ask for help, for it may teach both colleagues and clients the spirit of comradeship, all aimed at the goal of using the horse in the bettering of another person's life.

Remember, two heads are better than one. . . . . . .

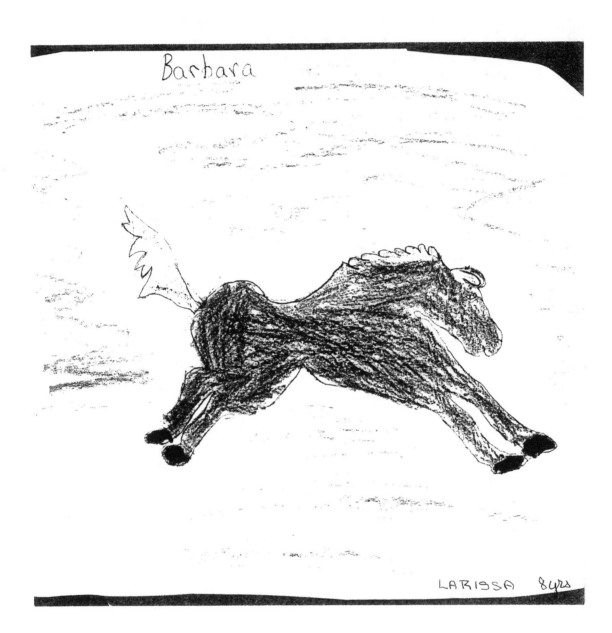

STUDENT INTERNSHIPS

Barbara T. Engel M.Ed, OTR

Incorporating student training within the therapeutic riding setting can have many advantages. Internship programs can add to the overall educational quality of the therapeutic riding program. Along with the fulfillment of course requirements, student programs help to keep standards high. Many college programs now include the treatment tools of hippotherapy as fieldwork experience.

Advantages of internships:
1. It helps to keep the standards of the program high to be in accord with the requirements of the student training program.
2. Provide extra staff with definite time commitments.
3. Help to bring fresh ideas into the program at a professional level.
4. Promote a community-based association with an institution of higher learning.
5. Educate future professionals in the value of equine assisted therapy, recreational and sports riding, and hippotherapy.

Student internships are set up for specific months or numbers of work hours. Different types of affiliation have different requirements. Some college courses require their students to perform pre-course volunteer requirements. Other programs incorporate internships within the curriculum for field work. Training of therapists usually requires internships at the end of the academic course work. Types of student programs which could fit within the framework of therapeutic riding include:

1. Occupational Therapy
2. Physical Therapy
3 Speech and Language Therapy
4. Psychology/psycho-educational intervention
5. Psychotherapy and Counseling
6. Recreation
7. Recreational Therapy
8. Special Education
9. Adaptive Physical Education.

Internship programs each set forth specific requirements. Most will require a formalized teaching program in addition to specific time requirements for hands-on participation. The teaching program must be either directly or indirectly taught by a qualified professional in the specific field being offered. For example: a rehabilitation center has a student training program for physical and occupational therapists. As a part of their training, each student spends four hours a week treating rehabilitation center patients at the therapeutic riding center. The physical therapy students are directly supervised by a physical therapist and the occupational therapy students are directly supervised by an occupational therapist in *equine-assisted and hippotherapy therapy*. Adaptive physical education students would be supervised and trained by an adaptive physical education teacher involved in the program. **It is important that those who are involved in training students in therapeutic** riding settings be trained and knowledgeable in the theory and application of principles of their profession as they relate to the use of the horse.

Within the internship program, the students would be instructed by the instructor and or stable manager on horse care, conformation requirements, training techniques and, possibly, riding lessons. The team approach can be taught by instructors or assistant instructors. The student might be exposed to special education, vaulting or any other approached at the center. Each of these fields can be taught by other then the supervising therapist. In the case of occupational therapy, only client treatment must be supervised by the occupational therapist. As we all know in using the horse as a treatment tool, our knowledge must extend far beyond the actual treatment session. By the end of the first month most students can begin to treat or provide intervention with indirect and occasional direct supervision. This allows the staff therapist time for other tasks or to take on an additional client. In this way the student pays for his or her supervisory time.

Despite the extra work for the staff, especially at the beginning of an affiliation period, students do contribute a great deal in working with clients. In addition, they enrich the overall therapeutic riding program and may bring to the program new techniques that they have studied. If the program is structured effectively, a student program can only add tonjy a therapeutic riding program.

WHERE DO I START? - A TRAINING MANUAL FOR NEW THERAPY STAFF AND/OR STUDENT INTERNS©

Lois Brockmann, RPT

Upon the arrival a new therapy staff member or student intern, the cry for organized orientation material can often be heard. The therapists currently working in the program struggle to gather important information such as: their therapeutic riding program structure, therapeutic riding techniques, safety and risk factors, documentation, etc. Time is short, schedules do not coincide; as a result, the new therapist or intern may enter into the riding program without an ideal or adequate orientation. An appropriate orientation with ongoing training is of major importance to the individual therapist and the entire therapeutic riding program. The format used in this training manual has been developed to promote a quick, smooth transition of the new therapist/intern into a individual therapeutic riding program.

Most of the informational content of the training manual can often be found within programs or organizations. The manual can, and should be, customized to concisely draw that information together into one readily available packet. The specific contents of the manual can also be individualized to meet the needs of a variety of "therapists" such as: physical therapists, occupational therapists, speech language therapists, or psychologists. Within our therapeutic riding program, the training manual developed from a need of the physical therapy staff to provide short term physical therapy student interns with a comprehensive orientation to a large organization working in nine barns or activity sites across two counties. As the manual has evolved over the past three years, new therapy staff have found it to be an excellent reference in addition to "hands-on" training from the other program therapists and staff.

When compiling the information for their training manual, each therapeutic riding program needs to decide on what sections are pertinent and functional for their organization. The training manual is divided into the following eleven sections: general program information, policy, staff information, directions to facilities/activity sites (in programs where more then one site is involved), documentation, volunteer responsibilities, disability descriptions and a vocabulary list, North American Riding for the Handicapped Association, American Hippotherapy Association, Special Olympics, and bibliography/selected articles. Any items requiring yearly updates are starred in the table of contents page for easy reference. (See Table of Contents - Figures 1 and 2) The manual information is introductory in nature. It is intended to bring the new therapist or student intern to a common background with other staff and to prepare them for additional technical training. Careful consideration to provide functional and concise information is important. A large, overburdened manual will most likely overwhelm even the most enthusiastic reader.

A training manual cannot substitute for ongoing training and education. It does provide an invaluable orientation tool to ease the transition of a new therapist or student intern into therapeutic riding. The manual format provides a structure for programs to meet their organization's needs and the needs of the individual therapist. By combining a training manual with ongoing education, the stage is set to send the new therapist or student intern on to a positive experience and/or a career in therapeutic riding.

NEW THERAPY STAFF AND THERAPY STUDENT INTERN
TRAINING MANUAL- 1997

TABLE OF CONTENTS

Figure 1.

TABLE OF CONTENTS (Detailed)

Section 1: General Information about the therapeutic riding organization
- History
- Mission Statement
- Executive Director's Report**
- Organization Yearly Goals**

Section 2: Policy Information
- Guidelines for Participants
- Contraindications for Participants
- Safety Standards,
- Fire and Emergency Drill Procedures
- Confidentiality Policy
- Guidelines for Reducing the Risk of Communicable Diseases

Section 3: Staff Information and "Chapter's"/Activity Site Information
- Staff Phone List**
- Staff listing including:**
  Addresses, phone numbers, staff position, level of NARHA instructor, certification, area of   interest, any additional training.
- E-Mail Directory**
- Pyramid Calling List**
- Chapter Chairmen Phone/Address List**
- Executive Committee List**

Section 4: Directions to each "Chapter"/Activity Site
  List of Chapters marked on local maps
  Individual Chapter written directions

Section 5: Samples of Current Documentation
- Daily Schedule
- Student Evaluation
- Instructor Report
- Therapist Report
- Progress Report
- Accident Report
- Program Horse Chart
- American Hippotherapy Association Hippotherapy Evaluation

Section 6: Volunteer Responsibilities
- General Information
- Leader Role- during mounting, halt, walk, trot, dismount
- Sidewalker Role- during mounting, halt, walk, trot, dismount
- Assisting with warm up exercises, games, lesson plans, back riding
- From a Student's Perspective...
- Basic Warm Up Exercises
- Articles on Sidewalking, Leading
- Diagrams of the Horse, Basic Riding Position, Saddles, Bridles

** Need to be revised yearly

Figure 2.

Section 7: Disability Descriptions and Vocabulary List
- Arthritis
- Autism
- Cerebral Palsy
- Cerebral Vascular Accident
- Developmental Disabilities
- Down Syndrome
- Emotional Disabilities
- Epilepsy
- Hearing Impairment
- Learning Disabilities
- Mental Retardation
- Multiple Sclerosis
- Muscular Dystrophy
- Polio
- Scoliosis
- Spina Bifida
- Spinal Cord Injury
- Traumatic Brain Injury
- Visual Impairment
- Please note- each Disability Description includes:
- Definition, characteristics, problems and benefits of riding, any associated problems.

Section 8: NARHA Information
- Committee List **
- Membership Application

Section 9: American Hippotherapy Information
- History and Functions
- Regional Network, Committees **
- Membership Application

Section 10: Special Olympics
- Regional Network, Committees **

Section 11: Bibliography and Selected Articles

** Need to be revised yearly

Figure 2. (Continued)

Lois J. Brockmann, RPT
Pegasus Therapeutic Riding Inc.
PO Box 2053
Darien, CT 06820 USA

RECOMMENCED READING FOR THERAPISTS:
REFERENCE TOOLS FOR SUCCESS

Barbara T. Engel, M.Ed., OTR

HIPPOTHERAPY, EQUINE-ASSISTED THERAPY, AND RELATED TOPICS

Bertoti, D.B. (1988). **Effect of Therapeutic Horseback Riding on Children with Cerebral Palsy.** *Physical Therapy* 68(10) 1505-1512. (Case reports by a physical therapists).

Bertoti, D.B. (1991). **Clinical Suggestions: Effect of Therapeutic Horseback Riding on Extremity Weight Bearing** in a Child with Hemiplegic Cerebral Palsy: A case Report as an Example of Clinical Research." *Pediatric Physical* Therapy. 3(4)219-222. (Case reports by a physical therapists).

Biery, MJ., Kauffman, N. (1989). *The Effect of Therapeutic Horseback Riding on Balance.* Adaptive Physical Therapy Activity Quarterly 6(3) 221-229.

Bennett, D. (1988). *Principles of Conformation Analysis*, Vol I Gaithersburg: Fleet Street Publishing Corporation.

Bennett, D. (1989). *Principles of Conformation Analysis, Vol* II Gaithersburg: Fleet Street Publishing Corporation Corporation.

Bennett, D. (1991). *Principles of Conformation Analysis, Vol III* Gaithersburg: Fleet Street Publishing Corporation. (These three small books cover different parts of the horse. Clear and easy to follow. Important information in understand the horse for therapists and instructors - may take the therapist back to his or her days college days- learning the bone and muscle structures which is the base of understanding conformation.)

Bennett, D. (1993). *Dr. Deb Bennett's Secrets of Conformation, Equus* Collection, 656 Quince Orcherd Rd, Gaithersburg, MD 20878 U.S.A. This is an easy to follow video which has been used in clinics and well understood.

Dietz, von S. *The Balance Seat.* Suzanna is a German physical therapist who has grown up with therapeutic riding under her Father's involvement. She is a dressage judge, teacher, and competitor. The English edition published in 1998 by AJ Allen, London.. This book is written for therapists but also for the German Riding Society. Important reading.

Engel, B. (1984). **The Horse as a Modality for Occupational Therapy.** In Cromwell (ed) *The Changing Roles of Occupational Therapists in the 1980s.* Haworth Press, New York.

Engel, B. (1997). *Therapeutic Riding I Strategies for Instruction* - Available from Barbara Engel Therapy Services, 10 Town Plaza, # 238, Durango CO, 81301. (This is the sister volume to this book. It provides the horse and instruction information and other aspects of therapeutic horseback riding.)

Engel, B. (1997). *Bibliography of the Federation of Riding for the Disabled* - 2nd Edition. Available from Barbara Engel Therapy Services, 10 Town Plaza, # 238, Durango CO, 81301. $21 USD pp [price US only- additional postage outside the US] . (Up dated to include material through April 1997.

Engel, B. (1997). *Rehabilitation With the Aid of a Horse: A Collection of Studies.* - Available from Barbara Engel Therapy Services, 10 Town Plaza, # 238, Durango CO, 81301. (The manuscript includes 20 studies - 300+ pages - some follow the research model, others are case reports.)

Engel, B. (2000). *Estrategías en Terapia Ecuestre.* Translated in part by Laura Campos Bueno. Available from Barbara Engel Therapy Services, 10 Town Plaza, # 238, Durango CO, 81301. (This manuscript is the Spanish translation of most of the book Therapeutic Riding Strategies in Rehabilitation.)

Fisher, AE; Murray, EA; Bundy, AC. 1991. *Sensory Integration - Theory and Practice -.* FA Davis Co. (An important book on Sensory Integration.)

Gurney, H. *Selecting your Dressage Horse.* Dwyer Production, 8430 Waters Rd, Moorpark, CA 93021. Available from tack stores and tack catalogue sales. Written by a leading American Olympian rider, judge, breeder, and trainer. An easy to view video describing characteristic of the dressage horse - not necessarily the top rider's horse but one that meets the requirement of dressage training and hippotherapy.

Harris, Susan E. (1994). *The United State Pony Club Manual of Horsemanship: Basic for Beginner.* Howell Book House, New York. (Basic level of Horsemanship written for easy reading [geared toward 8 to 12 year old] The knowledge is a must for therapists and instructors.)

Harris, Susan E. (1995). *The United State Pony Club Manual of Horsemanship: Intermediate Horsemanship* level. Howell Book House, New York. (This is the second level to the Pony Club series. It expands the information from level I, but does not duplicate it. Additional material and subjects have been added. Knowledge necessary for all equestrians, instructors and valuable for therapists.)

Harris, Susan E. (1994). *The United States Pony Club Manual of Horsemanship.* Level B, HA and A. Howell Book House, New York. (This book is the last in the serious of horsemanship written for Pony Clubbers. It is interesting reading and covers more medical and horse care information in addition to advanced combined training. Information an advanced instructor should know.)

Harris, Susan E. (1994). *Horse Gaits, Balance and Movement.* Howell Book House, New York. Basic level of Horsemanship written for easy reading.(This book is a must reading for therapists and instructors. Will written and easy to understand.)

Heipertz, Wolfgang, MD. (1981). *Therapeutic Riding.* Translated into English by Marion Takeuchi. Greenbelt Riding Association for the Disabled Inc., Ottawa. Available from CanTRA, PO Box 1055, Guelph, Ontario, Canada N1H 1J6. 519-767-0700. ISBN 0-969049-0-6. (An early book discussing therapeutic riding in sport. Education and medicine. A good reference book.)

Kuratorium für Therapeutisches Reiten. (1985). *The Horse in Medicine.*(video). Rental available from the Delta Society, PO Box 1080 Renton, WA 98057-1080. (An excellent video which reviews hippotherapy. Important to see.)

Lock, S. (1988). *The Classic Seat.* Horse & Rider Magazine - DJ Murphy Publishers, England. ISBN 0-9513707-1-5. *The Classic Seat* is also available on video. Available from your tack shop or tack catalogue. (A clear explanation of the seat - the same seat used in hippotherapy.)

MacKinnon, JR., Noh, S., et el. (1995). **A Study of Therapeutic Effects of Horseback Riding for Children with Cerebral Palsy.** *Physical & Occupational Therapy in Pediatrics.* 15(1)17-34.

MacKinnon, JR., Noh, S., et el. (1995). Therapeutic Horseback Riding: A Review of the Literature. *Physical & Occupational Therapy in Pediatrics.* 15(1)1-15.

NARHA GUIDE. North American Riding for the Handicapped Association Inc. PO Box 33150, Denver CO 80233. Phone 1-800-369-743.

Riede, Detlev, MD. (1988). *Physiotherapy on the Horse.* Translated into English by Angela C. Dusenbury, PT. Available from The Delta Society, 321 Burnett Avenue, South, Renton, WA 98055. U.S.A. Tel. 206-226-7357. (A major book for any therapist using hippotherapy.)

Schusdziarra, H., Schusdziarra, V. (1985). *An Anatomy of Riding.* Briarcliff: Breakthrough Publications. (This book is written by two physicians who are riders. Excellent book for all therapists and instructors.)

Smyth, RH., Goddy PC. (1993). *The Horse Structure and Movement.* Revised by P Gray. JA Allen London. A classic in anatomy and movement - important reading.

Spencer, Nancy. (1993). *Basic Equine Stretching.* VHS video demonstrates important stretching and conditioning for the horse.

Spink, J. (1993). *Developmental Riding Therapy.* Therapy Skill Builders, Tucson AZ. (The principals of several disciplines can be incorporated within the developmental riding therapy framework. An important book on the therapy horse and other aspects of equine-assisted therapy.

Strauss, Ingrid, MD. (1996). *Hippotherapy: Neurophysiological Therapy on the Horse.* Translated into English by Marion Takeuchi. Available from OntRA, Mrs. Helen Brcko, 19 Alcaine, Thornhill, Canada. (Dr. Strauss is a neurologist with extensive experience in hippotherapy - a must for all therapists. Very clear and easy to understand.)

Swift, Sally. (1985).*Centered Riding.* Book or video I & II. Trafalgar Square Farm Book, North Pomfret VT U.S.A. ISBN 0-312-12734-0. Available from any bookstore or tack shop that carries equestrian books. (An excellent source for classic dressage techniques and methods of developing posture. - a must for therapists to read)

Tellington-Jones, L. *Tellington-Touch video series*. From your local tack shop or tack catalogue store. Provides helpful handling and training material.

Proceedings of the International Congress on Therapeutic Riding:

4th Cngress: Kurtorium fur Therapeutisches Reiten, eV., Freiherr-von Langen strasse 13, 4410 Warendorf, Germany.

5th Congress: From Therapeutic Riding Service, Riderwood MD - $27.

6th Congress in Canada - out of print - must be borrowed from your friend.

7th Congress: Danish Sports Organization for the Disabled, Idraeeens Hus, Brondby Stadion 20, DK 2605 Brondby, Denmark.

8th Congress: RDA Monpgraph, National Training Resource Center, Private Bag (6) 368 7131. $112 New Zealand dollars.

9th Congress: North American Riding for the Handicapped Association Inc. PO Box 33150, Denver CO 80233. Phone 1-800-369-743.

10th Congress: Handi Cheval, France. Email:HANDI-CHEVAL@district-parthenay.fr

MOTOR CONTROL AND MOTOR LEARNING BIBLIOGRAPHY
SENSORY INTEGRATION AND RELATED SUBJECTS.

Contributed by Jane Copeland Fitzpatrick, MA, PT; Nancy McGibbon MA, PT and AHA

Abernethy B. Sparrow W.A. (1992). **The rise and fail of dominant paradigms in motor behavior research.** In J,J,Surnmers Ed. *Approaches to the study of motor control and learning.* Amsterdam, the Netherlands: Elsevier Science Publishers BV; 1992.3-46.

Dismuke-Blakely P.& Kranz K. (1992). **The sensory integration -cognitive/linguistic connection.** In Engel, B. ed. *Therapeutic Riding Programs: Instruction and Rehabilitation. Barbara Engel Therapy Services,* 10 Town Plaza, Suite 238, Durango CO, 81301.

Carr 3. & Shepherd, P. (1982). *A motor relearning programe for stroke.* London England: William Heinemann Medical Books Ltd.

Cart, 3. &. Shepherd, P. (1987). **A motor learning model for rehabilitation.** In Cart, J., Shepherd, P., Gordon, J., et al (Eds.) *Movement Science Foundations for Physical Therapy in Rehabilitation.* London, England : William Heinemann Medical Books Ltd; 1987: 31-91.

Colborn, AP. (1993). **Combining Practice and Research.** American Journal of Occupational Therapy. 8 (47)693-702.

Copeland, J. (1991). **A challenge to therapeutic riding.** *Anthrozoos ,* IV. 21 0-211.

Fisher, AE., Murray, EA., & Bundy, AC. *(1991). Sensory integration theory and practice.* F.A. Davis Co.,

Goodgold-Edwards, S A. (1993). **Principles for guiding action during motor learning: a critical evaluation of neurodevelopmental treatment.** *Physical Therapy* 1993(2)30-39.

Gordon, J.(1987). **Assumptions underlying physical therapy intervention: theoretical and historical perspectives.** In Cart, J., Shepherd P. Gordon, J., et al, eds. *Movement Science Foundations for Physical Therapy.* London, England: William Heinemann Medical Books Ltd; 1987: 1-30.

Giuliani,C. (1991). **Theories of motor control: new concepts for physical therapy.** In M.J.Lister (Ed.) *Contemporary management of motor control problems Proceedings of the II Step Conference.* Alexandria; VA. Foundation for Physical Therapy; 29-35.

Glasow, B.L.(1996). **Sensory integration and riding - part three - the tactile, proprioceptive, and vestibular systems.** Presented at R.I.S.E. Continuing Education Workshop, E. Stroudsburg, PA.

Haehl, V.(1994). **A dynamic systems approach to the use of hippotherapy.** *AHA News.* 3:1-4.

Haehl, V. (1996). **Exploring the influences of hippothearpy on the kinematic relationship between the rider and horse.** Unpublished master's thesis, Univ. Of NC, Chapel Hill.

Haley SM. (1994). **Our measures reflect our practices and beliefs: a perspective on clinical measurement in pediatric clinical physical therapy.** *Pediatric Physical Therapy.* 1994(6) 142-l43.

Heriza CB. (1991). **Implications of a dynamical systems approach to understanding infant kicking behavior.** *Physical Therapy.* 199(71)222-235.

Heriza CB. (1991). **Motor development: traditional and contemporary theories.** In M.J.Lister (ed.) *Contemporary management motor control problems proceedings of the II Step Conference.* (pp.121-126). Alexandria, VA: Foundation for Physical Therapy.

Horak, FB. (1991). **Assumptions underlying motor control for neurological rehabilitation.** In M.J.Lister (ed.) *Contemporary management motor control problems proceedings of the II Step Conference.* (pp.11-27). Alexandria, VA: Foundation for Physical Therapy.

Ingvar, DH. (1993). **Language functions related to prefrontal cortical activity: Neurolinguistic implications.** Annals New York Academy of Science. 240-247.

Jarus, T. (1994). **Motor Learning and Occupational Therapy: The Organization of Practice.** *American Journal of Occupational Therapy.*48(9) 810-815.

Kamm K., Thelan, B., & Jensen, J. (1990). **A dynamical systems approach to motor development.** *Physical Therapy* (70) 763-775.

Keshner, E A. (1991). **How theoretical framework biases evaluation and treatment** In: M.J.Lister (ed.) *Contemporary management motor control problems proceedings of the II Step Conference.* (pp.37-47). Alexandria, VA: Foundation for Physical Therapy.

Lewthwaite, R. (1990). **Motivational considerations in physical activity involvement.** *Physical Therapy.* (70) 808-819.

Mathiowetz, V., Haugen, BJ. (1994). **Motor behavior research: implications for therapeutic approaches to central nervous system dysfunction.** *The Journal of Occupational Therapy,* (48)733-745.

McGibbon, N. (1994) **Motor learning: the common denominator.** *Proceedings of the 8th International Therapeutic Riding Congress.* pp 63-69. Levin, NZ National Training Resource Center.

Morris, ME., Summers, JJ., Matyas, TA., Iansel, R. (1994). **Current status of the motor program.** *Physical Therapy.* (7)738-746.

Mosey, AC. (1986). *Psychosocial Components of Occupational Therapy:* Raven Press, NY.

Proteau, L., Marteniuk, RG., Levesque, L. (1992). **A sensorimotor basis for motor learning: evidence indicating specificity of practice.** *The Quarterly Journal of Experimental Psychology.* (44)557-575.

Schmidt, RA. (1991). *Motor control and learning: a behavioral emphasis.* 2nd ed. Champaign, Ill. Human Kinetics Publishers Inc.

Shumway-Cook, A., Woollacott, MH. (1995). *Motor control: theory and practical applications.* Baltimore: Williams & Wilkins,

Stuberg, W., Harbourne, R. (1994). **Theoretical practice in pediatric physical therapy. past, present, and future consideration.** *Pediatric Physical Therapy:* 6:119-125.

Thelan, E. (1995). **Motor development, a new synthesis.** *American Psychologist.* 50.79-95.

Tscharnuter, I. (1993). **A new therapy approach to movement organization.** *Physical & Occupational Therapy in Pediatrics.* 13: 19- 40.

Vereijken, B., Whiting, HT., Beck, WJ. (1992). **A dynamical systems approach to skill acquisition.** *The Quarterly Journal of Experimental Psychology.* 45A: 323-344.

Voeller, KK. (1991). **What can neurological models of attention, intention, and arousal tell us about attention-deficit hyperactivity disorder?** *Journal of Neuropsychiatry:* (3) 209-216.

Windek. S L., Laurel, M. (1989). **A theoretical framework combining, speech-language therapy with sensory integration treatment.** *Sensory Integration Special Interest Section Newsletter.* AOTA. (12) 1-6.

Winstein, CJ. (1991). **Knowledge of results and motor learning: implications for physical therapy.** *Physical Therapy;*71:140-147.

Woolacott, MH. & Shumway-Cook, A. (1990). **Development of posture and gait across the life span.** Columbia, SC. *University of South Carolina Press.*

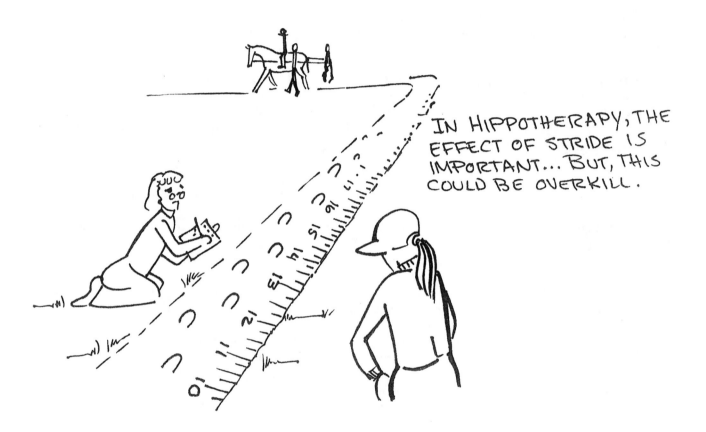

CHAPTER 8

THE THERAPY HORSE

CONFORMATION OF THE DRESSAGE HORSE

Hilda Gurney, "S" rated judge

KEY WORDS
    MOVEMENT
    CONFORMATION

Conformation in a dressage horse is important in how it relates to movement. A dressage horse should be built "uphill" so that it moves uphill. The neck should be set fairly high and right side up with a nice arch from the poll to the withers. Low set necks predispose horses to traveling on the forehand and to hanging in the rider's hands.

The hind legs should step well under the body of the horse. This makes engagement and balance easy for the horse. More muscling over the haunches and gaskins makes for power. The loin should also be well muscled, and the spine should not be higher than the back muscles.

Leggy, narrow horses perform better lateral movements. Long legs and a narrow body facilitate the crossing of the horse's legs in the half pass and in leg yields. Wide horses frequently become irregular and labored in movements requiring crossing of their legs.

The author feels that long backs are more supple and softer to sit, but horses with backs which are too long will have difficulty tracking-up, and in collection. Short backs are often associated with problems in bending and with tight hard backs which make the gaits hard to sit.

Free shoulders with the front legs carried more forward in front of the horse's body are best for dressage. Front legs carried back under the body make it difficult for the horse to balance itself with the haunches under the body, because the shoulders in this position are already carrying weight. Ideally, forelegs should be about the same length as the hind legs, and the dressage horse's elbow should be about parallel with the stifle. Horses with short front legs in relation to the hind legs look like wheelbarrows and are extremely difficult to balance. Front legs should reach forward. Extravagant knee action is not desirable. The hocks of a dressage horse should bend well at all gaits, even at the canter. Most good dressage horses have fairly well bent hocks. However, any snatching type of action will be severely penalized in competition.

Most dressage horses stay fairly sound if ridden in decent footing. As a result, conformation faults such as calf knees, crooked legs, too short or too long pasterns (though they may affect quality of movement if moderately severe), are usually **not as much** of a consideration as in horses **used for other** disciplines. Horses with injured tendons will often stay completely sound when used for dressage.

To conclude, conformation is important only in how it relates to movement and balance. Dressage horses do not have to have legs as straight as necessary for other disciplines, but must carry themselves in an uphill balance with engaged haunches and an elevated forehand with an arched neck. The strides need to be long and reaching with a good overstep at the walk and trot lengthening. Suspension and elasticity are important and the horse should appear to float above the ground in the trot and in the canter.

For further study of the conformation of the dressage horse, see the video by Hilda Gurney, *Selecting Your Dressage Horse*. Available through United States Dressage Federation, Dover Saddlery in MA; Millers Harness Co. in NY, or your equine tack and video companies.

CONFORMATION AND MOVEMENT OF THE
HIPPOTHERAPY HORSE

Nina Wiger, MA

KEY WORDS
 TEMPERAMENT
 GAIT
 TRAINING
 CONFORMATION

When selecting a riding horse we keep several general considerations in mind, the main ones being temperament, level of training and experience, gait, soundness and conformation. In many disciplines within disabled riding temperament stands out as being of overriding importance. In the hippotherapy horse, we require two main characteristics. These are **temperament and quality of gait.**

TEMPERAMENT
In addition to being kind, sensible, tolerant and unflappable, the hippotherapy horse has to have energy (to maintain quality of gait), and also be willing to accept constant instructions about position, carriage and stride length. This "ride ability through the long reins" is a different temperament characteristic from that of tolerance of equipment, erratic movements, and other unexpected occurrences on his back. An older dressage horse, who has proven through years of training that he can calmly accept endless corrections, is fairly sure to meet the temperament requirements. Horses from other backgrounds might have the required temperament, but often much additional training in carriage, figures and lateral work is needed.

QUALITY OF GAIT
As most hippotherapy horses perform almost exclusively at the walk, faults with the canter or increased gaits in trot are not too important. Two gait requirement are absolute: the walk must be **regular** and **energetic**. The natural walk of the most versatile, all-around hippotherapy horse would be rhythmic and elastic, **with a stride length** and **frequency as close to that of a typical adult person as possible**. If the walk is very big, it will have too much movement for some clients. The shorter walk that swings freely through the body of the horse can be tolerated by most persons with disabilities, but **will still be therapeutic for a less involved client**. Ideally several horses, with walks of different frequencies and amplitudes should be available for hippotherapy programs.

TRAINING AND EXPERIENCE
A hippotherapy horse **must** walk on the bit with enough energy to round its back. This is a minimum requirement, and it is the main reason many very nice riding horses do not qualify to be a hippotherapy horse. Horses at second level dressage should be able to do this. Some horses are built to be round and on the bit, and, if ridden sensitively previously, will have sufficient self-carriage with a swinging back without extensive dressage training. These horses are few and far between; finding one would be pure luck. For maximally effective hippotherapy, the horse must also be able to increase the curve of its body (bend), to laterally displace either shoulders or haunches on a straight line, and to move the whole body laterally, all the while staying round, having impulsion, and remaining on the bit.

SOUNDNESS AND FUNCTION

The basis of hippotherapy is the walk, and any unsoundness that interferes with rhythm, stride length and/or the elastic swinging of the back is unacceptable. Unsoundness affecting the quality of the movement, how it is transmitted through the horse's back and how it feels to the rider, is not always visible from the ground. A rigid or saggy back is not to hard to detect, but a lack of symmetry in the swinging of the back, or a tendency to slight, constant crookedness are more subtle faults. An experienced, feeling rider must try the horse on the footing on which he is to perform.

If the normally used footing is soft, many concussion types of unsoundness may be acceptable in the well-trained horse, but time is wasted training such an animal. A therapy horse **must** be schooled regularly under saddle, not only at walk, but at all gaits, and therefore must be sound enough for these sessions.

CONFORMATION

Conformation is important only as far as it pertains to soundness and function. Crooked legs and deviate leg movements are of no concern unless severe enough to cause stumbling or interference. The hippotherapy horse needs to move with a round frame at the walk, and it is a definite advantage to have a horse with conformation that allows him to be "naturally on the bit". This would be a strong topline with well muscled back and loin, solid connection between neck and withers, good arch to the neck and an open, supple head/neck connection. If only one horse is available, some compromises must be made. The horse needs to be relatively narrow where the saddle sits, to accommodate spastic riders, but be deep enough in the body to let the whole leg lie on the side of the horse for a secure feeling. He must be stout enough to comfortably carry two people, a client and the back rider, yet be short enough that you do not have to hire a basketball team for sidewalking. Very small horses and ponies seldom have the length and elasticity of stride required in hippotherapy, but if such a gem can be found, life is much easier for therapists and sidewalkers. These horses are especially useful for children, and the shorter gait fits the smaller stride length of the child. The therapist might prescribe a walk with less elasticity and more impact in selected cases, and a horse that hits the ground a little harder can be used. Access to a wide variety of horses is a definite advantage, as long as the therapeutic impact of each horse is known.

Regardless of whether the therapist/instructor team can have one or several horses for the hippotherapy, remember temperament and the quality of gait are major factors in the success of the program.

SELECTING THE HIPPOTHERAPY HORSE

Patricia J. Sayler, MA

KEY WORDS
MOVEMENT
BALANCE
TRAINING

When considering the type of horse that is to be used in hippotherapy, it is essential to have a working definition of classic hippotherapy and American hippotherapy and an understanding of the requirements of the task to which the horse is to be put. As with other aspects of therapeutic riding the horse must suit the needs of the approach and the intent of the therapist's methodology or of the instructor's lesson. A horse may be quite suitable for work as a remedial vaulting horse, but be unsuitable for classic hippotherapy or hippotherapy and vice versa.

The current working definition of classic hippotherapy and hippotherapy, as stated by the American Hippotherapy Association, (4/97) is as follows:

Classic Hippotherapy, literally means "treatment with the help of the horse" from the Greek word, "hippos" meaning horse. Specially trained physical and occupational therapists use this therapy treatment for clients with movement dysfunction.

In Classic Hippotherapy, the horse influences the client rather than the client controlling the horse. The client is positioned on the horse, and actively responds to his movement. The therapist directs the movement of the horse; analyzes the client's responses; and adjusts the treatment accordingly. The goals of Classic Hippotherapy are to improve the client's posture, balance, mobility and function.

American Hippotherapy is a treatment approach that uses the movement of the horse based on principles of Classic Hippotherapy, neuromotor function and sensory processing. It is a treatment approach that uses activities on the horse that are meaningful to the client. Hippotherapy provides a controlled environment and graded sensory input designed to elicit appropriate adaptive responses from the client. It does not teach specific skills but rather provides a foundation of improved neuromotor function and sensory processing that can be generalized to a wide range of activities outside to treatment. Hippotherapy is used primarily to achieve physical goals but may also effect psychological, cognitive, behavioral and communication outcomes. Hippotherapy is used by licensed/credentialed health professionals who have a strong treatment background in posture and movement, neuromotor function and sensory processing.

As can be seen from the definition and purpose of classic hippotherapy, the horse's movement is the key to change for the client and the key to therapeutic value for the therapist. Any asymmetries arising from unsoundness or conformation faults, or tension in the back muscles from poor self-carriage will be imparted to the client. The nuances of movement shifts, most often carried out at the walk, are only attainable if the horse is sound, symmetrical, balanced and equally flexible to both sides. The horse must be able to walk forward with impulsion, with a long free stride that is ground covering and rhythmic. Ideally, training would create for the horse a relaxation in body from jaw to hindquarters, so that the engagement of the hindquarters would enable self-carriage with a round top line and a relaxed and swinging back. With the more severely involved client , the horse must have an even greater degree of balance as the horse is required to walk at a speed slower than its normal rate, for 10-15 minute periods of time. This careful, precise, slower rhythm increases the horse's stress and fatigue both mentally and physically, illustrating the need for appropriate training and conditioning for the horse.

While there is not a particular breed or age of horse that is ideal for hippotherapy, the horse must be conformationally sound, tolerant, and conditioned for the activity. The size and width of the horse used will depend on the needs of the particular client. In a "classic" hippotherapy approach, the client often faces forward the entire time. This position does not impose the extra stress of weight placement and weight shift on the horse required of other positions used in hippotherapy treatments. For example, sitting backwards is an alternative position used to facilitate increased mobilization of the client's pelvis. The weight shifts and changes to alternate positions create significant demands on the horse, both physically and mentally, and must be taken into consideration and monitored when selecting a using a horse for this type of therapy. The size of the client and severity of disability is another factor that enters into the tolerance equation.

Backriding is a technique sometimes used in hippotherapy when the client cannot maintain balance or postural control without the assistance of a therapist sitting behind the client. Backriding, while a most valuable tool when used appropriately, severely increases the stress on the horse. For this reason, NARHA (North American Riding for the Handicapped Association) has developed guidelines that will effectively deal with this important issue. Without going into detail regarding backriding standards, the technique should only be used by a therapist in a very carefully prescribed treatment protocol. The size, weight, height, and disability of the client is taken into consideration. A limited time period is placed on the number of times the client will need to be backridden in order to assist in developing functional sitting balance. If independent sitting balance is not achievable, other methods of treatment need to be considered. With the increased stress that backriding places on the horse, it is imperative that the horses chosen for such a treatment approach have particularly strong backs, be consistently maintained and trained, and be allowed periods of rest and relaxation through turnout and other riding experiences.

In the beginning of this article, I stated that a horse selected for a therapeutic riding activity must be suited to its task. The need for graded movements, changes of pace, and evenness of footfall required in the hippotherapy horse are much greater than the demands on other horses used in therapeutic riding activities. The success of hippotherapy is not only dependent upon a properly selected and trained horse, but upon the therapist/instructor team who need to be well trained in hippotherapy skills themselves. The trainer/instructor should be able to train and maintain the classic hippotherapy and hippotherapy horse at first level dressage at a minimum, and through third level dressage preferably. The instructor and horse must be trained in the use of side-reins, lunging and long-lining techniques. The instructor must be proficient in long-lining, therapeutic lunging and leading; able to respond immediately and smoothly to the movement requests of the therapist during a hippotherapy session. The therapist, likewise must be well-versed and trained in classic hippotherapy technique and equine movement in order to utilize the technique appropriately and beneficially for the client. Both the instructor and therapist must be alert and sensitive to any signs of stress or discomfort evidenced by the horse. Without the intuitive and trained component of the therapist and instructor team, the horse will be unable to perform its assigned task.

Without the intuitive and trained component of the therapist and instructor team, the horse will be unable to perform its assigned task.

The importance of the team approach of horse, therapist, and instructor to the success of classic hippotherapy and hippotherapy cannot be overestimated. The hippotherapy horse, classic or otherwise, is not "just any horse". He is carefully selected, trained and maintained by the trained therapist/instructor team. As the quality of hippotherapy depends upon the quality of equine movement imparted to the client, the successful performance of the hippotherapy horse is largely dependent upon our judgement and the correct utilization of the horses's attributes and skills. It is our moral and ethical responsibility to judge wisely.

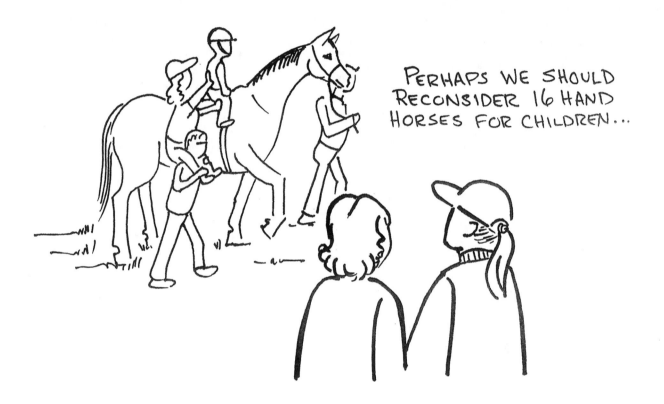

BASIC EQUINE STRETCHING

Nancy Spencer, CFI

In the past, when we spoke of equine fitness it usually referred to how well developed a horse looked and how fast he could run or how high he could jump. Aerobic or cardiovascular endurance is an essential component of a horse's health. However, flexibility, symmetry in muscular strength and development, and muscle endurance are of equal importance. Only through adequate fitness in all these components can a horse attain and maintain optimal fitness. Inadequate conditioning in any one of these components will not only affect a horse's performance, it will put him at a higher risk for over-use injury.

Before the evolution of equine sports medicine, horses were conditioned through trial and error, normally at the expense of the horse. Aerobic or cardiovascular endurance, flexibility, and muscle strength/endurance were not addressed as separate components of a horse's training and conditioning. Research found that in order to attain optimal health and fitness, as well as reduce the incidents of injury, and to safely and efficiently restore and maintain a horse's health, each of these components, being of equal importance, must be addressed separately.

Training a horse for skill-related components of fitness, flexibility, suppleness, balance, coordination, power, speed and reaction time is not the same as conditioning a horse for muscle endurance, strength and cardiovascular endurance. Sports experts discovered the key to developing all fitness and health related components regardless of discipline is flexibility. This is the ability to move a joint through full range of motion and recover without injury. Lack of flexibility is responsible for nearly 80% of soft injuries that occur during activity. Without flexible joints and the ability to move its body freely, a horse will never obtain optimal cardiovascular conditioning. Unfortunately flexibility is often neglected and seldom recognized as an important part of a horse's training program. It is the easiest component fitness to obtain, the least time consuming, and the number one component for improving a horse's performance and preventing injury.

Stretching is expected among human athletes to maintain maximum flexibility during performance, and to prevent injury should an unexpected movement occur. The same expectation is necessary for the equine athlete.
Equine sports medicine has kept pace in many ways with its human counterpart, yet emphasis on stretching has lagged behind. Passive stretching of our horse's muscles is a new concept to equine health and fitness thinking. The idea of a person stretching a thousand pound horse may sound formidable, but it can be done easily and effectively when proper techniques are used.

The Basic Equine Stretching program is designed to teach to riders, trainers, farriers and veterinans the principles and proper techniques to effectively stretch a horse's muscles to increase their flexibility, improve performance reduce injury and for use in restorative therapy during recovery and during confinement.

FLEXIBILITY DEFINED
Flexibility is the ability to move joints and recover without injury. The amount of flexibility a horse has depends on his body type, the elasticity of his muscles, tendons, connective tissue and the conditions of his joints. Limited movement caused by inflexible joint will prevent a horse from ever achieving optimal fitness.

It is the key to all skill and health related components. The good news is flexibility can be improved and maintained by incorporating a regular stretching regimen into a horse's training and conditioning program, regardless of his discipline.

COMPONENTS OF EQUINE FITNESS

Equine fitness is characterized by two components. The first are health related components: muscle endurance, strength, and cardiovascular endurance. The second are skill related components: agility, balance, coordination, power. speed and reaction time. Skill related components arise from the application of health related fitness components. None of these components of conditioning can be fully achieved without flexibility. Whatever level of fitness one seeks for his or her horse, these components will always apply. A horse's body will adapt to perform the work asked of it.

PRINCIPLES OF STRETCHING

Active Verses Passive Stretching

Lack of mobility or stiffness in one joint restricts movement and puts added stress on the joints above and below the restriction in an effort to achieve a desired action. A horse may warm out of a stiffness within to fifteen to thirty minutes of active stretching by walking and trotting. But unless this warm up period is followed with passive stretching, over time the cumulative effects of repeated stresses of poor alignment, inadequate muscle lengthening will eventually give rise to acute mechanical breakdown.

Active stretching more closely relates to the level of functional than passive stretching. However, passive stretching is necessary in order to assume an initial extended position. It is necessary for safety and effectively improving a horse's performance, permitting maximum strength output where the horse needs it most, in the lengthened position.

The first signs of muscle imbalance normally show up as chronic postural pain, compensation and poor performance. The rider and veterinarian are often left trying to figure out what is wrong with the horse and more often than not the farrier gets the blame.

Unlike active stretching, passive stretching is performed by an outside force acting on the horse such as the ground or a human. It is performed slowly and with purpose, after the muscles have been properly warmed up. We have all seen a horse do the "cat stretch" with his front legs extended out in front with a nice long arch in his neck and back. The outside forces the body in. In this case it is the ground. Humans will use a wall, or bench or position their bodies to perform a passive stretch.

WHY STRETCH A HORSE'S MUSCLES

Movement only occurs at a joint. If the muscles and connective tissue that surround the joint are short and tight, joint movement is restricted. To maintain a position of good alignment and smooth function between joints, there must be adequate muscle balance between opposing sets of muscles, and flexibility to allow full movement of the joint. Passively stretching the muscles takes each joint through its full range of motion, increasing the length of the muscle fibers and the connective tissue.

This maintains a balance of the opposing muscle groups and permits the greatest range of movement available during performance, enabling the horse to safely cover the greatest amount of distance with the least amount

This maintains a balance of the opposing muscle groups and permits the greatest range of movement available during performance, enabling the horse to safely cover the greatest amount of distance with the least amount of effort. It permits maximum strength output where the horse needs it most, in the lengthened position.

The skill level and amount of conditioning a horse gains from training is directly influenced by muscle function. Flexibility is responsible for quality of movement and plays a major role in injury prevention. Persistent faulty alignment results in uneven wear and undue compression of the joint's surface. This results in joint inflammation, arthritis, bone spurs, and bony changes seen in the hocks and fetlocks of horses.

When conditioning a horse that has habitual faulty posture, faulty body mechanics will most likely occur over a period of time. A well-rounded training and conditioning program should focus not only on increasing muscle strength and endurance, but more importantly on the symmetry of muscle development and structural alignment as conditioning occurs.

WHO SHOULD STRETCH

Every equine athlete, regardless of discipline or flexibility. If the horse is healthy and without specific physical problems, stretching is safe and enjoyable and will enhance his overall performance, health and well-being. Very young horses usually under the age of six months, do not need stretching unless under the direction of a veterinarian for a specific problem. Yearlings whose bones are still growing do not need to hold a passive stretch more than 7-10 seconds. When teaching a very young horse to be handled, hold the limbs in the stretch position without applying tension or short periods of time while grooming. If a horse has any physical problems, consult the veterinarian before starting a stretching program.

WHEN TO STRETCH

When a muscle is inactive for a period of time, it will generally shorten about 10% of its normal resting length. When properly warmed and stretched, a muscle will lengthen an average of 10% beyond its normal resting length. This represents a 20% change it muscle length between an active and a chronically inactive muscle.

Daily stretching keeps muscles supple and ready for movement, Maintaining muscle length and elasticity by stretching during inactive periods can narrow the 20% gap considerably, reducing the risk of soft tissue injuries. Stretching should be done following a 10-15 minute warm-up of easy active stretching, walking and trotting to prepare the muscles for movement prior to activity. Passive stretching should be done following an activity cool-down of easy walking and trotting to maintain circulation in the muscles and reduce the risk of stiffness and cramping. Leaving the muscles long will minimize the occurrence of stiffness the following day.

HOW TO STRETCH

Stretching is performed gently and slowly when the horse's muscles are relaxed. Stretch position is important for the effectiveness and the safety of a stretch. Proper position isolates the particular muscle group that one is trying to stretch without having to worry about resistance offered by the surrounding muscle groups. Body position of both the handler and the horse is important for safety and to provide the greatest mechanical advantage over the muscle group being stretched. Position of the handler provides maximum control of the intensity and the speed of the stretch. A slight change in the handler's position or the angle t of the limb, can make a significant difference in the effectiveness of the stretch.

Stand far enough from the horse so that you can properly and safely position the limb. Make sure to allow space for the movement of the stretch to occur. This distance will vary depending on one's own body size and the size of the horse. Never stand directly behind the horse while performing a stretch.

When stretching a limb, always support it with two hands: one above the joint, the other below the joint. To prevent twisting or torquing the limb force should always be applied from the upper hand, guiding the stretch with the lower hand. Always stretch muscles in their natural line of movement which is in line with. the muscle.

Apply force gently until resistance is felt. Hold the position maintaining easy tension. As the tension diminishes, gently take up the slack, applying new tension. Hold time starts now. Lengthening of the muscle occurs during this hold time. This new tension may slightly diminish or stay the same.

HOLD TIMES
7-10 seconds = Yearling
8-20 seconds = Beginning
20-30 seconds = Maintenance
No more than 30 seconds

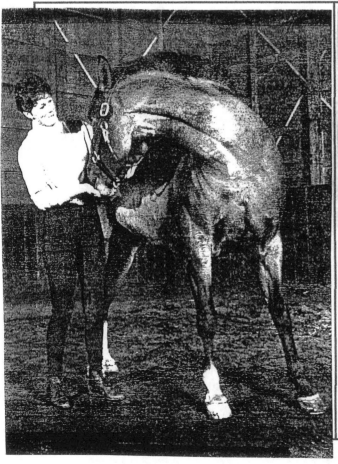
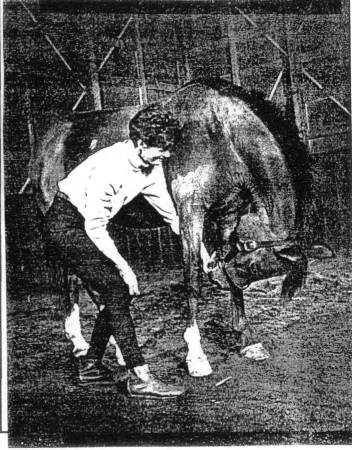

When first starting this stretching program, count the seconds for each stretch. This will ensure that you hold the proper tension long enough. If the horse is unusually tight, start by holding for shorter periods of time. Increase this time as the horse becomes accustomed to being stretched and becomes more flexible. When a horse resists being stretched, move slowly and do the relaxation exercises. Allow him time to relax; otherwise, you will be tightening the very muscles you are trying to lengthen. <u>The key to successful stretching is to keep the horse relaxed while concentrating on your own breathing and the area being stretched.</u>

Care should be taken never to jerk, hyper-flex or over-extend a limb. Movement should never be forced. It may take several sessions to loosen tight muscles and their surrounding tissue. Horses that are stretched, however, progress faster with less stiffness and fewer problems.

> THE KEY TO SUCCESSFUL STRETCHING IS TO KEEP THE HORSE RELAXED WHILE CONCENTRATING ON YOUR OWN BREATHING AND THE AREA BEING STRETCHED.

RECOMMENDATION:
It is best not to use food as encouragement when stretching the neck and poll region. A carrot is good in the beginning to teach a horse the desired movement. However, if used over a period of time it elicits only a reaction in response for food and will not produce muscle lengthening. Gently tickling the muzzle works well, with more control and better results.

CARE OF YOUR OWN BACK
At no time should you allow your own back to support the weight of the horse. Lifting should always be done using your upper legs and buttock muscles, keeping your lower back muscles extended and straight. To do this, broaden your base of support by spreading your feet apart, placing one slightly in front of the other. When it is necessary to lower your body, increase flexion at the knees and hips. Place the elbow supporting the horse's weight onto your knee. This creates a new line of support, avoiding strain on your back. This position provides stability and resilience for both you and the horse.

ORDER OF STRETCH
A stretch is never performed for the benefit of only one muscle. Not only is it very difficult to do, it could cause the muscle to be overstretched. Muscles function in groups and are layered on the body, overlapping in

their functions. For this reason the order in which these stretches are performed plays an important role in their effectiveness. As a general rule when stretching a horse, each region should be stretched in the following order:

1. Thoracic Limb - shoulder and front leg
2. Pelvic Limb - hip, thigh and hind leg
3. Poll - neck
4. Trunk - back

Always stretch both sides of the horse in one region before moving to the next region.

Once you learn to do the stretches correctly you can optimize your time by modifying your routine to selected stretches that apply to the horse's particular discipline. However, regularly stretching the entire horse is recommended to maintain a balanced muscle function.

CONCLUSION

To maintain a position of good alignment and smooth function between joints, there must be adequate muscle balance between opposing sets of muscles and flexibility to allow full movement of the joint to occur. Regular stretching can play a vital role in maintaining muscle balance good posture alignment, and flexibility necessary to attain optimal health and performance.

QUESTIONS MOST FREQUENT ASKED

Can I hurt my horse if I do the stretches wrong?
No, what will happen is the stretch will be ineffective, or the horse will pull away from you.

Can I hurt myself?
Not if you use the proper technique. Just as with learning to ride, move forward slowly. Concentrate on one stretch at a time. Remember you and your horse will be using your muscles in new and different ways. Your muscles will become stronger as they adapt to doing the stretch routine. As with any activity, the more you do it, the easier it gets! If you have any physical problems, it is best to check with your doctor before starting any riding or exercise program.

I have a busy schedule and limited time to ride. How long does it take to stretch my horse's muscles?
After learning the proper techniques you can incorporate the stretching exercises into your grooming routine They take about 10-15 minutes before and after activity Taking a few minutes to properly warm-up, cool down and stretch out your horse's muscles is the least time consuming and the easiest way to improve his performance and reduce the incidence of injury.

The bottom line - will my horse like having his muscles stretched?
Yes, after several sessions, he will be greeting you at the gate. Horses love being stretched and will eagerly look forward to participating once they understand the routine.

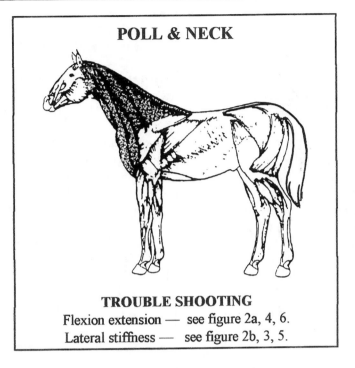

POLL & NECK

TROUBLE SHOOTING

Flexion extension — see figure 2a, 4, 6.
Lateral stiffness — see figure 2b, 3, 5.

Figure 1.

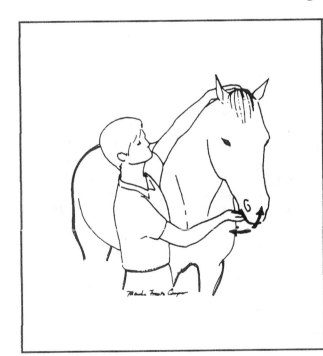

Relaxation Exercise:
to be done before stretching the neck and poll. Stand at the head of the horse opposite his cheek. Place one hand on his poll just behind the base of his skull bone and the other hand under his chin. Stabilize the poll area with your upper hand and slowly extend the neck by raising the chin outward and upward. As the horse relaxes, gently raise and lower his head in a nodding motion - five to ten repetitions.

Important: Movement in this area should only come from the head moving on the neck.

Figure 2a

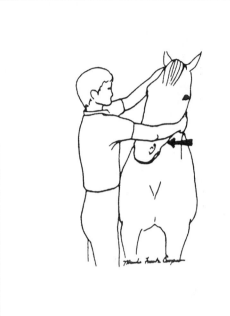

Relaxation Exercise:
to be done before stretching the neck and poll.

Stand at the horse's head opposite his cheek. Place one hand on his poll about four inches behind the base of his skull bone.

Place the other hand on the opposite cheek. Depending on the size of the horse, this is done either over the bridge of his nose or under his jaw. Stabilize the poll area with your upper hand and gently draw the cheek toward you rotating the head on the neck.

IMPORTANT: This movement is often very small, but it is very important. Try to keep the head as vertical as possible and hold.

Figure 2b.

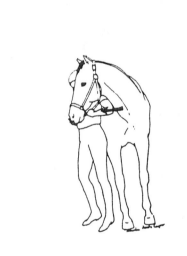

Before starting his stretch, make sure the horse is standing with his shoulders and feet squarely in front of him.

Stand at the front end of the horse with your back against his shoulder and face outward.

Hold the cheek piece of the halter with the hand closest to the horse's head. Slowly bring his head and neck around and toward you, while making sure his head remains vertical and his shoulders remain level. Light tickling on his muzzle will encourage him to follow your hand. Never force this stretch. When resistance is felt, stop and hold.

IMPORTANT: The position of this stretch is necessary for maximum affect. If the horse twists his head and neck as in stretching #5, "the carrot stretch" or raises his shoulder, this stretch has little benefit.

Figure 3.

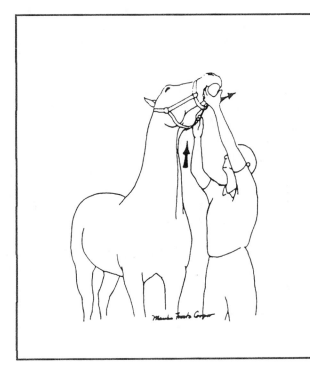

Before starting this stretch, make sure the horse is standing with his shoulders and feet squarely in front of him.

Stand directly in front off and face the horse. Place both hands under his chin. Slowly raise his head upward and slightly turned to one side while making sure his shoulders remain level and both front feet are squarely on the ground.

IMPORTANT: Never raise the horse's head straight upward. Shoulders must remain level with both feet on the ground for maximum benefit.

Figure 4.

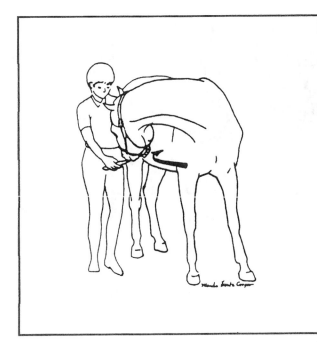

Before starting this stretch, make sure the horse is standing with his shoulders and feet squarely in front of him.

Stand at the belly of the horse facing his head. Hold the neck piece of the halter with your inside hand. Slowly bring his head and neck around toward his belly. Light tickling on his muzzle will encourage him to follow your hand. Guide his head with the halter. This stretch is done slowly and never with force. When resistance is felt - stop - hold.

IMPORTANT: Correct position and technique of this stretch is important. Never ask the horse to touch his hip or belly. To do this he must rotate his shoulder, in which case this stretch is ineffective.

Figure 5.

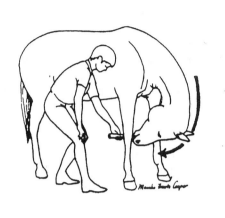

Before starting this stretch, make sure the horse is standing with his shoulders and feet squarely in front of him.

Stand at his belly, facing forward. Begin by tickling the horse's nose with a carrot to encourage him to bend his head and neck downward between his front legs, about 6 to 8 inches from his chest. (After he has the idea of what you want, encouragement should be done by tickling his muzzle.)

This movement is done slowly while maintaining level posture. When resistence is felt - stop - hold.

IMPORTANT: Never ask the horse to touch his chin to his chest. This can result in hyper-flexing the base of the neck and throat latch area.

Figure 6.

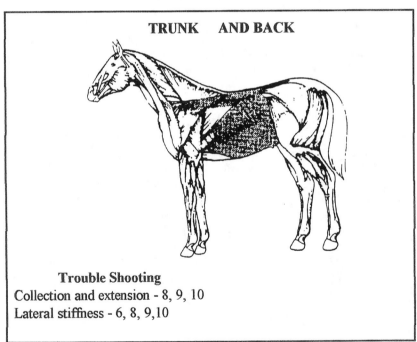

TRUNK   AND BACK

Trouble Shooting
Collection and extension - 8, 9, 10
Lateral stiffness - 6, 8, 9,10

Figure 7.

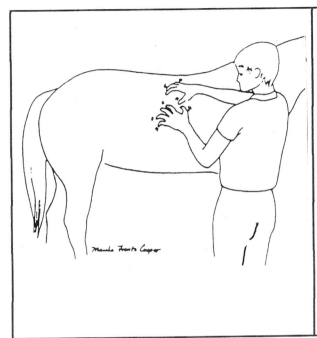

This technique is designed to strengthen the muscles on the side of the belly that assist in holding the back up for posture and movement.

Stand next to the horse, facing his belly. Place both hand approximately two inches down from the spine and six to right inches apart on the side of the horse.

With your fingers spread, stimulate the underlying muscles with little back and forth movement of the finger tips. Keep both hands on the side of the truck, gradually move downward. You will see the muscles contract under your fingers.

Figure 8.

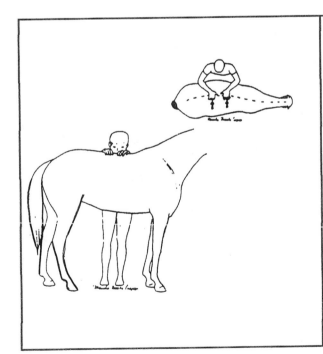

Stand next to the horse, facing his belly.

Place both hands on the horse's back about two inches from his spine on the opposite side from where you are standing.

With the tips of your fingers, gently pull toward the spine from the opposite side. Your will see the spine bend toward you like a crescent. Move downward toward the tail two to three inches and repeat. Repeat this exercise on both sides of the horse two to three times.

IMPORTANT: Make sure the horse's back remains up during this stretch.

Figure 9.

117

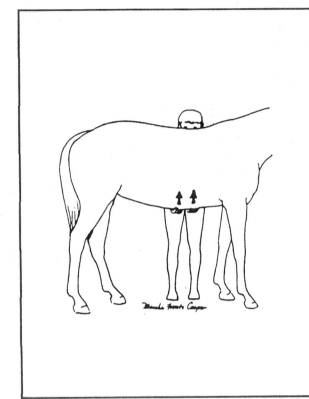

Stand next to the horse facing his belly.

To begin, gently stroke both the back and the belly of the horse, allowing them to relax.

Place both hands on the midline)center of the belly) and just behind the girth area.

Give a quick poke upward with your finger tips then immediately flatten your hand and hold to the count of eight. Move five to six inches toward the rear of the horse and repeat.

IMPORTANT: If the horse is short, support your body weight with your upper legs and buttock muscles to protect your lower back. To do this, spread your feet and flex your knee and hip joints keeping your back extended and straight.

Figure 10.

CHAPTER 9

THE THERAPY ENVIRONMENT

THERAPY ARENA REQUIREMENTS

Barbara T. Engel M.Ed., OTR

KEY WORDS
    SAFETY
    POINTS OF REFERENCE
    SCHOOLING FIGURES
    THERAPY
    TRAINING

The riding arena is an enclosed area in which hippotherapy or equine-assisted therapy takes place. Normally the size is that of a dressage arena that is either "small" - 20 x 40 meters (66 x 132 feet) or standard 20 x 60 meters (66 x 198 feet). The ideal dressage arena for hippotherapy is an indoor arena that is at least 20 x 40 meters. This provides the therapy team (horse, an instructor, a therapist and possibly helpers) a non-distractable environment where the team has full focus on the client. For those who provide group sessions, as may be true in psychology or with a sensory integration group, the arena may need to be 100 X 200 feet.

If an indoor arena is not available, an outdoor arena can be used. The outdoor arena must be fenced with safe and secure material such as pipe, wood, or plastic fencing material. It must be high enough so that a horse will not attempt to jump the fence. There should be one or two secure gates. The fence not only provides a safe boundary but excludes others from interfering with the therapy focus. The horse must be totally accustomed to this environment and its natural changes - temperature, wind, sounds and shadows allowing it to maintain a focus on the task at hand that decreases the changes of spooking.

The arena must have good footing. Footing should have a solid level base of natural dirt. This is covered by sand, peat, sand/shaving mix, tire shavings/sand, or synthetic materials about 2 inches deep. It should be dust free and easy to walk on. Soft footing is important to maintain the health of the horse and to allow the spring from the legs to transmit to the client. A hard surface will cause the percussion of the horse's hoofs to vibrate to the client's spine. A hard surface is also hard on older horses whose muscles, tendons and ligaments are not as resilient as those of the young horse. A wet surface or dry on top and wet on the bottom surface can cause a horse to slip. Too deep or an uneven surface is also undesirable. It is hard on the horse's legs and will affect the quality of the treatment. The rubber shredded footing dries easily but in very hot climates such as Las Vegas, Nevada the footing will be very hot.

A dressage arena normally has letters around its walls or fences. They are used in dressage as points of reference. In dressage, one learns to train both horse and rider to go forward in a supple, balanced and rhythmic manner while maintaining a straight, forward frame. Gymnastic exercises, or schooling figures as they are called in dressage, provide exercises to increase lateral bending to supple and strengthen the horse and in turn, to go straight. These exercises strengthen the hindquarters that allows the horse effectively to carry the client, rider or trainer.

The letters are used for changes in gait -, i.e., halt at "B" for two seconds then walk to "C" - or to begin a turn. In hippotherapy the dressage arena provides the instructor the same advantages as it does to the dressage rider. The instructor will be driving the horse in straight lines, in circular movements, and on two tracks (a lateral movement) to facilitate the postural reactions in the client requested by the therapist. Working with children who have directional problems, the therapist might use a game - for example: going on a trip. At "A" we must turn left to go to Monroe "M." Then we are going to right to go to forest at "F," and so on.

The following figures (Figure 1 and Figure 2) will describe exercises within the standard 20 X 60 meter dressage arena. The arena is divided lengthwise by three lines into four quarters. The center line runs lengthwise from the letter "A" to the letter "C." The quarter lines run parallel to the center line halfway between it and each of the long sides.

The basic patterns of dressage are described here. These patterns can be used during therapy when appropriate or combined in many ways to help the instructor or therapist to school the horse before the therapy session and after the last session.

When a horse is being ridden often by riders with disabilities or inexperienced or stiff riders, special care should be taken to see that it gets regular schooling by an experienced rider to keep it properly "tuned" and in balance.

STRAIGHT FIGURES:

These all incorporate straight lines and are often the most difficult to do correctly. The most common fault, besides crookedness and weaving, is having the haunches to the inside of the shoulders when following a certain track. Any of the figures that are executed away from the fence line will be more difficult for the horse and rider as the fence is no longer there to help guide them.

Outside track: Follows the fence line of the arena all the way around. It should be ridden or driven as four straight lines with four corners. The corners must be ridden with the same attention as with circles (Figure 3).

Inside track: This track parallels the outside track about 1½ meter (four to five feet) to the inside of the arena (Figure 3).

Permanent quarter line: The rider takes each of the quarter lines as his track down the long sides (Figure 4).

Diagonal change of a rein: A change of rein using a diagonal line from one corner across to the opposite corner. On the right track these are done from the letters "K" to "X" to "M" or "M" to "X" to "K." On the left track they are done "FXH" or "HXF." They may also be done across the half arena, starting in the corner and ending at "B" or "E" (Figure 5).

Simple turns: a simple turn is a 90-degree turn to the right or left. These turns always end with the same turn with which they were started. They can be done across the width of the arena, as in a turn from "B" to "E," or they may be done down the center or quarter lines (Figure 6).

Turns with a change of rein: the same as the above only these end with a change of rein (changing directions across the arena) by turning in the other direction as one meets the far side (Figure 7).

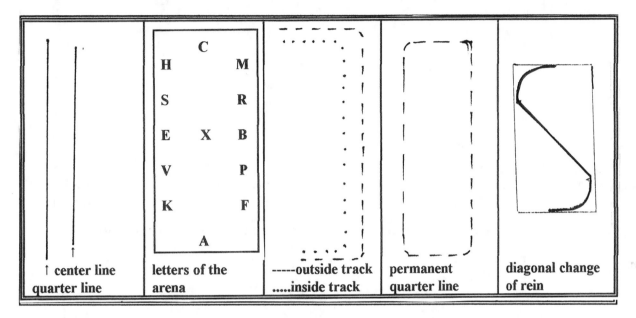

	letters of the	-----outside track	permanent	diagonal change
↑ center line quarter line	arena	.....inside track	quarter line	of rein

Figure 1.   **Figure 2**   **Figure 3**   **Figure 4**   **Figure 5**

SCHOOLING FIGURE

Broken lines: In this movement one rides two or more diagonal lines joined by a quick turn. For one broken line the rider would ride "M" to "X" then turn and ride to "F"; for two broken lines he or she would ride from "K" to "L," turn to "E," turn to "I" and then turn to end at "H." If the rider softens the turns then they are known as "loops" and is more of a round figure. Loops are excellent for helping to soften and relax the horse (Figure 8).

*Oblique***:** This is a 45-degree line from one track to another, or attaching to another figure (Figure 9).

ROUND FIGURES:

These are figures made up of curved lines, ridden with a consistent bending of the horse's spine throughout the entire movement. These are good for improving the lateral suppleness of horse and rider. They increase the rider's torso rotation and can be used to facilitate changes in the way that the rider positions and carries his or her weight.

Circles: An excellent movement to flex the horse laterally and loosen and supple him. A novice rider may incorrectly lean inward on the circle, collapsing the inside hip and pushing all the weight to the outside. This can be corrected by encouraging him or her to ride on his or her inside seat bone somewhat forward and push the inside knee toward the ground.

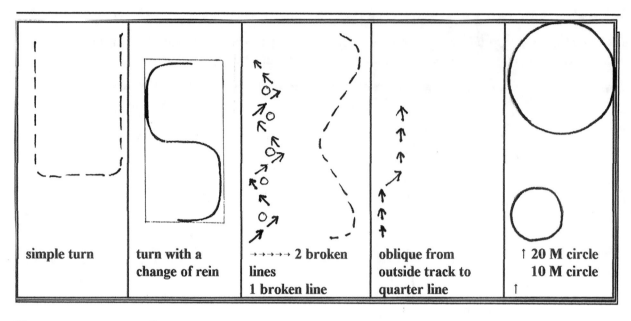

| simple turn | turn with a change of rein | →→→→→ 2 broken lines
1 broken line | oblique from outside track to quarter line | ↑ 20 M circle
10 M circle
↑ |

| Figure 6 | Figure 7 | Figure 8 | Figure 9 | Figure 10 |

SCHOOLING FIGURES

Voltes: These are circles of exactly 6 meters in diameter, the smallest circle that a horse may do. They should be ridden only at the collected gaits (Figure 13, 14).

Serpentine: These are a series of alternating half circles joined by a short straight line. The longer this connecting line and the larger the half circles the easier the movement is. The constant changes of flexion are beneficial to both the horse and rider (Figure 11).

Figure 8's: This is simply two circles of equal size joined at the center of the figure (Figure 12).

Half Volte: A half circle ending with an oblique back to the track. Results in a change of rein (Figure 13).

Reverse half Volte: An oblique away from the track ending with a half circle back to the track. Results in a change of rein (Figure 14).

Change of rein through the circle: Two alternating half circles within a larger circle that result in a change of rein (Figure 15).

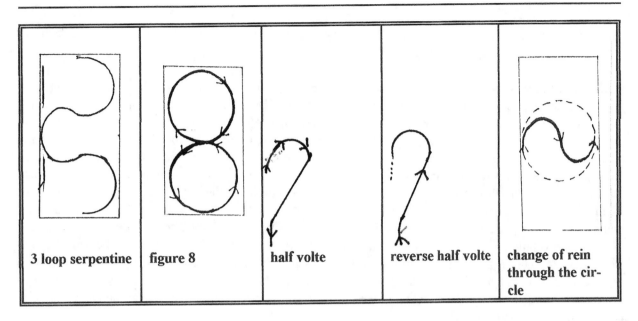

3 loop serpentine	figure 8	half volte	reverse half volte	change of rein through the circle
Figure 11	Figure 12	Figure 13	Figure 14	Figure 15

SCHOOLING FIGURES

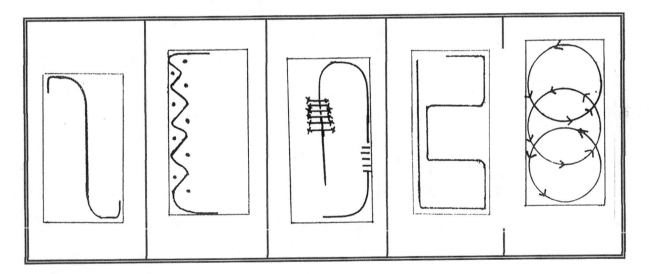

Simple patterns
SCHOOLING FIGURES

The exercises that strengthen and supple the horse also help the rider to become straighter, more evenly coordinated with better balance and greater trunk control. Due to limited space the purpose of this discussion will be to consider only those school figures consisting of work on one track. These figures are universal and can be practiced by anyone whether they ride "dressage" or not, although anyone training a horse to move in balance under the rider is doing "dressage."

Before beginning, a few general thoughts should be considered. The horse should always move forward in a straight manner even when bending through the round figures. By straight we mean that the hind legs of the horse should always follow the line of the front legs exactly. The rider should aim to ride in a balanced and upright manner, avoiding as much as possible any deviation from the correct position. The use of these patterns should help decrease, not increase, any unilateral tendencies in both the horse and rider. Generally work on straight lines will encourage the horse forward, while any work that is not on a straight line will tend to slow the horse. This principle can be used to your advantage in conditioning the horse. The work on straight lines is also a measure of how successful training is and helps to restore forwardness after a demanding bending exercise. Generally one can expect clients to experience a decrease in skill and coordination as the gaits are increased in riding the figures. Work that was good in the walk may need improvement at the trot, although forwardness in all gaits always improves things. Proper visualization of the patterns is important in executing them correctly. To aid the rider, props such as traffic cones may be helpful. They may be used by placing two to form a "gate" that the rider passes through at certain key spots, or single cones may be used as a point around which the rider forms his figure.

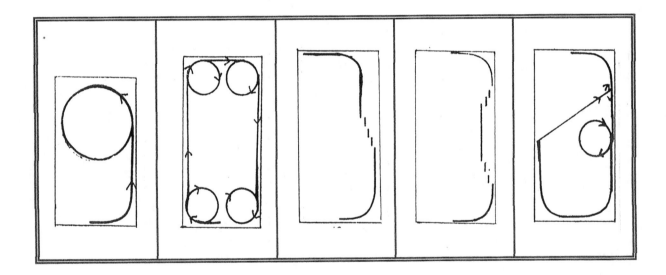

CHAPTER 10

TREATMENT PROCEDURES
INSURANCE REIMBURSEMENT FOR HIPPOTHERAPY-
AN EVER CHANGING PICTURE

Barbara L. Glasow, PT

One of the fastest areas of change in the 90's is the health care field. The field of therapeutic riding and hippotherapy are also changing and evolving. Many therapists and therapeutic riding programs are seeking third party medical insurance reimbursement for the provision of hippotherapy. This is no longer a simple process and will continually change from region to region and from one insurance policy to the next. Anyone venturing into the area of third party reimbursement needs to be both a good clinician and knowledgeable in reimbursement processes. The following provides only a brief overview of the basic points that need to be considered before trying to pursue reimbursement for treatment that includes hippotherapy.

Hippotherapy as a Treatment
Hippotherapy is a treatment tool that uses the multi-dimensional movement of the horse and activities on the horse as a means of achieving measurable functional outcomes in clients. It is used by a growing number of licensed/credentialed health professionals that include physical therapists, occupational therapists and speech pathologists. Hippotherapy is used primarily with clients that have movement dysfunction but it can also be appropriate in helping to achieve sensory processing, psychological, cognitive, behavioral and communication outcomes.

Hippotherapy should always be one part of a comprehensive treatment plan that integrates gains made during hippotherapy into functional activities. Treatment should be based on a thorough evaluation, the establishment of goals and a treatment plan that results in the achievement of functional outcomes off the horse. The goal should never be an improvement in functional riding skills. Rather, the horse is used in hippotherapy as one means of assisting in achieving functional outcomes in the client's daily life.

The Changing Health Care Field
Since the late 1980's the health care field in the United States has changed more and more rapidly from insurance policies that were based on a "fee for service" plan to one of managed care.

Major medical insurance policies (i.e., indemnity plans) traditionally paid for outpatient services on a fee for service basis. The medical provider provided the service and either billed the insurance company directly or asked the patient to pay for the service at the time of delivery. If the patient paid at the time the service was provided then the patient submitted the bill to their insurance for reimbursement. The patient was responsible for a yearly deductible (a sum of money that typically must be paid every year before the insurance policy began to pay. For example, a $250 deductible per family member per year or a $1000 total deductible per family). The patient also was responsible for a co-insurance payment. (If the insurance paid 80% of a service charge then the patient was responsible for the remaining 20%.) As long as the treatment was prescribed and was considered "medically necessary" there was seldom much difficulty in a patient obtaining reimbursement for treatment, even for a long-term or chronic problem. Treatment strived to achieve a return to a prior level of function (if the problem was an acquired one) or to achieve an optimum level of function if the patient had a congenital or developmental diagnosis. Some of these policies still exist but in an ever decreasing number.

As health care costs escalated more and more, insurance companies began to use some type of managed care system in order to control costs and achieve more efficiency and consistency in patient outcomes. Managed care systems attempt to control costs through a variety of means. Some of these means include placing price controls on their providers, requiring preauthorization before services are rendered, using primary care "gatekeepers," and regulating which providers the patient can go to.

In some regions of the country the majority of people are enrolled in **HMO's (Health Maintenance Organizations)**. In HMO's the insurance company contracts with employers (or Medicaid or Medicare, etc.) to provide a predetermined set of services to its members on a prepaid basis. Insured patients are usually assigned to a specific primary physician who acts as a "gatekeeper" for any other services that the patient may need. The intent is to focus on preventive care so that the patient will not need more costly services in the future. The reality often is that the more chronically ill or disabled person does not get the needed specialty services that are required. Utilization management (a review process that a service is " medically necessary" and requires pre-approval) is needed for any referrals to neurologists, orthopedists, physical therapy, occupational therapy, speech therapy, etc. HMO's contract with their own set of providers. If a patient goes to a provider outside of the HMO, the service will not be reimbursed unless it has been pre-approved.

Preferred Provider Organizations (PPO's) lie somewhere between major medical policies and HMO's. PPO insurance company plans contract with a variety of providers that agree to provide specific services for a discounted fee structure in return for having a preferred status in treating the group's members. Some companies limit payment for service only to providers that belong to the PPO. Others, allow patients to seek services outside of the PPO network but will then reimburse for services rendered at the lower rate of return. (For example, it will pay 100% of the negotiated rate for providers in the network but maybe only 70% of the fee for someone outside of the network.)

Focus on Managed Care
All types of insurance providers (HMO's, PPO's and Major Medical Policies) are involved in various types of managed care regardless of the type of reimbursement. Most policies are no longer interested in their patients receiving physical therapy services with goals that include decrease pain, increase range of motion or increase muscle strength which are considered impairments with no limits to the length of time or frequency of service. Instead, insurance companies now want the patient treated in order to eliminate or minimize specific functional limitations and disabilities whether it is through a return to prior level of function or through learning a compensation. For example, a person who has had a stroke may have an impairment of decreased hand motor control and coordination. He may have a resulting functional limitation of being unable to put on a button shirt which results in a disability of being dependent in dressing. However, occupational therapy treatment could quickly eliminate the disability in dressing if the patient is either coached to change their type of clothing (eg. wearing pullover shirts) or is taught how to dress with a one handed technique of dressing and use of a button hook. Learning how to dress in the traditional manner may take months or years of therapy. However, learning to dress through the use of compensations would probably require fewer than ten treatment sessions before discharge. In the same manner of thinking, a person who has had a stroke could return to functional walking much more quickly if given a brace for the ankle and taught how to use a quad cane versus developing the ankle motor control and dynamic balance responses necessary to walk independently without any assistive devices.

Outpatient rehabilitation services of physical therapy, occupational therapy and speech therapy are changing in their orientation of treatment. In general, therapists can expect to receive less reimbursement per visit, much more case management, fewer approved visits, often a shorter time period per visit and decreased frequency of treatments per week. Insurance companies are interested in having their patients achieve functional outcomes in the quickest, most efficient manner possible. Insurance companies often no longer pay whatever fee for service that the provider charges. Instead, payment can take many forms but there is often room for negotiation.

Some types of payment include:
- a negotiated discounted fee for service
- a per diem rate (a fee per day for a total rehabilitation program of PT, OT, SP)
- a case rate (eg. A case rate of $900 may be the going rate for outpatient PT treatment for a stroke. This could be negotiated as 20 visits of 30 minutes at $45/visit or you might ask for 10 visits at $90/visit if you can achieve equal functional outcomes.)
- an HMO may have a policy of 20 visits in 60 days. You may be able to negotiate 20 visits but ask for the visits spread over 6 months to a year.
- major medical/PPO's policies often have caps of a particular number of treatments/year.

Hippotherapy as a Viable Option
Therapists wanting to provide hippotherapy as part of a treatment plan need to be fully aware of what the local insurance market is in their territory. Is it dominated by HMO's? Is it a mix of HMO's, PPO's and major medical policies? Are there only a few large therapy practices that are providing all the HMO contract therapy services? Is there still room for negotiating contracts with individual insurance companies or does the therapist need to negotiate subcontracts with larger therapy practices with the offer to treat the more difficult neurologically involved patients?

The therapist getting involved in offering hippotherapy as part of a total treatment plan MUST have a good depth of existing clinical knowledge and experience with the patient population that is going to be treated with hippotherapy. The therapist must have an existing track record in achieving measurable functional outcomes with the proposed patient population off the horse as well as on. Hippotherapy should only be used a part of a total treatment plan. It should be used in the treatment plan where and when it can be most effective and efficient in achieving the desired functional outcomes. Treatment plans need to be developed with the knowledge that the number of treatments are apt to be limited; the goals should be functionally oriented; a home program should be part of the plan; and the patient and family should be instructed in self management.

The use of hippotherapy as a treatment tool is at a crossroads in the field of health care. There is presently little written research to support the efficacy of using it as a treatment tool. However, clinicians are empirically well aware of how efficiently functional outcomes can be achieved when hippotherapy is used judiciously within a total treatment plan. Managed care plans are also sometimes more open to innovative treatments that can be expected to achieve desired functional outcomes in an optimum amount of time or with the least cost.

Payment Options for Hippotherapy

There is presently no such thing as payment for the therapy called "hippotherapy". The client does not go to a hippotherapist[1] to receive hippotherapy. Instead, the client is in need of services that may include physical therapy, occupational therapy and or speech therapy in order to achieve certain functional outcomes. The licensed/credentialed health professional, when performing the evaluation, may determine that the use of the horse as a treatment tool through hippotherapy would be an appropriate part of the total treatment plan. Depending on the state in which the client lives a prescription may be needed before the evaluation and/ or treatment can be provided. The prescription for the service will state physical therapy, occupational therapy or speech therapy and may state the desired goals, number of visits, frequency of treatment, etc. As discussed above, the type of payment for therapy depends on what kind of insurance plan the client has. Payment options for therapy that includes hippotherapy can come from a wide variety of sources including:

- private pay
- family support service dollars that are available in some states to disabled children
- school contracts (eg. part of the child's IEP (Individual Education Plan)
- contracts with Department of Human Services
- contracts with state & county MHMR (Mental Health/Mental Retardation) Dept.
- Medicaid waiver programs
- Medicaid/Medicare
- fee-for-service payment from major medical insurance
- provider contracts with Preferred Provider Organizations
- provider contracts with Health Maintenance Organizations
- subcontract with a provider in a PPO/HMO

Options for payment all depend on what part of the country the therapist is in and what type of contracts the provider has negotiated with local insurance plans. It is up to the provider to decide whether hippotherapy is used as a marketing option through education of insurance companies or if it is discretely used within the treatment plan.

Unless a per diem rate, case rate or fixed fee per visit is established, billing for treatment normally involves the use of recognized CPT-4 codes for the services provided (in 15 minute increments) and ICD-9 diagnostic codes for the diagnosis of the client. Billing for services needs to be submitted on an invoice (Many states require a standardized HCFA-1500 form be used.) that includes:

1. The agency's name, address, phone number, Business EIN Tax ID#
2. The therapist's name, profession and license number
3. Client's name, diagnosis (with ICD-9 code) and referring physician's name
4. A list of the services provided (with CPT-4 codes) with the charges for each.

---

[1] On 2/28/92 the American Hippotherapy Association (AHA) Board of Directors passed a resolution to "**discontinue the use of the term,** *Hippotherapist.*" It was agreed that (AHA) did not intend to create a new filed of hippotherapy, therefore, it was not creating a new profession of hippotherapists. Instead, each professional involved in hippotherapy, occupational therapy, physical therapy, and speech therapy, would use hippotherapy within the context of their own State Practice Act. So, for example, an occupational therapist may be treating with sensory integration. As of April, 1997, AHA nor any other agency or association in the U.S. offers certification in hippotherapy; there is at present no such entity as a "**certified hippotherapist.**"

Hippotherapy does not have its own CPT-4 code number. Many treatments used by physical and occupational therapists do not have separate code numbers for many of the legitimate treatments that are used in pediatrics and rehabilitation. So a number of different treatments are clustered under the existing codes that best reflect what the treatment is. When the horse is used in treatment it is often used for different purposes depending on the client diagnosis and the goals that are trying to be achieved. The horse can be used to provide sensory input; arouse the limbic system; facilitate postural and balance responses, strengthen muscles, change breathing patterns; enhance motor learning; assist in developing motor planning; etc., etc. Speech therapists use their own designated speech code numbers regardless of how the horse is used. Physical and occupational therapists are most commonly using the following CPT-4 codes when the horse is used in treatment, with the choice of code determined by how the horse is being used in that particular session.

CPT-4[2]

CODE	PROCEDURE	UNITS	COST/UNIT	SUBTOTAL
97110	THERAPEUTIC EXERCISE			
97112	NEUROMUSCULAR EDUCATION			
97150	THERAPEUTIC PROCEDURES TWO OR MORE INDIVIDUALS			
97530	THERAPEUTIC/FUNCTIONAL ACTIVITIES			
97770	SENSORY INTEGRATION			

Presumably during the same treatment session the client may also receive manual therapy off the horse, gait training, training in activities of daily living, wheelchair training, etc. as part of a total treatment.

The Decision to Use Hippotherapy

For therapists who are presently in private practice or working in a pediatric or rehabilitation agency the addition of hippotherapy as a treatment tool may prove to be very advantageous. Many specialty practices are trying to position themselves as providers of choice for niche markets. The use of hippotherapy for the correct clients and at the right point in their treatment plan has the potential of optimizing the functional outcomes that can be achieved.

However, for therapists or therapeutic riding programs that are contemplating entering the area of third party reimbursement for the first time they face the need to become thoroughly familiar with their local market and the process of reimbursement. As soon as you begin to bill insurance companies for treatment that includes hippotherapy you are putting your organization into a whole different level of professional obligation and scrutiny. You are providing a professional service with the need to follow professional standards and ethics for physical, occupational and/or speech therapy. Appropriate evaluations, treatment plans, goals and progress notes need to done for each client. Professional medical liability is now an issue with a need for good risk management. Health insurance companies more and more often will ask for documentation to prove that therapy is "medically necessary" and to prove that progress is being made. Clients often need assistance in appealing denials for coverage by insurance.

[2] CPT-4 codes-1996. These codes can be obtained from you professional association or the American Medical Assoc. or hospital.

Being involved in the health care field at this time of rapid and constant change is a daunting process. However, it is also an exciting time. Managed care is forcing therapists to seriously look at their treatment protocols and to create treatment plans that are much more timely and cost effective than those of the past. It already has made better clinicians of many of us. The horse, used in hippotherapy, can play a valuable part in helping our clients to achieve the best outcomes possible with the more limited financial resources that are available today. We just need to do our homework up front in order to manage the maze of managed care.

References
Abeln, S. & Stewart, D. (1993). *Documenting Functional Outcomes in Physical Therapy.* St. Louis, MO: Mosby-Year Book, Inc.
American Medical Association CPT-4 Codes.
Crispen, C. & Hertfelder, S. Editors (1990). *Private Practice - Strategies for Success.* Rockville, Maryland: American Occupational Therapy Association, Inc.
Gorman, I. (1996). Notes from presentation: *Treating and Managing the Adult Neurological Patient in a Managed Care Setting.* July 26-27, 1996, Arlington, Virginia

TREATMENT PROCEDURES AND DOCUMENTATION

Barbara T. Engel, M.Ed., OTR

Occupational and physical therapy have historically documented treatment sessions. This is a requirement for members of the medical and para-medical professions. Traditionally, a treatment begins with an initial evaluation and ends with an outcome evaluation. The evaluation states the clients diagnostic codes (ICD-9 codes), the specific problems the client has, recommended therapy goals in measurable terms, and a time frame when these goals will be met. Treatment noted follows each therapy session. The degree of detail required by agencies, states, Federal, insurance companies, and/or physicians will vary. K. Ottenbacher (1987) states "without assessment expertise, rehabilitation practitioners will be unable to meet the demands for efficiency, accountability, and effectiveness that are certain to increase in the future."

In the Joint Commission of Accreditation of Health Care Organizations publication of 1994, it stated that among the importance for establishing an outcome assessment initiated in the health care setting is to establish an accurate and reliable basis for clinical decision making, and to evaluate the effectiveness of care, and identify opportunities for improvement. It also states that how the delivery of care impacts the clients life - stated in quantitative term is important. From my experience, this means that the delivery of care has caused improved functional ability in how the client can care for him or herself, can hold a job, or a decreased degree of needing assistance. The pleasures of life like a full bath or shower, being happier or having more self-esteem may not qualify for meaningful life improvement under how the delivery of care impacts the clients life.

In the United States, the occupational and physical therapists are responsible for their choice of treatment tools with a referred client. The physician may say the patient who has had a stroke needs physical therapy, occupational therapy, and speech therapy. These are the accepted treatment methods for such a diagnosis. The therapists must then evaluate the client to determine the need for their expertise and the outcome the therapist expects. It is important to use standardized assessments appropriate for the specific disability and the hippotherapy setting. One might refer to a new book - *Assessment in Occupational Therapy and Physical Therapy* edited by J. Van Deusen and Denis Brunt for a review of currently acceptable assessment tools. A clinic therapy session, a home therapy session or a hippotherapy session does not change any aspect of the documentation. The therapist uses the standards of practice related to his or her profession regardless of the location of practice. All aspects of treatment are the same.

For insurance purposes, a referral from the physician must be obtained. If the therapist decides that hippotherapy would be the best method to treat for the client, he or she will need to obtain an approval from the physician that the client can safely ride a horse. The physician must approve the appropriateness of hippotherapy. This is a standard of the industry. This has nothing to do with a prescription for treatment or the tool the therapist chooses - it just states that "there is no reason that Johnny can not ride a horse."

To solicit physician approval, we must demonstrate by documenting procedures and results that hippotherapy is an effective treatment tool . Evaluations stated in quantitative terms are the only way therapist can show this to be an effective method of treatment. Not only must we document evaluations in measurable terms but we must show that this method of treatment is superior to the more typical clinical method.

When using the horse as a tool in rehabilitation, documentation becomes immensely important. Hippotherapy and equine-assisted therapy as a treatment tool are still a relatively new method of treatment. In many parts of the world, as in Germany, physicians are either directly involved in hippotherapy treatments or involved by specifically directing the physical therapist in the treatment of their patients. They are required to document their findings in journals. As a result this method of treatment has become widely used and accepted.

As therapists we need to clearly show that what we do on the horse differs, and has increased benefits with what a riding instructor does with a client. A riding lesson may cost from zero to twenty-five dollars in the United States while occupational, physical and speech/language therapist may charge from fifty to one hundred and twenty -five dollars for a session. The difference in fees needs to be reflected in the difference in skills. What is being referred to here are statements from instructors claiming the same type of changes occurring during a riding lessen as that which are addresses in therapy. For example if one can obtain functional sitting balance during a series of riding lessons costing $20 each - why would one need a therapist at one hundred dollars a session? Something to think about.

Reference:
Van Deusen, J. PhD. OTR/L & Dennis Brunt, PT EdD. (1997). *Assessment in Occupational Therapy and Physical Therapy*. Philadelphia: W.B. Saunders Co.

ACTIVITY ANALYSIS

Barbara T. Engel M.Ed, OTR

KEY WORDS

TEACHING TECHNIQUE
SIMPLIFIED--BREAK DOWN
DECREASE FRUSTRATION

Task analysis is used by occupational therapists to examination the components of a task in order to determine its use as a treatment modality or to teach a client an activity of daily living skills (Hopkins & Smith, 1978). Llorens (1978) states in occupational therapy "Activity analysis is usable to determine the most utilizable properties of an activity or task to accomplish a specific treatment objective." In this setting the properties to be considered can influence physical, psychological, or cognitive-perceptual-motor deficits. As examples, tasks may be selected to:

- Provide increased range in the shoulder-arms area.
- Allow for expression of independence.
- Provide an outlet for aggression.
- Allow for socialization.
- Provide tactile stimulation.
- Provide a variety of movement experiences for vestibular stimulation.
- Provide fine-motor manipulation of the fingers and hand-eye coordination.
- Increase problem solving skills and motor planning.
- Allow for repetitious arm movements.

Snow (1985) describes task analysis as breaking down the total task into small components and then forward or backward chaining the steps. Forward chaining is more common with occupational therapists. Each step is practiced and mastered before the next step is attempted. Many times intervention must occur in order that a task can be performed. For example: motor planning has its basis of function in sensory awareness and processing. The right hemisphere appears to be involved in the processing aspect. If Jessie has a deficit in sensory processing, this needs to be addressed through a treatment technique. All the practice in the world will not allow Jessie to motor plan if the neurological mechanism for motor planning is not there. In forward chaining, the first step is mastered before the second step is attempted and so on. Wallace & Kaufman (1978) state "Task analysis may be viewed as a sequence of evaluative activities that pinpoint the child's learning or processing problem and guide the therapist in planning an effective remedial sequence of instructional tasks." This approach uses a step-by-step process of breaking down the activity a child is doing to **find** the **problem**. The activity may then be broken down into sub-skills if necessary. Each sub-skill is tackled separately. For example, Christy is have trouble putting the saddle on her horse. The therapist performs a task analysis of the task Christy is having problems with.

- To find the right saddle in the tack room.
- To carry the saddle to the hitching post.
- Find a rack to place the saddle on.
- Go back to the tack room to find the saddle pad
- Find the girth that goes with the saddle

- Take the pad and girth to the hitching post
- Place the saddle pad on the horse with the front of the pad on the neck of the horse
- Slide the pad to its proper position.
- Pick up the saddle and lifts it up to place it on the saddle pad.
- Pick up the girth to attach to the saddle.
- Attach the off side of the girth to the saddle.
- Attach the near side of the girth to the saddle
- Tighten the girth.

The therapist examines each step to see which one is causing Christy to fail this task. She finds out that Christy has trouble knowing which goes forward and which is the back. She can not distinguish front from back and she does not have the strength to lift the saddle.

Activities are analyzed for the selection of age-appropriate work/play categories in order that the skills involved are meaningful to the client's needs (Clark 1985). Following the suitable selection of the activity, a task may be analyzed to determine if it needs to be adapted in order for Jake (who has cerebral palsy) to do it successfully. If Jake cannot pick up the brush, he will not be able to perform the next task, brushing the horse. This example breaks down the activity so that it can be examined for the components of normal physical function. For example--picking up a brush while standing in front of the table requires the following movements:

- Turning around to locate the brush by looking toward it on the table.
- Taking several steps toward the table.
- Raising the arm at the shoulder.
- Activating an arm in extension to reach for the brush.
- Lowering the arm toward the brush.
- Extending the wrist and fingers to open the hand.
- Lowering the arm till the extended hand touches the brush.
- Grasping the brush with the hand and closing the fingers.
- Flexing the elbow and bringing the brush to the midline of the body.

This analysis breaks down the physical movements required in this task only. The next step would be to analyze Jake's ability to perform each movement and how he can perform the tasks to gain the best range of motion in body and limbs. In this example the task analysis may help the therapist identify a movement that a rider may have trouble doing, such as reaching with the arm and hand, because of the inability to inhibit flexion of the shoulder/elbow and wrist. The task may need to be altered in order for the person to grasp the brush effectively and use it in brushing the horse. For example, the therapist gives Jake a brush with a velcro strap that holds the brush securely in his hand--he does not need to concentrate on clinching the fingers which increases the strong flexion tendency. Jake will be able to extend his arm more easily without tightly flexing his hand and wrist to hold the brush--which in turn may cause his elbow and shoulder to flex. Jake will stand on a mounting block, eliminating raising his arm, to make it easier for him to extend the arm outward. In this way Jake can independently brush the horse with good arm motion.

In a treatment situation, an occupational therapist may use these activities to develop normal motor function while performing a functional task. He or she would stand next to Jake and would assist him to move his hand and arm (using positioning and facilitory techniques) while maintaining a balanced body posture. Jake would learn both balance and function by allowing the therapist to assist when he cannot make the appropriate movement--in essence Jake and the therapist are working as one--as his body learns new motor behavior. The therapist has used the activity analysis to isolate the areas that need her assistance.

Lilly wants to ride the horse and is motivated to accomplish the task but is having trouble climbing up on the mounting block. Once she has mastered the mounting block, she does not have the concept of how she might get on the horse. In therapeutic riding, the therapist needs not only know the sequential development of riding skills but must also be able (Lamport et al., 1989):

- To recognize the physical, mental, and emotional requirements of the task.
- To recognize the rider's physical, mental and psychological limitations.
- To recognize the cognitive skills necessary to carry out a task.
- To recognize the processing skills required in the cognitive area.
- To recognize the areas where assistance is beneficial.
- To recognize the areas where the client needs intervention and by what means.
- To recognize supplies, equipment and environmental requirements.
- To recognize precautions, contraindications, indications associated with the task.

Activity analysis helps the therapist to understand how to proceed with the motor problem that Lilly is having in order that she will be successful with her task.

References

Clark, P.N. (1985). *Occupational Therapy for Children.* St. Louis: The C.V. Mosby Co.

Hopkins, H.L., Smith, H.D. (1978). *Willard & Spackman's Occupational Therapy.* 5th ed. New York: J.B. Lippincott Co. 102-105.

Lamport, N.K.; Coffey, M.S.; Hersch, G.I. (1989). *Activity Analysis.* Thorofare: Slack Incorporated.

Llorens, L. A. (1973). Activity Analysis for Cognitive-Perceptual-Motor Dysfunction. *AJOT*, 27:8: 453-56.

Snow, B.S. (1985). Children with Visual or Hearing Impairment in Clark, PN & Allen, AS: *Occupational Therapy.*

Wallace, G., & Kaufman, J.M. (1978). *Teaching Children with Learning Problems.* (2nd ed) Columbus: Charles E. Merrill Publishing Co. 105.

GROUP DYNAMICS-GROUP INTERACTIONS IN A THERAPY GROUP

Barbara T. Engel, M.Ed, OTR

KEY WORDS:
SUCCESS
PLEASURE
TEAMWORK

A group consists of two or more people who are motivated to deal with a common goal or task. There are many types of groups and types of leadership styles. A collection of people can become a group. At a social gathering a common goal can be identified, such as playing bridge. The group then forms around this common interest. There are social groups, family groups, and business groups, like a board of directors. There are horse groups such as the U.S. Pony Club, American Horse Show Association (AHSA), 4-H clubs and therapeutic riding programs. Therapeutic riding programs require a group concept. One cannot work with a rider with a disability without a group even if it is just the therapist ,the client, and the horse. The therapy group is affected by other groups in the program. Programs have several types of groups. There is the board of directors for all non-profit programs, the program management, the riding program group and the riding session group. Each of these groups has different tasks to perform and requires different styles of leadership. They must interrelate and work together. Mary, the psychiatric occupational therapist, needs the three Haflingers for her group therapy with three hyperactive teenagers. If the riding instructor does not cooperate with Mary's timing of her therapy session and takes two of the horses for her lessons, Mary can not carry out her session. Mary needs these horses because of their low-keyed temperament, their size and their smooth gait.

Other influencing groups may be:

- The **board of directors** whose main purpose is to secure and control funds, set and carry out policy, and promote the health of the organization. Within the board group, group process is very active and its health can be determined by the fulfillment of the group process. To the organization, its purpose is administrative, and therefore, collectively has an **authoritarian leader** role.

- The **program management group** whose main purpose is to carry out the administrative functions of a program. This role may be held by the head instructor or may be a coordinator in a large program. Tasks could involve scheduling, securing appropriate forms, ordering supplies and paying bills. These are administrative tasks and the leadership is **authoritarian.**

- The **riding program group** that involves all the people that work with the riders and teaching staff and volunteers. The main purpose of this group is to promote growth in both students/clients and staff/volunteers. The task of this group is dynamic and requires **dynamic leadership**. The healthier the group process, the more productive and cohesive the group will be.

Why Some Groups Succeed and Others Fail

In order for a group to succeed it must (Hall, 1961):
1. Have stated goals with changing objectives to continue the group's purpose.
2. Have leadership.
3. Have maintained the group process.

Groups fail when (Hall, 1961):
1. The group is composed of the wrong combination of people.
2. The organizers have a faulty purpose.
3. The atmosphere does not promote organizational growth.
4. The members lack skills in playing the necessary group roles.

For instance there are five members of a group intending to develop a summer camp program. Two members have dominant personalities and determined to be the leader of the group. The group may be overshadowed with the leadership battle and other group skills are not workable not will the goal of the group be reached.

5. All persons are not included in the group, causing subgroups.

Four members of this group are personal friends and the other three members are new to the area and do not know each other. The four friends marginally include the new members so that the group is not a cohesive working group. All members are not involved in the group process and decision making.

How a group functions depends a great deal on its purpose and the type of leadership.

Tammy, a young occupational therapist in her first job, wanted to run a summer sensory integration group. She is well trained in sensory integration skills and feels confident in her ability to do group treatment. Five children ages seven to nine years sign up for the group. The first three sessions went very well. After the fourth group session, Tammy is in tears. "I can not get the children to listen or work together in any activity. They are just out of control." What has happened - the children have made their own group but have not included the therapist. Tammy did not have the leadership skills to keep the group process going and to maintain control. Since one or two the children could sense this, they took over, leaving Tammy out. The children had no goal or direction so the activities got out of hand.

Basic Leadership Styles
1. An **authoritarian leader** directs his or her group with little input from its members. This leader takes his or her task and establishes goals and expectations according to his or her perception. If his or her **leadership** skills are more like a dictator, members will be expected to do as they are told. He or she does not want to give others too much responsibility for fear of losing control of the group. This leader is power-driven and has little if any concern for the members, or in the case of a therapeutic riding program, the rider participants and families. Members gain little satisfaction and volunteers do not remain with this type of a group very long. Authoritarian leadership is appropriate to administrative roles but poor for "leading people."

2. A **laissez faire leader** guides his or her group in such a way as to maintain an equilibrium, avoiding problems with the group and his or her superior at the possible expense of the group goals or its members. A small therapeutic riding program with few changes would suit him or her the best. Whether or not the riders were gaining from the program would probably be of little concern. His or her focus is on a social and happy environment with no pressures.

3. A **democratic leader** is group oriented and involves the members in decision making and goal setting. This leader is as concerned with satisfying the needs of the group members as he is with reaching objectives. The instructor, leader, sidewalker team should be a democratic group with the instructor maintaining the leadership role but involving each member of the team in a fully participatory role with equal responsibility to the rider.

4. A **dynamic group** (shared leadership) is a participatory group in which members share in the problem solving process and **share leadership responsibilities**. The leadership role can actually emerge from within the group even when a person initially pulls the group together, or it may be shared by two or more people. The leadership role includes the facilitation of the group process as the group fulfills its purpose. A dynamic group has two major functions. One function is to focus on its major purpose and goals. The second function is to develop group objectives and deal with the group maintenance roles. In a dynamic group, people are willing to listen, understand, consider the merit of a statement from other members, and draw a conclusion based on its evidence. The group thrives from members' different viewpoints. The group members and the group tasks are of equal importance.

Successful leadership is dictated by the group, for one cannot lead if members refuse to follow. The authoritarian and laissez faire groups are not as original or efficient in their work as democratic or dynamic groups. The latter groups will have less deviant members, role conflict, or search for sub-leadership. The democratic and dynamic groups put their energy into meeting objectives and group needs. Members are cohesive, gain a feeling of fulfillment and feel responsible for the group productivity. They have an investment in the life of the group, provide support and rewards for each other, and therefore prevent "burn out."

A group needs to understand its purpose, focus on its overall goals, and set objectives. It needs to recognize its unhealthy elements, clear them up, and move on toward becoming a healthier group. Members need to develop trust in each person in the process. The group process is a movement which passes through various phases. As long as the process moves forward toward its objectives and develops new objectives as old ones are met, the group will become stronger and develop into a mature functional group. A mature group is a self-directing, self-controlling body in which *every member* carries his part of the responsibility for developing and executing the group's plan. (Hall, 1961)."

Your program's group is mature if:
1. Its leader fosters growth of all participants.
2. There is intelligent management of its environment
3. It understands the group process and has the ability to make appropriate adjustments.
4. It is skilled at problem-solving.
5. It has full quality participation of its members.

Since therapeutic riding programs have several types of groups who interrelate at different levels, it is important that each group is clear about its purpose and goals. If they overlap in purpose and in control, they can not establish realistic and obtainable objectives and maintain a growth-oriented environment. For example, the lesson group selects teaching methods, matches riders with horses, determines training needs and decides on volunteer and staff tasks. The board of directors sets budgets, selects the program director, makes policies and directs fund raising. Some people may be members of more than one of these groups. When one group interferes with the other's roles and objectives, the group growth process breaks down, for the internal control of the group is lost.

Task-Oriented Team Building Groups
The advantages of a functional group are (Rogers, 1970):
- To create an open problem-solving climate.
- To increase the knowledge and competence of the people in authority roles.
- To build trust among all members.
- To recognize achievement and acknowledge it.
- To increase the sense of "ownership" of the group project.
- To help manage the project toward relevant objectives rather than "historical" practice.
- To increase self-control and self-direction of each group member.
- To increase success of the group.
- To increase the joy of working together toward a common goal.

The Group Process: Its Importance
When people get together for the purpose of accomplishing something, they need to become acquainted, to "feel each other out. As people within the group test each other, and explore their feelings and attitudes toward each other, their facades begin to disappear. Trust increases and the "real" person begins to emerge. At this point one begins to gain a true sense of communication. People may wall themselves off initially, showing their "public self". They may feel their *real self* may not be as acceptable because they do not want to get too involved. They may have had difficulty in the past with relationships and thus avoid new ones. Some people will leave the group rather than get *involved* or show *themselves*. As group members become more open they find that their *real self* is more accepted by others and a sense of trust and warmth builds for each member with open communication. Open communication increases group cohesiveness which in turn develops group pride.

During the process of forward movement of the group, there will be times that specific issues regarding each member must be dealt with while still maintaining a focus on group objectives. The group will also establish its own specific goals even though the overall goal of therapeutic riding will be maintained. Each group needs to have the ability to plan for and develop growth. A board of directors which interjects their own ideas or special controls into the program group may squelch the whole group process and set up a "fight or flight" process.

Group cohesiveness depends on the willingness of each member to play his or her role or roles in such a way as to foster the success of **others** (Kemp, 1970). The group develops through building and maintaining roles. These roles must be carried out by a group member. Many times one person will take on numerous roles. Group members will take on these roles as the group develops.

Group roles include:

1. Initiator--contributor
2. Information seeker
3. Opinion seeker--encourager
4. Information giver
5. Opinion giver
6. Elaborator
7. Coordinator--compromiser
8. Orientor
9. Evaluator--critic
10. Energizer
11. Procedural technician
12. Recorder
13. Harmonizer
14. Standards and limit setter

Negative behaviors in groups include:

- Splitting the group by developing opposing methods or not including all members.
- General disagreement.
- Absence of real leadership or a leader who is less skilled than the group members.
- Lack of interest of members, causing their partial or full withdrawal.
- Interpersonal aggressiveness.
- Break-down in overall communication.
- Lack of clear objectives and problem-solving ability.
- Failure to include some members.
- Blocking of the group growth.
- Diverting group direction.
- Focusing attention on self.
- Playboy--diverting attention away from task and group growth.

Therapy groups always begin with a designated leader which is the therapist. Group roles are shared among members and one person may fulfill several roles. Assigned leader is the initiator of the group process and may begin by giving information and seeking opinions. The leader's ability to communicate and reinforce group problem solving and objectives will have a strong influence on the initial success of the group.

Groups need time and patience to develop. This does not distract from the program's function since group growth develops best with a task-oriented focus. The growth of the **group process** is like the growth of any relationship. As it grows, it changes. Change is stressful but necessary for growth. Growth in turn develops strength and a feeling of accomplishment. The process may be stressful at times but its rewards are everlasting--both in the development of meaningful relationships and in the productivity of the group. The clients gain a feeling of bonding with the group and the horse(s). They gain independence and feeling for their group members as they develop skills in the task area and a feeling of accomplishment.

References:

Bonner, H. (1959). *Group Dynamics*. New York: The Ronald Press Co.

Hall, D. M. (1961). *The Dynamics of Group Discussion*. Danville: The Interstate Printers & Publishers, Inc.

Kemp, C. G. (1970). *Perspectives on the Group Process*. Boston: Houghton Mifflin Co. 25-26,36,48,62.

Luft, J. (1970). *Group Processes*. Palo Alto: National Press Books.

Rogers, C. R. (1970). *Carl Rogers On Encounter Groups*. New York: Harper & Row.

Reeves, E. T. *The Dynamics of Group Behavior*. American Management Association.

Walport, G. (1955). *Becoming: Basic Consideration for Psychology of Personality*. New Haven: Yale University Press.

INDIVIDUAL VERSUS GROUP TREATMENTS

Barbara T. Engel M.Ed, OTR

The present environment for treatment has changed drastically in the last forty years. The advancement of medical information, research and data collection plays an ever mor important role in how we treat our clients. In addition to being more knowledgeable in why, what, and how we treat, we are now facing another new dimension. Health care is not necessary under the direction of a physician who might determine the needs of the client but under the direction of 'managed care'. This system many or may not be interested in the best way to rehabilitate the client in his or her best interest. The system may be based on the minimum cost of treatment, that is states for an individual with a given diagnosis for maximum benefits within stated number of visits, or other such criteria.

As therapists we are obligated to treat our client in the best way we know to bring them to a higher level of function. We therefor must look at the most cost effective treatment method that produces best results in a minimal amount of time. A solution to this problem maybe group treatment. Group treatment has advantages and disadvantages to situations. Some clients must obviously be treated on a one on one basis. Others do better in a group.

There has been some discussion that the more skilled would supervise the less skilled to treat their clients. This has already occurred with the use of trained assistants. One therapist could work with two clients during the same period if he or she had well trained assistance to help her. The level of direct help from the therapist would determine the feasibility of this situation.

Group advantages with individuals with physical disabilities (not including time saving for the therapist) includes:
▸ More interesting and social.
▸ Peer pressure can be stimulate achievement.
▸ Clients helping each other.
▸ Clients coping each other.
▸ Increase motivation as a support group.
▸ Client working for self instead of producing for the therapist.
▸ Group treatment may be longer (one & a half hours instead of 50 minutes but cost less then the 50 minutes treatment).

The therapist places the client in a session that is learning to take direction while performing specific riding skills. Should Thomas be in a group class or in a class by himself? There are a number of considerations which need to be made regarding the best environment for the client and the program's ability to meet Thomas's needs. There are positive and negative considerations for both individual and group sessions. Individuals in groups affect each other in positive and negative ways. One must also remember that equine-assisted therapy is always a "group" experience. The group is always the rider-horse-instructor/therapist, the rider-horse-leader, the rider-leader-sidewalker(s)-instructor. To this core group can be added more assistants and then more horses, riders and helpers. This can produce an overwhelming amount of activity to some people. For persons who have difficulty attending, who are hypersensitive to noise or movement, or who have difficulty making their own nervous systems and bodies perform basic skills, groups can distract from the value of gaining the facilitation from riding a horse. Groups also can add to the experience.

Advantages of Group Lessons:

- More economical than individual sessions
- Can accommodate school and association groups
- More efficient use of the therapist's time
- Staff can reduce the hours they work
- Provide a social environment
- Can use the group for peer pressure or stimulation
- Horses like to work together and are less likely to become bored
- Clients can copy or learn from each other
- Clients learn social skills
- Games can be incorporated into the session

Disadvantages of Group Lessons:

- Individual analysis and intervention is limited.
- Needs may be overlooked.
- Fewer choices of horses.
- Clients are given stimulation from all the other clients--may overwhelm them.
- May be difficult to understand instructions in group setting.
- Independent riding may be less because or more horses are in the arena.
- Less independent thinking and riding skills - all clients do the same task.
- Communication is more difficult
- Need for a large staff and volunteer group.
- Need for more horses.

Group lessons are not <u>functional</u> <u>working</u> <u>groups</u> (where members interact to problem solve); rather they can be a <u>parallel</u> <u>interaction</u> <u>group</u>--members copy each other or perform a task at the same time. These clients are generally not involved in developing group objectives and maintenance roles. The group meets for shorter periods (the lesson period). The therapist is in control of the group in an authoritarian role in order to carry out his or her treatment plan (authoritarian role is used here -one person leadership). The client may be allowed some decision-making but the therapist will make this determination and set limits.

Any time two or more people get together, even for short periods, dynamics do occur. In a group of children or adults one can observe people who:

- Seek to identify with others.
- Copy others' actions.

◘ Please the leader.
◘ Try to be the best in the group.
◘ Get the most attention
◘ Take over the session
◘ Avoid being noticed.
◘ Refuse to participate in the group.
◘ Disrupt the session.

These acts are the result of social interaction and pressures. All social beings must find their place in the social structure and will react to it in various ways. Peer pressure and group interaction can be used by the leader to foster an individual's progress. One must remember that some people do not tolerate groups well or cannot learn in a group setting.

The therapist in the authority role is able to make his or her clients do only what they are already willing to do (Cumming & Cumming, 1963). But instructors can manipulate *groups* to pressure clients into actions they would otherwise not take. A social person wants to be accepted by his or her peers and will therefore do something to be accepted which he or she would otherwise not do. This manipulation can be carried out through riding exercises and games which make the experience pleasant and, in turn, productive. The Client is not aware of the manipulation and gains a good feeling from a new or improved experience. An example is the use of **Simon Says** with children. They will most often do what the game **Simon Says**, especially when the other children are doing it.

The Need for Individual Sessions
Children or adults who have an attention-deficit disorder, language processing disorder or who have an autistic disorder may need to work on a one-to-one basis in a quiet environment. Stimulation needs to be at a minimum in order for them to focus and attend for even short periods. Children and adults with closed head trauma and attention difficulties also profit from a quiet environment. Learning disabled people who must concentrate very hard on instruction and performance work best on a one-to-one basis or in small groups of two to three people.

Is it helpful to "challenge" a rider with attention deficits, some emotional disorders, language processing disorder, autism or head injury (all have degrees of learning disabilities) to be gradually moved into larger group classes? The answer depends on the **goal** for the rider. If the major purpose of the session is **to integrate sensory-motor and communication processes**; in turn to **increase learning** (understanding of riding skills) and to **develop a true communication with the horse** (execution of riding skills), the answer is "no" since the additional stimulation would distract from the initial goal. The ability to concentrate to a high degree in a stimulating environment for a person with learning disabilities is not possible. This is so for even an adult with relatively good functional skills (able to hold a professional job). On the other hand if the **goal** is to **increase the rider's social skills and tolerance for environment stimuli** then increasing the group size is useful and challenging.

In determining the advantages and disadvantages of individual or group sessions, both on and off the horse, one must consider many factors. What are the rider's most pressing needs? Can these best be carried out in a group or individual setting? Which tasks should be on a group level or on an individual level? What is the best size of the group--two, three, four, six or? Is the therapist skilled as a group leader? Program considerations must also be weighed since time factors and labor are always pressing in a therapeutic riding program.

Cumming, J., Cumming, E. (1963). *Ego & Milieu*. New York: Atherton Press.
Rogers, C. R. (1961). *On Becoming a Person*. Boston: Houghton Mifflin Co.

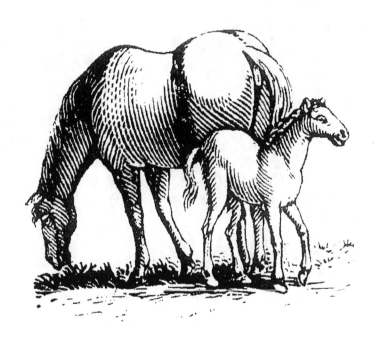

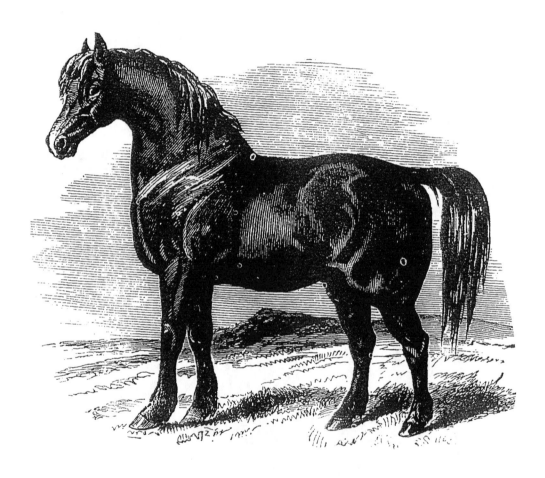

CHAPTER 11

HANDLING THE THERAPY HORSE DURING TREATMENT

MOVING THE HORSE TO INFLUENCE THE RIDER

Marcee Rosenzweig, PT

The horse's movement can be beneficial for a rider; however, it can also be detrimental (Heipertz, 1977). Moving the horse to specifically influence the rider should be supervised and/or performed by a therapist with the knowledge and understanding of the horse's movement and its effect on the rider. However, **everyone** working in the field of riding for the disabled will benefit from understanding which movements are creating the changes one sees in **all** our riders.

The first factor to consider when moving the horse to influence the rider is the quality of the horse's movement. A balanced, symmetrical gait is necessary for the rider to perceive symmetrical movement of his or her own pelvis and trunk. The quality of the horse's movement is also affected by the method in which he is engaged into all movements. When driven on long reins, the horse is allowed to maintain a natural freedom of movement. Long-reining also provides the opportunity for the therapist or instructor to control the horse as if it is being ridden and make any necessary changes in motion without disturbing the rider.

The first component of the rider's movement which can be influenced by the horse's motion is the anterior/posterior pelvic tilt. All riders should begin to ride on long straight lines at the walk with low impulsion. Gradually the impulsion and/or stride length is increased and this stimulates the anterior/posterior pelvic tilt and also trunk control. To further enhance the rider's trunk control, transitions from low impulsion to a higher impulsion combined with the lengthening and shortening of the stride can be performed by the horse. Transitions from walk to halt to walk **will** also improve anterior/posterior trunk control. Walking in straight lines, varying impulsion, varying stride length, and acceleration, elicits a flexor/extensor response of the trunk. **All** upward transitions stimulate a flexor (bending the trunk) dominant response. **All** downward transitions stimulate an extensor dominant (straightening the trunk) response.

The second component of the rider's movement which can be influenced by the horse's motion is lateral (side to side) trunk control. The horse progresses from walking in straight lines to walking in a large circle, serpentine, and figure eights. Movement through these figures produces increased rotation of the horse's pelvis, facilitating the rider's shift in weight and promotes lateral flexion of the trunk. The therapist must be careful to avoid collapse of the trunk instead of active lateral flexion. School figures should be performed in both directions to encourage symmetry.

The third component of the rider's movement, rotation, can be elicited when the horse's trunk moves laterally through the movements of leg yielding and shoulder in. All three components of movement can be influenced simultaneously with the increase and decrease of impulsion, stride length and acceleration while moving through the school figures and lateral movements. Straight lines can be used to connect the movements as a baseline for the rider to return to before attempting more difficult tasks. The therapist or therapist/instructor team must constantly evaluate and re-evaluate the rider's responses to the horse's movement. It is their responsibility to make the necessary changes which will provide a safe and therapeutic program for the rider.

Reference

Glasow, B. (1984). *Hippotherapy: The Horse as a Therapeutic Modality*. New York: Warwick.

Heipertz, W., Heipertz-Hengst, C., Kroger, A, & Kuprian W. (1977). *Therapeutisches Reiten* [Therapeutic Riding]. Stuttgart, Germany: Franckhische Verlagshandlung.

Hippotherapy Curriculum Development Committee. (1991). *Introduction to Hippotherapy - Module C Instructor Resource Book*. Maryland: Riderwood.

Reide, D. (1988). *Physiotherapy on the Horse*. Maryland: Therapeutic Riding Service.

TECHNIQUES OF LONG-REINING DURING HIPPOTHERAPY AND THERAPEUTIC RIDING SESSIONS

Carolyn D. Jagielski, MS, PT

The use of long reins (sometimes called longe lining) is not a new concept. Man has been working the horse from the ground on long reins for centuries and "work in hand" was part of the training methods used by the European schools of equitation. This technique was found to build the horse's muscles and increase suppleness. Long-reining helped to develop a good mouth and good manners and had the added benefit of allowing the trainer to see what was happening. Although ``work in hand" was difficult for even an experienced trainer, the use of the long-reining technique may be modified, and this simplified form may be learned within a few weeks. The purpose of this chapter is to familiarize the reader with the equipment, technique and benefits of long-reining the therapeutic horse.

FITTING THE TACK

Long-reining equipment requires proper fit and should not be "make-shift." The horse should have a snaffle bit and bridle with side-reins adjusted to the same length. Correctly fitted side-reins position the horse's head at least one hand width in front of the vertical. The long reins are approximately 3 meters long and are attached to the bit above the side-reins. For safety, the long reins must **NOT** be joined at the ends. The line will thread through a low ring on the surcingle or through a loop (spur strap) attached to the girth. The reins must not be so long that they drag on the ground (Figure 1).

TECHNIQUE

When tracking to the right, the horse handler walks one step behind and just to the inside of the horse's right hind leg. This location allows the handler a less restricted view but facilitates leg yields without interfering with the horse's legs. During a change of rein, the handler should switch position so that he or she is behind and just to the inside of the other hind leg of the horse. This move requires a shortening of the left rein and a lengthening of the right rein as the long-reiner (horse handler) first steps directly behind and then just to the inside of the horse's left hip. The horse handler must be close enough to the horse's hind quarters to avoid the impact of a kick. The horse's movements are controlled through the use of the long reins, the handler's voice commands and the whip.

As the horse walks forward, the handler must match his or her own stride with the tempo of the horse's stride. This technique decreases the likelihood of interfering with the horse's mouth and allows the handler to time his or her rein aids in synchronization with the horse's movement. The handler must be careful not to drop back a step or two as this position will place him or her in a dangerous situation--the center of the kick zone. A side-aid will walk beside the rider next to the rider's legs. The number of necessary side-aids will depend upon the rider's ability. The rider sits on the horse in the normal position. The long reins pass under his or her lower leg so that the reins are not trapped against the horse's flank.

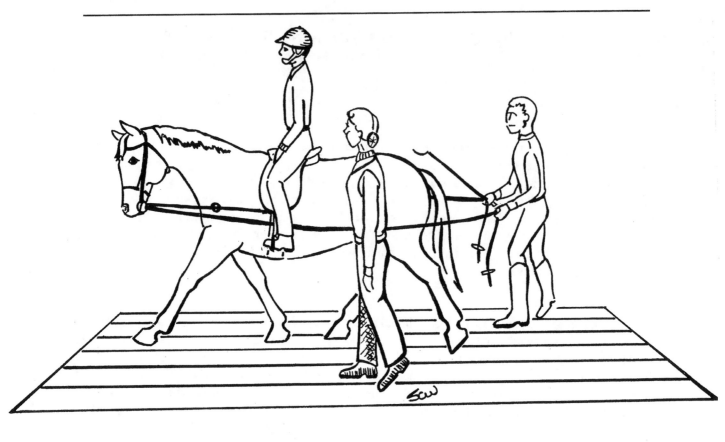

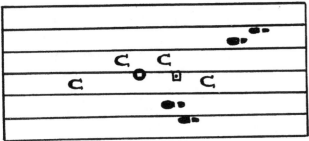

FIGURE 1.

THERAPEUTIC LONG REINING HORSE WITH EQUIPMENT AND POSITION OF THE HANDLER

BENEFITS

Therapeutic long-reining has developed as an alternative to leading the horse. Leading is not always an adequate solution for treating a rider's needs. For example, working the horse on long reins allows the horse to move through a variety of school figures, lateral movements, and rein-backs as well as straight lines and circles in a straight and collected frame. Unlike in traditional leading, the horse does not need to be pulled forward in an attempt to urge it to walk. When long lining, transitions from walk to halt or halt to walk can be done with precision and with immediate response to a therapist's request.

The quality of the horse's movement is improved when long-reins are used. The horse can move from a collected walk to an extended walk when needed and with more impulsion. The horse carries itself in a better frame when it is long-reined than when it is being led by a lead rope or bit lead. When performing a curved figure, bending occurs through the length of the horse with the hind legs following into the steps of the fore legs. This bending promotes better weight shifts and more appropriate equilibrium responses in the rider as his or her body adapts to the horse's bend.

Although used primarily for hippotherapy and equine-assisted therapy, long-reining is an effective tool for the riding instructor in therapeutic riding. Long-reining allows the horse handler to be "invisible" to the rider. The rider feels that he or she alone is in control of the horse. The handler is always present as a back-up should the need arise. The riding instructor may also use long-reining as a way of isolating a task the rider is learning. By having the horse perform a leg yield in long lines, the rider can improve his or her weight shift or coordinate leg aids without needing to concentrate on rein aids.

THE IDEAL HORSE
The horse chosen for long-reining should have a wealth of abilities. As with any therapy horse, temperament is foremost. He must be friendly, trusting, responsive and intelligent. A suitable height is between 14 and 15.3 hands. This height range allows the rider to be guarded adequately by side aids. **The horse must be sound. Asymmetry in the horse's step length will be transmitted to the rider.** If the rider already has a postural asymmetry, an uneven stride could increase his or her difficulties rather than improve them. Good conformation is also a requirement for the long-lining horse. Conformation faults in the horse's legs may predispose the horse to injury or progressive lameness; muscle weakness in the animal's back could develop into a sensitive and painful back or progress to a swayed back. As faults in conformation may negate months of training, the horse should be evaluated carefully for weak body structures.

Lastly, the horse's quality of movement is important. The following abilities are necessary to achieve peak performance:
1. **To move in straight lines with even strides**
2. **To track-up at the walk with the hind foot stepping into or beyond the imprint of the forefoot**
3. **To move symmetrically**
4. **To be able to bend laterally through the length of his body in both directions**

However, **good movement does not come from good conformation alone; the horse also needs good training.**

The horse needs specific prerequisites before long-reining training begins. Training in longeing or therapeutic longeing makes the horse responsive to voice commands and familiar with a longe line and a whip. The horse should accept the bit with flexion at the poll and a yielding of the jaw. Either ground driving or double longeing will acclimate the horse to contact from an outside line and to the feel of the line behind its hind legs. (Some horses never accept this feeling and therefore cannot be used for long reining). Training the therapy horse to long rein is not within the scope of this article. Information on this procedure can be found in detail in the texts listed in the bibliography.

THE RIDING INSTRUCTOR

With most programs, the person most qualified to long rein is the riding instructor. Long-reining the horse requires more horse expertise than leading. Several weeks of practice are required for the horse handler to learn the technique correctly. He or she must know the equipment and the proper way to fit it on the horse. The horse handler needs a good following hand so that he or she does not interfere with the horse's mouth. Other important abilities for the horse handler are to know the horse's gaits and to have experience working with long reins.

Since the therapeutic riding instructor is knowledgeable about horses and client disabilities, he or she is a good liaison between the physical or occupational therapist and the horse. The riding instructor must be familiar with any ground figures or activities the therapist may request.

THE TEAM

The primary benefit of long-reining is that the effectiveness of the entire team is increased. The horse is capable of better movement patterns and more complex figures. The riding instructor has greater control over the horse's collection, impulsion and direction of movement. The therapist can control the horse's activities through the horse handler and thus can influence the rider's responses with greater precision. All of these benefits are provided to the rider when the horse is long-reined.

References

Heipertz, W., et al. (1981). *Therapeutic Riding*. translated by Marion Takeukchi. Available from Canadian Equestrian Federation, 1600 James Anismith Drive, Gloucester, Ontario, Canada KlG 5M4.

National Hippotherapy Development Project.(1990). *The Horse as a Facilitator*-A Workshop in Hippotherapy.(1990). Warwick,NY.

Stanier, S. (1972). *The Art of Long Reining*. J. A. Allen and Company Limited. London, England.

LEADING THE HORSE TO MAINTAIN SELF-CARRIAGE

Barbara T. Engel, M.Ed., OTR

The rhythmic movement of the horse and its influence on the rider is a major factor in the value of hippotherapy and therapeutic horseback riding (Heipertz, 1981; Riede, 1988; and others). Physical and occupational therapists study hippotherapy theory to understand the horse's movement and how it can be enhanced to affect the client to achieve specific changes in function. Heipertz, Reide and Strauss have found that the gait of a 15 to 16 hand horse is very similar to the gait of the adult human transferring 110 impulses per minute to the rider's pelvic and spinal region. This movement pattern influences the human adult's walking gait. A good rider knows that the rhythm of the horse must match his or her rhythm to gain the feeling of *going with the horse or being one with the horse.*

There is a need for the horse to be trained to be in self-carriage to accommodate the dynamic weight of a rider. (Self-Carriage-The relationship of the hooves of the horse to the mass of his body providing the horse with stability (Swift, 1985) to adjust his balance to accommodate a rider astride. See definitions, pp 53-60.) This remains true whether the horse is ridden, driven, or lead with rider astride. One, therefore, leads a horse with a rider astride somewhat differently then leading him from his stall to the tack-up area. The normal method of leading a horse out of his stall is to walk next to the horse at his shoulder or behind the head. If the horse is well trained he will walk with you at your pace, turn as you turn and stop when you stop without a tug on the leadline. This is a safe way to lead a horse since one can observe the horse and allow him to move forward freely. He will most likely tend to overload his forehand since this is where most of his weight is. The horse need not adjust his balance to carry the extra weight of the rider since there is no rider astride.

If a person astride a horse is a rider and not just a passenger, he or she will drive the horse forward from behind with pulsing pressure of his or her legs and using the pressure of a deep seat. This allows the impulsion to come from the hindquarters, the driving force of the horse's motion. When leading a horse from the ground with a rider astride the horse leader can apply the same principles. Drive the horse forward encouraging engagement of the hindquarters by asking him to come from behind using the hand or whip as the leg aid. A horse whose hindquarters and hocks have been strengthened enough to allow him to balance the rider's weight will generally assume a frame of self-carriage naturally. The horse leader must then be careful not to encourage the horse to fall on his forehand by tugging on his bit/head.

An effective method of leading a horse is using a longe line and whip (the longe line as the rein--the whip as the inside leg.) The longe line is passed through the near bit ring, over the poll and snapped to the far bit ring as in longeing but the line remains short, three to five feet from the bit. The leader drives the horse forward by walk a few feet from the horse and by or behind the rider's leg using the line as a rein and the whip as a leg. In this position one can observe both horse and rider, yet maintain full control of the horse and encourage a rhythmic forward gait in self-carriage (Figure 2). This position can be used effectively when working as both leader-therapist for a rider who needs minimal help but may need to have the security of having someone controlling the horse.

There is an art to leading a horse safely. It requires undivided attention. If a horse is lead in the traditional manner during a therapy session it must be well-trained and attend to the leader in the same manner that it attends to a good rider. The horse becomes aware and responds to the leader's body language and voice aids. The lead line is used with the same lightness as one would use the reins. The horse should be led from the shoulder (Figure 1). The leadline needs to be long enough so that it does not restrict the function of the head and neck or restrict the forward motion. A well-trained horse does not have to be pulled or tugged to move or halt - rather the leadline is there **only** as a safety measure. The leader and horse should work together until effective communication and a working relationship is established. Horses are not always secure with someone they do not know or trust.

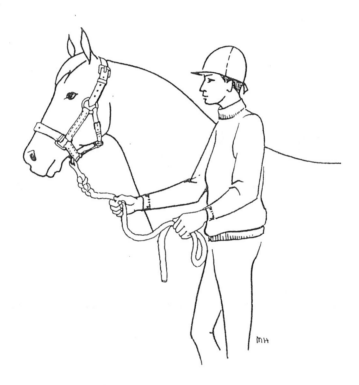

POSITION OF THE LEADER TO THE HORSE

Figure 1.

The horse and leader should be able to lengthen and shorten strides as needed. It is important when trotting the horse with a rider astride to synchronize the leader and horse's movements with that of the rider. If the leader moves the horse forward without this consideration, the rider will no doubt bounce and feel out of control, gaining little from the experience. Leading the horse from the front should never be done. Not only is this an unsafe practice (since the leader cannot communicate or read the horse's communication), but it totally destroys the horse's stride and forward motion.

AN ALTERNATIVE LEADING POSITION

Figure 2.

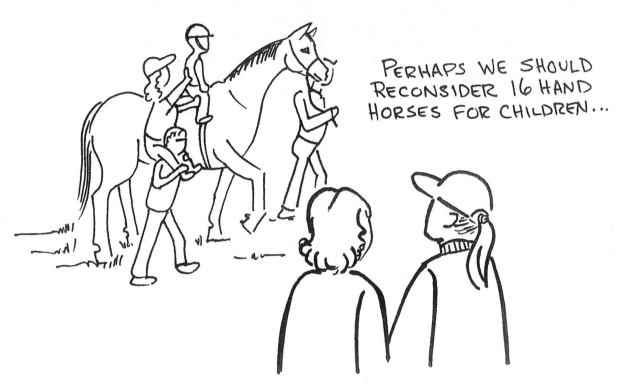

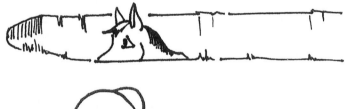

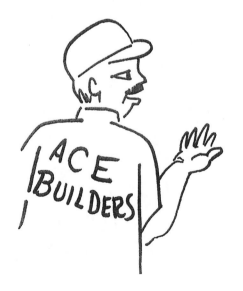

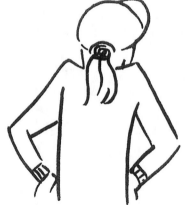

CHAPTER 12

MOUNTING THE CLIENT ASTRIDE A HORSE

MOUNTING METHODS FOR THERAPISTS

Joann Benjamin, PT

The process of getting a client on and off the horse, mounting and dismounting, is an essential part of the hippotherapy treatment. Careful consideration should be made in several areas in order to make this event safe and therapeutic.

Safety is the most important consideration when mounting and dismounting the horse, as this is the most dangerous part of the hippotherapy treatment. First, the process consists of moving a client from a stable surface, such as a platform, ramp or the ground, to an unstable surface, the horse. Every precaution should be taken to avoid movement by the horse. This is achieved by a stationing a person, sometimes called a header, on the ground in front of the horse, holding onto the horse's head by a lead rope or reins. The header must stay in the horse's limited field of vision; the horse has a blind spot directly in front of him. The header does this by standing slightly to one side yet still in front of the horse. The header must avoid pulling on the lead rope as this could accidentally give the horse a cue to move or cause the horse to throw his head.

Second, the process of mounting is hazardous when using a ramp or platform because of the potential of falling from the raised surface; falling directly to the ground, or worse, getting caught between the horse and the raised surface. Specific ramp or platform guidelines must be followed to minimize the hazard of falls. The therapist should be familiar with the safest designs of this equipment (see Therapeutic Riding Volume I) and with the periodic evaluation of its condition.

Third, the dynamics of the mounting process pose a risk because the client is moving onto an uneven surface. The contours of the horse's back or the saddle are stable when the client is centered, yet unstable in the process of moving onto it. There will be a moment during the mount in which the client is unstable and at risk of losing his or her balance.

The dismounting process is also risky. Gravity causes momentum to be gained and a client dismounting to the ground may end up with greater impact than is safe for him. Also, an uncontrolled dismount to the ground could result in the client falling underneath the horse.

Safety is always the primary consideration when planning and executing the mount or dismount with the horse. These few minutes of mounting and dismounting can make or break the hippotherapy treatment session.

When mounting and dismounting in the therapeutic setting, it is important to use the safest procedure available while also maximizing the client's independence and control. If, for instance, a client can be safely assisted in mounting the horse from a platform using a pivot transfer with minimal assistance, this sequence may be preferable to using a lift from the ground. This client would be practicing a transfer which is functional for on and off the horse.

The type of mount or dismount should be chosen with consideration of the effects it may have on the client. The mount is part of the treatment and will set the stage for the hippotherapy session. The dismount will determine whether the client will leave the arena with the therapeutic benefits to the hippotherapy session. A transfer which is extremely difficult can increase the client's muscle tonus significantly. Ideally, the mount or dismount should be as effortless for the client as possible while still promoting independence. Therapists should consider potential fears and anxieties when doing the mount or dismount. If the client becomes fearful, the hippotherapy session will be adversely affected.

How the therapist handles the client during the mount or dismount is just as important in hippotherapy as in any therapeutic session. The therapist should anticipate changes in the client's muscle tonus, motor control, and sensation when choosing how to perform a particular mount or dismount. The therapist needs to ensure that the staff assisting the mount or dismount is proficient in handling the client. Training may need to be done on handling skills, transfer techniques and body mechanics.

Consider staff safety when choosing a mounting or dismounting technique. The staff must be able to safely manage the client for the client's safety as well as their own safety. Re-balancing a client who may lose balance while mounting takes much more strength then in the clinic. A particularly heavy client or one who is difficult to move due to poor motor control will necessitate more work by the staff. Be judicious in the type of mount used. Consider assistive devices, use of the ramp or other means to make the mount easier and safer for all involved.

Mounting and dismounting can be difficult for the horse for several reasons. Consider the amount of time needed to complete a mount or dismount for a client. The more time standing, the more likely the horse will become impatient with the mounting procedure. Also, consider the physical strain on the horse's body. Mounting and dismounting from the same side all of the time may cause undue stress on the horse asymmetrically. Mounting a horse from the ground, even with a very agile rider, causes strain on the horse's back from the downward and sidewards pull. Frequent repetitions of this type of mount can cause the horse back problems. An uncontrolled mount from a platform or tall ramp may cause a significant pressure on the horse's back due to the downward forces. The client must come down upon the horse is a gentle and controlled manner. Be humane in your evaluation of the mount and dismount that you use. Remember that this horse may be subject to many mounts and dismounts in the course of a day. Consider his overall workload and not just the mounting or dismounting procedure for a single client. Use devices such as a step or ramp if these will alleviate some of the strain usually encountered in the mounting process.

There are many mechanical lifts available for mounting and dismounting the client who is very large or who has significant physical disability. Some considerations when using these lifts are:
- ▸ Is the device reliable?
- ▸ Is the horse, and are the staff, extremely comfortable being around the lift?
  Is the staff able to safely assist this client during the hippotherapy session on the horse considering size? disability?
- ▸ Is there a safe way to abort a mount or a dismount if something should happen

AT ANY TIME during the mounting or dismounting process?
- Is the staff capable of handling this client in an emergency dismount without the device?
- Is this method the best option to help the client achieve therapeutic goals?
- Is the client able to gain total or more independence with this lift?

More centers are using mechanical lifts to decrease the strain that mounting and dismounting takes on the horses and staff. Mechanical lifts should be thoroughly evaluated. Therapists need to be able to satisfactorily answer all of the above questions and possibly using the lift his or her self before using a lift with a client.

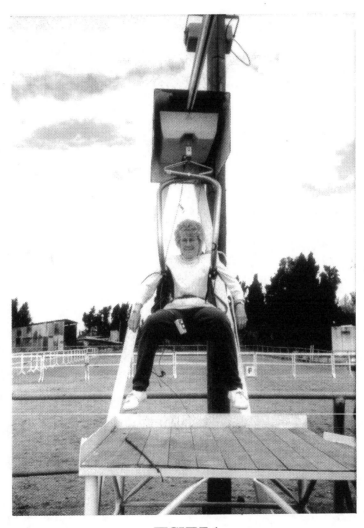

FIGURE 1.

A MECHANICAL LIFT USED INDEPENDENTLY BY RIDER (switch to maneuver the lift lays on riders leg-lift is the Handi-Move.)

During the hippotherapy session, the therapist is ultimately responsible for everything the client encounters. The therapist must be intimately familiar with the mounting and dismounting process in order to choose the procedure which is safest for the horse, client and helpers:

▸ Which is the most therapeutic for the client regarding the client's goals in the hippotherapy session

▸ Which is most humane for the horse.

The therapist should consult with the horse expert to ensure that all aspects of the process are considered. The therapist can then be assured that the hippotherapy session will start off and end in the safest and most enjoyable way for all involved.

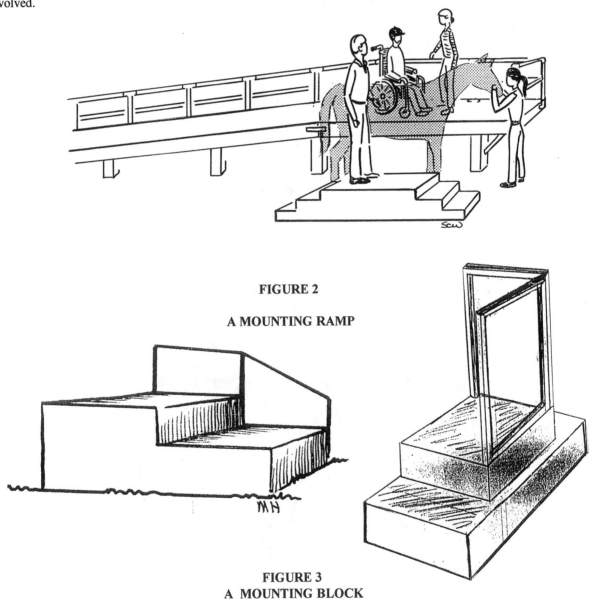

FIGURE 2

A MOUNTING RAMP

FIGURE 3
A MOUNTING BLOCK

For additional information on mounting procedures, please refer to the *Therapeutic Riding I Strategies for Instruction..*

CHAPTER 13

IMPROVING THE CLIENT'S POSTURE

FROM EXTERNAL TO INTERNAL POSTURE

Susanna von Dietze, PT

INTRODUCTION

I WOULD LIKE YOU TO LOOK at this picture; I brought it back with me from a visit to Australia and New Zealand ten years ago. It fascinated me, how different and strange such a common picture as the map of the world could look when it is put upside down. Nothing is wrong on this map; every country stayed in its place and remained as big as in the 'normal' map. Still, to me it looked like a complete new world, and of course the Australians and the New Zealanders liked to place Europe "down under" on the right end of the map.

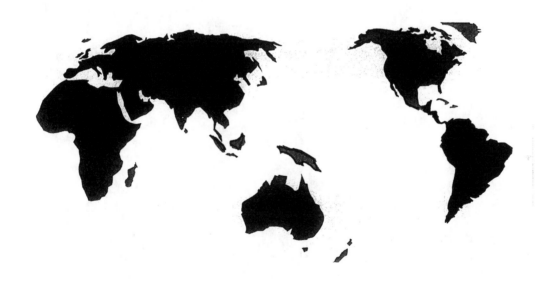

FIGURE 1.

What happened was that looking on a common picture from a different angle showed me new ways to look at the world. The main stress lies suddenly not on Europe but on Australia and New Zealand. I brought it as a poster and it is hanging in my flat, reminding me that I want to try to keep looking at the world from more than one direction.

Observing things from various angles shows deeper sense, comes closer to truth, and helps to understand various positions. I want to look at riding not only from the point of riding but also from the view of physiology and psychology to find connections and links between.

LIFE IS MOVEMENT
a) Physiology
Life is movement! The truth of this statement becomes more and more obvious to me during my physiotherapy training and my work with patients who lack movement or mobility. The way someone moves is always his or her own individual style. It depends on his or her body's own individual structure, his or her constitution, his or her training, and his or her whole personality. As long as we live there is movement. Even in sleep, breathing, heartbeat, and blood flow are movements.

When you say a person is standing still, it is not true. It just appears as if there were no movement because the movements are so tiny that they cannot be seen. You can feel it when you stand up and shut your eyes. You can feel how much you move over your feet and how different muscles have to work and relax again to support your balance. This is very important.

I want to talk about movement and posture. Posture is movement. It can be so small, you can hardly see it. Because posture is movement, you can easily change from posture to movement and back again. Someone's posture can already tell you a lot about his or her movement because it is part of his or her movement. The way someone sits and stands is equivalent to the way he or she moves and walks. In walking, all the muscles and joints have to coordinate in an optimal way. This is the reason many therapy techniques like PNF, Voita, and Bobath, concentrate on analyzing and correcting the way of walking.

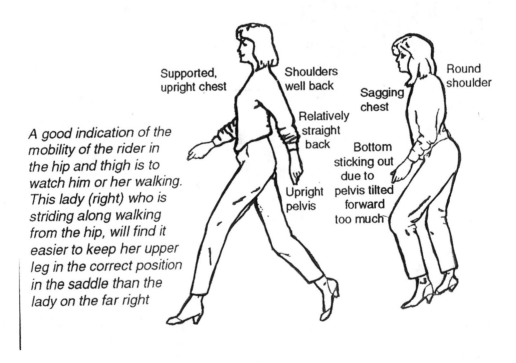

A good indication of the mobility of the rider in the hip and thigh is to watch him or her walking. This lady (right) who is striding along walking from the hip, will find it easier to keep her upper leg in the correct position in the saddle than the lady on the far right

Supported, upright chest

Shoulders well back

Relatively straight back

Upright pelvis

Round shoulder

Sagging chest

Bottom sticking out due to pelvis tilted forward too much

FIGURE 2

162

If you want to analyze a movement, you have to know how a movement is developed and how it can be learned and trained. How does movement develop and how is a precise movement learned?

Children learn movement more easily than adults. It is because of a special function of the brain that children can learn a whole sequence of movements as a whole complete term; whereas adults have to gain the same movement step by step. Adults have to combine movements that they already know until they are able to achieve the new movement. This is a longer but not impossible process.

Learning a movement always follows three basic criteria:
1. First movement then posture.
   A child learning to crawl will start rocking on hands and knees before it will be able to keep the position that appears to be still. Walking is easier than standing.
2. From the truck to the extremities.
   The development begins from head to feet, from the trunk to the extremities. First they learn to rest on the shoulders, then on the elbows, then on the hands and then they learn to use their fingers.
3. From a big rough movement, to a fine precise movement.
   A refined or precise movement is found only by staggering or swaying from one side to another until the center balance of the movement is found. This balanced movement appears easy and smooth. Trying to start to learn the refined movement right away will always end in a stiff unharmonized motion.

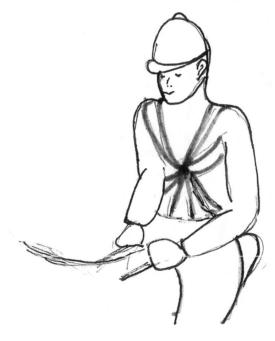

FIGURE 3

b) Psychology

Everything I have said above about movement is linked closely to mental development. Because I am not a trained psychologist I do not want to go into deep theories, but I would like to describe some examples out of everyday life.

A child learning to talk will do so in combination with movement. They run around and speak in funny but not always understandable words, listening to the sound and the rhythm. Their own rhythm of movement helps them to keep on talking.
And very often one will find the same thing when learning a poem by heart. It is helpful to recite by walking or at least by moving your head or hands in the rhythm to the poem. If you stop moving you are often not able to continue.

In many words the link between mind and movement can be shown plainly. One can talk about a flexible minds, versatility, balanced people... you jump out of joy or you crouch down when you are sad....
Your state of mind influences your movements and your movements influence your mind. It works both ways.

In learning a movement, the state of mind can be of enormous importance. Being afraid or under stress will provoke automatic reactions and one will not be able to keep suppleness which is of essential virtue for many tasks.

And if you talk about someone having a stable mind, it is only seemingly stable; it is not fixed it is balanced in the way posture is developed by balancing movements of different extremes. Balancing in different ways can lead to a stable mind, but a stable minds is always able to move, to react, and to change when necessary.

Mental development, just like physical development is never ending. You are a learner for your entire life.

c) Riding

Riding is movement with the horse. A rider is always in movement with the horse. Two movements, horse and rider, harmonize in a way that it seems to be one. This harmony explains why even non-horsy people can

FIGURE 4

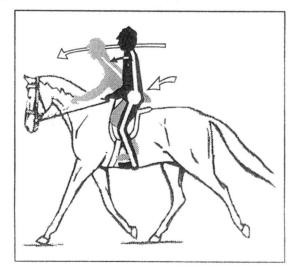

distinguish between a good and a poor rider, because of the harmony of movement. When the harmony is disturbed you can see the movement on the horse and you can see the physical strength it costs the rider to work the horse. Good riding always appears smooth and easy, not showing the real effort.

Knowing that riding is movement, I want to talk deeper about the rider's seat, how it is learned, and what other achievements, other than good riding can be obtained.

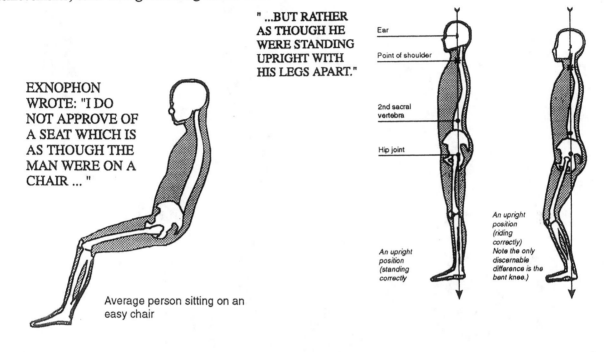

" ...BUT RATHER AS THOUGH HE WERE STANDING UPRIGHT WITH HIS LEGS APART."

EXNOPHON WROTE: "I DO NOT APPROVE OF A SEAT WHICH IS AS THOUGH THE MAN WERE ON A CHAIR ... "

Average person sitting on an easy chair

Ear
Point of shoulder
2nd sacral vertebra
Hip joint

An upright position (standing correctly

An upright position (riding correctly) Note the only discernable difference is the bent knee.)

FIGURE 5   FIGURE 6

RIDING

1) The Seat

The rider's seat is inseparable from the idea of movement. One does not need to be a rider to know that a rigid body on top of a moving, bouncing body will be banged and jarred unless there is a mechanism which can give elasticity. This is the hip joint of a rider.

The basis of your seat is the pelvis on which the rider has to balance his or her upper body. The relaxed hanging leg can help to support balance. You can compare it to a bicycle artist on a rope.

Riding can be compared more to standing and walking than to sitting on a chair. In fact it is similar to walking as we use it in hippotherapy.

The pelvic position has an important influence on the whole body. Without a correct pelvic position, a correct posture is impossible. You cannot correct chest or shoulders when the pelvis is tilted the wrong way.

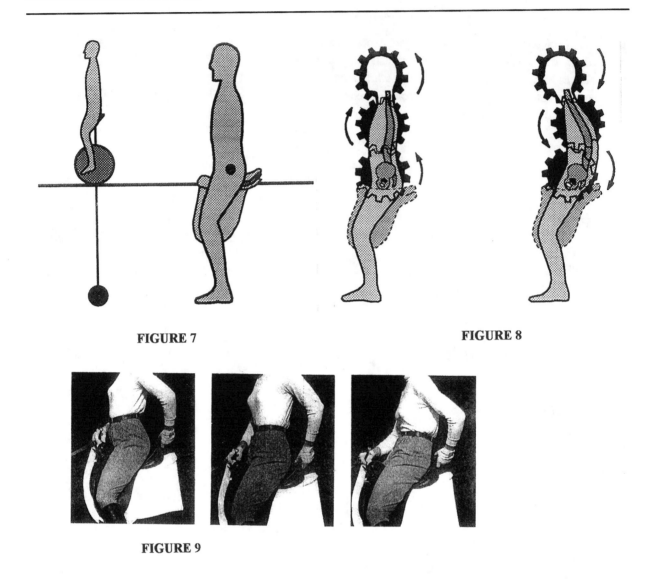

FIGURE 7

FIGURE 8

FIGURE 9

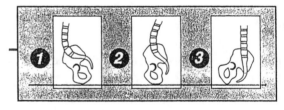

FIGURE 10

In riding the pelvic position has an important influence on the whole seat, the leg position and the upper body. As you can see in the picture, the main seat faults can be caused by an incorrect pelvic position.

You can see that the curve of the spine can be influenced by the pelvic positions as well. For riding you want a normal upright spine which needs an upright pelvis. The normal S-shaped curve of the spine gives all small joints freedom to move. No joint will be in a locked position, so the movements of the horse can be absorbed economically; there is no stress on any one point.

The last part of the chain of joints is the head. You can compare it to a ball being batted on the top of a flexible stick. The head can be quite heavy (depending upon how much is inside) and just looking down can disturb the whole balance enormously.

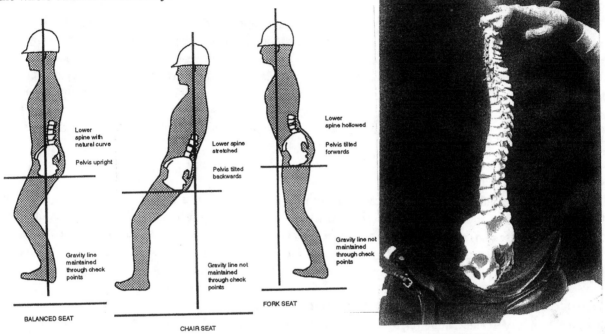

FIGURE 11

Lower spine with natural curve

Pelvis upright

Gravity line maintained through check points

BALANCED SEAT

Lower spine stretched

Pelvis tilted backwards

Gravity line not maintained through check points

CHAIR SEAT

Lower spine hollowed

Pelvis tilted forwards

Gravity line not maintained through check points

FORK SEAT

FIGURE 11

FIGURE 12

The eyes are linked closely to movement. They can initiate movements. If you start looking to your left your whole body will follow turning left. In riding, when you look down you encourage your whole body to bend down, but at the same time you try to sit upright. These two inharmonious movements meet in a joint which has to cope with that stress and mainly it gets stiff.

The tummy and back muscles will work automatically and help to maintain balance. Only in the upright position can the diaphragm work efficiently. And good breathing is of essential value for good relaxed movements.

In physiotherapy we talk about a dynamic stabilization of the spine. This is a good and stable posture, which is supported by good muscular control. Everything is balanced, no joints are stiff, different groups of muscles (agonist and antagonist or flexors and extensors) work together and no single muscle works on its own. The whole body should be balanced and in harmony with itself.

LEANING TO RIDE

When you watch someone learn to ride, you can immediately start noticing faults. It is important, especially for instructors, not to regard a beginner as a mixture of different faults, but as someone being capable of achieving and with encouragement working on a method of progression best for that particular rider. One must also be aware that the talent displayed may fall short of an ambitious dream. I want to show the main steps which you have to follow in learning to ride. These are balance, suppleness, giiving aids/influencing the horse, feeling or being aware, and reaction.

BALANCE

The first thing you have to do on horseback is balance. To sit upright and square on the horse's back and to stay with its movements in every gear is of great importance for all riding disciplines. Riding can be compared more to standing and walking then to sitting on a chair. The basis of your seat is the pelvis on which the rider has to balance his or her upper body. The relaxed hanging legs can help to support balance. You might campare this to a bicycle artist on a rope. In fact it is nearly the same as walking as we use in **hippotherapy**. It sounds so easy but in fact most of the faults, even in international standard dressage or show-jumping, are caused by balance problems. Whenever balance is lost, it can only be compensated for with strength which disturbs the harmony of the horse and rider.

SUPPLENESS

Once balance is achieved, the muscles can work economically. Suppleness is a balanced phase in between tension and relaxation in the form of a pulsation which allows momentary relaxation for re-oxygenation. And as the pace increases, so does the workload carried by the agonist and antagonist muscles increase accordingly. In this way the muscles develop unhindered and without undue stress. Likewise, muscles have less tension in walking than in running. It will be the same for riding in walk or in a collected trot.

GIVING AIDS AND INFLUENCING THE HORSE

This will be a very technical undertaking at first. Applying aids is learned as a technique: how to place the leg or how to shorten the reins. At first these aids will be rough until the rider learns to measure out the required dose.

FEELING, AWARENESS AND REACTIONS

A good feeling is called the crown of riding. There is no magic about it and everyone can learn feeling up to a certain degree. A sensitive understanding between horse and rider should and can be trained right from the beginning. The rider will have to learn to listen to his horse. He or she has to be aware of everything concerning his horse and the surroundings to be able to change the severity of his aids to the requested situation.

LEANING TO RIDE - *LEARNING TO LIVE*

As you may have noticed there is a direct comparison; in learning to ride there are many points you need for living as well.

M. Scott Peck wrote in his book;

> "*Balancing is the discipline that gives us flexibility. To be organized and efficient, to live wisely we must daily delay gratification and keep an eye on the future; yet to live joyously we must also possess the capacity, when it is not destructive, to live in the present and act spontaneously.*"

Balancing yourself and your life is the foundation on which your inner suppleness is built. This suppleness is necessary to be able to open one's eye and observe one's self and one's surroundings, to be aware and able to react when it is required. This is the only way you can influence your life or yourself to achieve something and get on in life.

The rider's seat with its healthy upright position demands the same rules as life. The upright sitting rider can become an upright person, i.e. it can mirror one's personality. And put into practice or movement, riding a horse and applying aids to get a certain reaction encourages one to be more aware and to react sensibly in everyday life. This is a very daring task. Many are afraid to trust their own awareness. In riding the rider has to learn to trust the horse, and sometimes this trust in a horse compensates for lack of knowledge or skill.

Whenever you have to cope with a problem in riding, you get taught to solve it by riding forward. Straight forward people, that's what we need! People being upright, aware and reacting forward, daring to trust in their own or the capabilities of others, daring to act, daring to change situations, balancing one's life in a forward attitude with flexibility; and taking the road less traveled can make all the difference!

The whole part of responsibility and discipline the horse teaches his rider. This paper can not discuss all these points, but you could easily carry on drawing lines between riding and living. I do hope that riding instructors become aware of what a wonderful task they have, how much responsibility and capacity they have to help their riders develop, not only in riding.

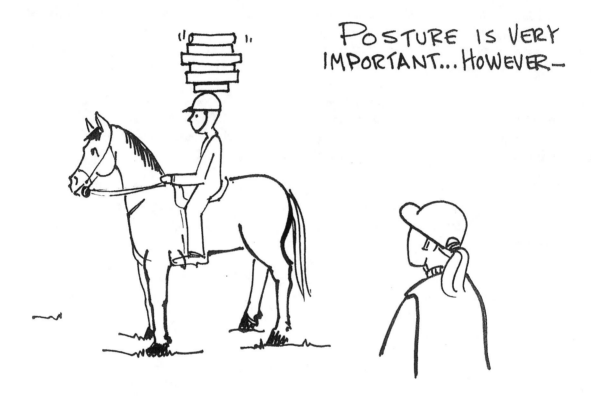

STABILIZING THE RIDER - HANDLING TECHNIQUES TO
IMPROVE THE BASE OF SUPPORT IN SITTING

Jill Strandquist, OTR/L

This article will address methods and assistive handling techniques to be used with the neurologically atypical rider to promote dynamic sitting balance and improve upper body control for more efficient visual-motor (eye-hand) coordination. By activating balance reactions in the pelvis and trunk during assisted riding, dynamic sitting balance is promoted and the upper body, head, and arms are freed for more efficient visual motor activity.

Sitting Balance: Stability vs Rigidity

It is well known that sitting balance is achieved through progressive development of the musculature surrounding the lower trunk and pelvis. In a typical child, gross movements needed for one to stay upright (righting reactions) are replaced eventually with minute muscular adjustments (equilibrium reactions) giving the appearance of a rigid, static position. Such a position, while stable, is not rigid, and the normal child learns to constantly monitor and adapt to kinesthetic, vestibular and proprioceptive stimuli with balance reactions.

Dysfunctional Sitting Balance: The Prospective Rider

Normal children, if challenged, will generally be able to sustain or regain their balance without falling. Atypical children lack the ability to adequately control muscle tone for smooth, dynamic balance in sitting/standing/walking. These prospective riders have achieved sitting through rigidly "bracing" their muscles or by relying on external support. They cannot sustain or regain dynamic balance in unsupported sitting.

The prospective rider with inadequate postural control generally also displays impaired visual regard and tracking, impaired visual-motor coordination and poor attention and/or endurance. Common diagnoses of such children include cerebral palsy, head injury, encephalitis, learning disability, developmental delay, Down syndrome, and neurological impairment.

The Seated Posture, Corrected Base of Support:

Correct sitting alignment and muscular balance can rarely be achieved or sustained in most chairs/wheelchairs due to their inherent design. In the typical chair the seat is flat or curved up on the sides and tilted toward a concave backrest. Thus a slouched, flexed posture (Figure 1) with the pelvis tipped backwards and the trunk rounded forward is nearly unavoidable. With the center of gravity behind the person's base of support and his or her hips/upper thighs close together with no stabilization (a typical sitter will frequently cross his or her legs in an effort to rigidly stabilize the pelvis), the sitter has little opportunity for dynamic sitting balance. Attempts to perform functional eye-hand activities cause further stress and fatigue.

A review of literature (Heipertz, 1977; Reide, 1986) has indicated that the position of a rider astride a horse best promotes correct postural alignment and more evenly activates and strengthens trunk musculature for dynamic balance in sitting (Figure 2). Some innovative chair designs have attempted to improve sitting posture (Scandinavian kneeling or posture chairs and bolster chairs) but cannot provide the 3-D movement of the horse's walk which continuously encourages dynamic sitting balance. The shape of the horse's back and rib cage

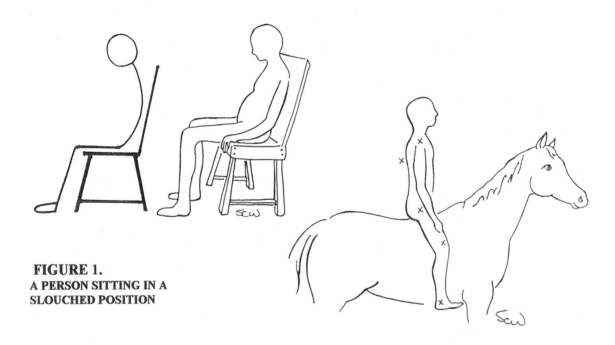

FIGURE 1.
A PERSON SITTING IN A
SLOUCHED POSITION

FIGURE 2.
SITTING ASTRIDE A HORSE

provides a wide, naturally contoured base of support for the pelvic "seat bones" (ischial tuberosities) and improved stability for the very mobile ball-and-socket joint of the hip and upper thigh. With continuously corrected sitting posture through supportive handling, while astride, muscle tension becomes balanced, endurance and strength for independent sitting is improved and stress is reduced to the shoulders, neck and arms for improved visual-motor activities.

For Those Without Stable, Sitting Balance: Handling and Stabilizing Strategies.
Following medical/therapy evaluations to determine whether therapeutic riding is appropriate, a trained occupational and/or physical therapist should determine initial postural goals for the prospective rider. (Riders requiring backriding support will generally lack trunk and head control or be too difficult to support from the side. The backridden rider is always handled by a trained therapist.)

Handling/supporting techniques following *neurodevelopmental treatment* (NDT) principles, for example, enable the rider to modify muscle tone and posture and respond to a weight shift or movement with a righting

Handling/supporting techniques following *neurodevelopmental treatment* (NDT) principles, for example, enable the rider to modify muscle tone and posture and respond to a weight shift or movement with a righting or balance reaction. This author feels that NDT training should be strongly recommended for all therapists involved in riding programs. Therapists should then train their instructors/volunteers in these techniques.

The principles of sensory integration affect a rider's response and progress. Occupational therapists are trained in the processing of sensory information by the brain and its effect on behavioral and motor responses. A basic premise of occupational therapy is that active participation in a functional (meaningful) activity always yields the best progress. Riding on horseback is a functional activity which is usually inherently motivating to the prospective client. During riding, strong vestibular and proprioceptive stimuli are produced by the horse. Active participation of the rider means he or she is actively responding to the vestibular and proprioceptive stimulation with an adapted motor response. It is the job of the therapist/instructor/volunteer to assist the rider as he or she responds to these stimuli with improving adapted responses, through handling and activities, in combination with the horse's movement. Repetitive, non-purposeful or stereotypical motor responses are not active participation as they are not modified (adapted) in response to the stimuli.

Facilitating Change: Helping The Rider To Feel A Stable Base Of Support
The initial goal is to achieve a stable, secure base of support from which the rider can learn to better control his or her trunk and upper body. The base of support for the rider is formed by the shape of the horse's back, the pad, or the saddle chosen for the rider to sit on **and the hands-on support provided by the sidewalkers**. Selection of the horse is critical for the entry level rider. A horse which is too narrow or who has an erratic, weaving walk will not provide a stable base of support. A medium sized horse (14.2 to 15.2 hands) with solid bone structure, good conformation, well muscled, and with a straight, smooth movement and a freely swinging back has proven very successful for the average child or smaller adult. It is easier for sidewalkers to reach the rider if the horse is not too tall but the size of the rider must be considered, and occasionally a taller horse is needed to balance a tall or heavier rider. Usually a natural fleece pad is the first choice for the rider to sit on. The fleece allows direct contact with the horse's back for transmission of stimuli and allows unrestricted positioning of the rider's body. A surcingle/vaulting surcingle secures the fleece and provides rigid hand holds for the very unstable rider. If a saddle is used, it should fit the horse and rider and not interfere with efforts to modify the rider's posture and balance.

Supportive Positioning and Handling To Establish Initial Base of Support:
Position and center the rider on the horse as well as possible after he has mounted and before moving the horse away from the mounting device. The rider should be checked from the side as well as from behind. Have someone check during the riding session to maintain the centered position. Stabilize the rider at key points (Figure 3) before moving off. Once walking, adjust supportive handling until the rider accepts and responds to the motion. It is important not to encourage the rider to brace or hold tightly to the hand holds (handles) of the surcingle as this will block his or her body from responding to the movement stimulation. Encourage the rider to hold lightly and release hands from the hand holds and move them to his or her thighs, as soon as he or she is comfortable. Sidewalkers should provide enough support to secure the rider, and to allow him or her to feel comfortable without the need to hold on tightly or brace his or her body.

The most secure contact given by the sidewalker is made by walking very close to the horse, next to the rider's side and maintaining contact with the rider's leg with both hands. An insecure rider with poor sitting balance will generally respond to secure and appropriate handling by becoming more relaxed.

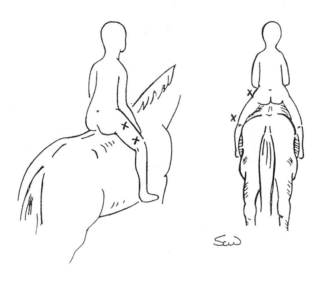

FIGURE 3.

STABILIZING THE RIDER AT KEY POINTS

Facilitating Changes in Muscle Tone and Pelvic/Trunk Alignment

Frequently the movement of the horse alone will accomplish much of the muscle tone adjustment **if** correct supportive handling is provided. Each session should begin with several minutes of supportive riding without requiring challenging efforts, to allow the rider's body time to organize and respond to the stimuli. As the rider begins to accommodate to the movement of the horse during these initial minutes (changes in muscle tone can be observed or felt by a trained person), handling techniques should continue to offer dynamic support (not static holding) while gradually shaping the pelvis and trunk into correct alignment (Figure 1 & Figure 2). Key points of control help to support the rider and diminish the need for rigid bracing. Be careful not to grab or pinch soft tissue with the fingers but rather to use a widely spread hand to deliver support evenly through palm and fingers while grasping the bony "handles" of the pelvis, shoulders, knees, feet, elbows and hands when moving the rider into position.

Facilitating Change: Helping The Rider To Mobilize The Pelvis

The horse must be able to walk with a smooth, free-flowing, rhythmical gait to stimulate the rider's pelvic movement and help him or her to accept the motion without bracing or resistance. The leader must make every effort to lead or drive the horse in a straight path with a consistent pace which stimulates pelvic movement but does not overly challenge the rider and cause increased bracing or tense holding. **It is extremely important when providing supportive handling that the sidewalker follow the movement of the horse with his or her body and hands to allow the rider's body to move in response to the horse's movements.**

Dynamic balance requires a state of constant muscular activity, and supportive handling must be adjusted continually. However, handling which is too rigid will block the rider from responding to the movement and will not encourage the rider to make balancing efforts. Handling which is erratic or not secure enough will not produce the desired changes in the rider's posture or muscle tone.

Facilitating Change in the Stiff Rider:
Poor sitting posture is frequently accompanied by strong muscle tension (particularly in extremities), making it quite difficult to mold a rider into the correct posture. While the most noted postural defect may be the position and/or abnormal muscle tension of the head and neck, arms and hands or legs, poor control of the pelvic and trunk musculature is generally the cause (Figure 4). If after a reasonable time of 5 to 10 minutes, with appropriate supportive handling in upright sitting position, the rider has not "softened" or has become more rigid it will be necessary to modify the movement of the horse, the position of the rider and/or handling techniques. If the rider needs to use his or her arms to stay upright he should do so by leaning on them with hands open rather than hanging onto the handhold or sidewalkers (Figure 5). Weight bearing on hands (or forearms) increases proprioceptive input into the upper trunk, shoulder girdle and neck, and assists to modify tone. Supportive handling may be necessary to stabilize the shoulder and arm during weight bearing.

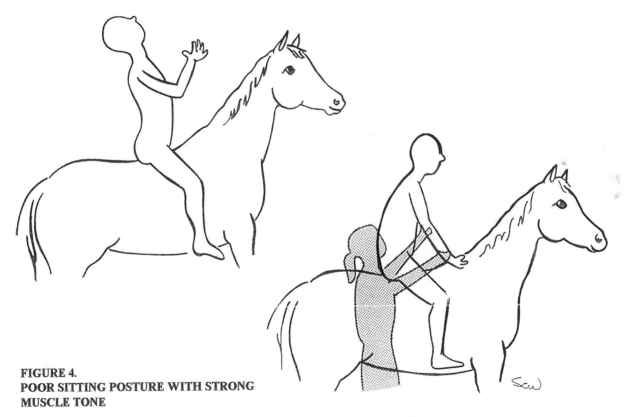

FIGURE 4.
POOR SITTING POSTURE WITH STRONG
MUSCLE TONE

FIGURE 5.
WEIGHT BEARING ON HANDS AND ARMS

It is frequently effective to facilitate increased muscle tone even in a child with stiff extremities because the muscle tone in the trunk is generally inadequate. Once the trunk has become more active, it is generally easier to maintain corrected posture. The improved trunk control will soon allow the tension in the extremities to relax and they can be molded into corrected positions.

Facilitating Change In The Floppy Rider

Some riders will have too much movement and be difficult to hold in position. Their muscle tone seems too weak and they frequently hold onto or collapse onto available support (Figure 6). It is often easier to mold this rider into position but more difficult to keep him there without strong support. It is particularly important to provide graded supportive handling for this rider (gradually increasing or decreasing in response to rider's control) to develop strength and endurance and reduce reliance on external support. Increasing the sensory input of proprioceptive and vestibular stimuli through strong movement of the horse (active walking, trotting, stop and start) and weight bearing (rider leaning on open hands and extended arms rather than holding on to hand hold) is quite effective in increasing muscle tone.

Facilitating Changes In Alignment And Stability of Shoulder Girdle, Neck and Head.

Once the pelvis and lower trunk have been stabilized and are moving with, rather than braced against the horse's walk, it will be easier to help the rider to unblock his shoulders, neck and extremities. He may show rigidly braced postures such as elevated shoulders, head locked in a chin down position, arms tightly flexed against the body or the upper trunk and head. Weight bearing on extended arms and open hands will help to increase

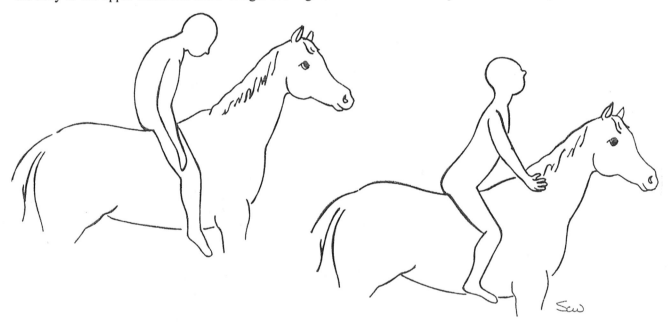

FIGURE 6.
RIDER COLLAPSES ONTO SUPPORT

FIGURE 7.
HANDS SUPPORTED TOO FAR FORWARD

stability in upper trunk, shoulders, and neck. Supportive handling is needed to achieve and maintain corrected alignment. In the forward sitting position, supporting on hands too far to the front will encourage over extension of trunk and neck (Figure 7). Placement of the hands on the thighs encourages more correct alignment, by supporting the rider's arms in extension, (Figure 5) weight bearing is felt in the palm and transmitted to the shoulders, improving muscle tone and head righting. Even a rider with very poor trunk control can be stabilized in this manner and be helped to develop shoulder stability and head control.

Sitting backwards provides a wider base of support for the unstable rider and forearm weight-bearing is a good starting position for those with very poor trunk and shoulder girdle strength (Figure 8). Placement of hands behind the back will encourage trunk extension, chest expansion, neck flexion and opening of the shoulder/arm joints in preparation for reaching (Figure 8). Supporting the rider's upper body is facilitated by stabilizing at the shoulders and elbows, externally rotating the arms to a "thumbs out" position and creating a direct line of weight bearing input from the open hand to the shoulder.

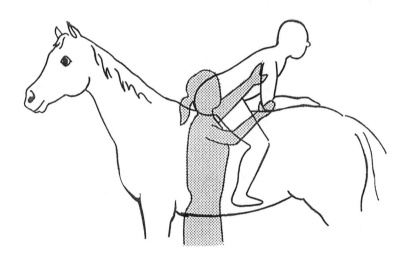

FIGURE 8.
SITTING BACKWARD WITH FOREARM WEIGHT BEARING

As the rider's control increases, supportive handling is withdrawn and returned smoothly, as needed, to guide the rider back into correct alignment. Increasing challenges of quick stops and starts, trotting, changes of direction or lateral work can be introduced to improve balance reactions. Riding time can be increased to promote endurance but not so long that the rider fatigues and again requires maximum support or frequent postural corrections.

With each new challenge it may be necessary to return to more supportive handling temporarily until the rider achieves a greater level of control. When the rider is able to maintain a correct sitting posture (Figure 2) with his or her hands resting lightly on his or her thighs and only intermittent or minimal supportive handling or correction, visually-directed reaching should be introduced.

Facilitating Visually-Directed Reaching/Functional Eye-Hand Activity

Dynamic sitting balance is necessary for efficient visual-motor activities. The arms must be freed from supporting the body, and the head must be able to move independently of the upper trunk for tracking of a moving object, visually-directed reaching, and two-handed manipulations. When the rider is able to maintain a corrected upright posture with only light support on his or her hands and minimal support/facilitation/correction from sidewalkers, it is time to begin freeing the hands from supporting and begin visually directed reaching (Figure 2).

It will usually be necessary to increase supportive handling temporarily when introducing reaching in order to promote correct patterns and maintain good alignment of head and trunk. Initially the rider should be directed/assisted to "unweight" one arm at a time by shifting weight to one arm/hand in preparation for lifting the other arm. With prompting as needed to make and maintain visual contact, the rider should be assisted to reach up, forward, and away from the body toward the target. Generally, forward reaching is easiest while reaching out to the side; crossing the body and overhead are more difficult. Reaching behind may be difficult for those with restricted range of motion but is very effective in encouraging rotation of the head and trunk.

When facilitating reaching, support is given to stabilize the shoulder and extend the arm by pushing from behind the elbow, to guide the arm toward the goal, rather than pulling from the hand or forearm. For a rider who is beginning steering control of the horse as a visually-directed reaching activity, it is extremely important that the arms not be held tightly flexed against the body or turned palm down and brought up against the body. Rather the rider should be assisted (as described above) to move the extended arm away from the body in a thumb-up position (direct reining) for turning and to move the arms backward and down along the sides for halting. Reins should be short enough that it is not necessary to over-flex the arms during steering or halting.

Limited ability to stabilize the lower body while turning the upper body and/or head inhibits (discourages) crossing the midline of the body and two-handed visual-motor activities. Stabilization of the pelvis may be needed to assist with body on body rotation (when part of the body turns but the other remains as is). For example, resist the pelvis from following the trunk's movement, and assist the upper trunk to rotate independently. Assist the upper trunk rotation by guiding the shoulders and upper arms across the body while maintaining an upright and stable base of support.

If head alignment and visual regard/tracking are poor during reaching, present objects for grasping at midline and at eye level. When alignment and visual regard are good in midline, move the object to the side gradually, assisting with trunk rotation as needed. Objects grasped in midline can then be released to the side. Be sure to achieve controlled release first with visual regard rather than just dropping or throwing. If necessary, leaning the hand on a support will provide better control for accurate placement. Objects can then be grasped at the side and released in midline. Once reaching to both sides is accomplished with good head alignment and visual regard, reaching across midline can be initiated.

Children with poor postural control will avoid crossing midline and body rotation by transferring objects from hand to hand. Objects which must be held with both hands can be presented in midline and released to the side with gradually increasing rotation as postural control improves. Choosing objects which encourage two handed grasping at shoulder-width apart, as well as presenting them at or near shoulder height and encouraging release at or near shoulder height, will improve postural strength and control.

References

Ayres, A.J. (1972). *Sensory Integration and Learning Disorders*. Los Angeles: Western Psychological.

Boehme, R. (1988). *Improving Upper Body Control*. Tucson: Therapy Skill Builders.

Bobath, B. (1985). *Abnormal Postural Reflex Activity Caused by Brain Lesions*. Rockville: Aspen Systems Corp.

Bly, L. (1983). *The Components of Normal Movement During the First Year of Life and Abnormal Motor Development*. Chicago: NDT Assoc. Inc.

Chakerian, D. (1991).*The Effect of Upper Extremity Weight Bearing on Hand Function in Children with Cerebral Palsy*. NDTA Newsletter 9/7

Dowler, L. (1991). Seated Work Positions. *Occupational Therapy Forum*, August.

Heipertz, W. (1977). *Therapeutic Riding*. Greenbelt Riding Association for the Disabled (Ottawa) Inc. Canadian Equestrian Federation, 333 River   Rd., Ottawa, ONT K1L 8B9,

Riede, D. (1986). *Physiotherapy on the Horse*. Delta Society, 321 Burnett Ave. So., Renton WA

Scherzer, A.L.; Tscharnuter, I. (1982). *Early Diagnosis and Therapy in Cerebral Palsy*. New York: Marcel Dekker, Inc.

Swift, S. (1985). *Centered Riding*. New York: St Martin's Marek.

DEVELOPMENTAL SEQUENCE ON HORSEBACK

Colleen Zanin, M.Ed,OTR

DEFINITION OF DEVELOPMENTAL SEQUENCE

Developmental sequence is a term commonly accepted for describing the normal sensorimotor progression of development in the first few years of life. Neuromotor development is concerned with this maturation of the nervous system and the parallel acquisition of control over the muscular system. (Banus et al, 1979). There are four principles concerning the "anatomical directions of development". First, maturation starts in the head region and proceeds toward the feet (the cephalocaudal direction). Control of the joints closest to the central axis of the body occurs before control of the joints farther away from the body (proximal joints develop before distal joints; the shoulder joints develop before hand control). Maturation proceeds from the front surfaces of the body, expanding to the back surfaces (ventral to dorsal). Finally control spreads from near the midline in the anatomical position outward or in the ulnar to radial directions. (Banus, 1971). This neuromotor maturation can be regarded as the acquisition of postural control against gravity and balance which seems to follow a definite sequence relative to the planes of the body, i.e., sagittal, frontal, and transverse. (Scherzer & Tscharnuter, 1982). The normal transition between these stages of neuromotor development occurs in a smooth and overlapping fashion.

As control over the muscular system is achieved, different postures emerge, i.e., front lying, back lying, sitting, crawling, standing, and walking. Again, the anatomical direction of development is repeated in each of these positional levels. In abnormal development (as in a child with cerebral palsy), the sequential development of postural control in the normal anatomical direction is arrested at the initial phase. Therefore, the smooth transition between stages of development is interrupted and faulty movement patterns emerge which prevent control over the muscular system. (Conolly, Montgomery, 1987).

THE DEVELOPMENTAL SEQUENCE ON HORSEBACK

Just as the traditional treatment of clients with movement dysfunctions has been strongly influenced by the work of the Bobaths (1979), the emerging field of *equine-assisted therapy* also draws from the treatment principles of the Bobaths' Neurodevelopmental Treatment (NDT). The scope of this paper is not to compare and contrast the use of these techniques in the clinic to their applicability on the horse. (Refer to Glasow, 1984, 1985 for material on this subject). However it is to discuss how the use of developmental positioning and handling on the horse of the client with movement dysfunction can be an effective form of assessment and treatment. For further information on the use of developmental positions with clients with psycho-social, sensory integrative, or educational impairments, please refer to Chapter 26 in this book by Spink which discusses *Developmental Riding Therapy*. (Tebay, Rowley, 1990).

Throughout the years, several misunderstandings have arisen regarding the use of developmental positions on horseback. Occasionally, these positions are used as a "cookbook approach" and each rider is routinely moved in and out of the designated positions with limited regard to purpose, quality, or individual treatment goal. Stanford, Glasow, and Spink stressed in early seminars the need for an experienced therapist to assess and direct treatment for the client. This principle is reinforced today through the development of the Hippotherapy Competency Guidelines (Tebay, Rowley, 1990).

Therapy goals on horseback are the same as accepted neurodevelopmental techniques (techniques used by physical and occupational therapists to treat clients with movement disorders): the reduction of spasticity and reduction of postural compensations with subsequent facilitation of normal movement skills such as improved posture, balance, trunk control, weight shift, rotation through the body axis, and dissociation at the shoulders and pelvis. (Bertoti, 1988). The use of developmental positions coupled with the movement provided by the horse and the graded handling by the therapist helps to achieve these goals.

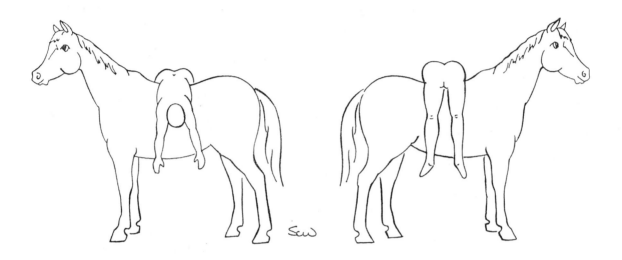

FIGURE 1.
PRONE OVER HORSE'S BARREL: POSITION TO NORMALIZE AND DEVELOP EXTENSOR CONTROL (MOBILITY).*

I. CLIENT LYING PRONE OVER THE HORSE'S BARREL

Lying prone over the horse's barrel may be very uncomfortable for the client. The position should be used sparingly (Figure 1). The speed of the horse's walk should be carefully monitored, as well as the length of stride. As long as the client is not experiencing discomfort, this position provides the therapist with an opportunity to mobilize the clients's pelvis and scapulae, to improve symmetry throughout the body, and to promote generalized relaxation throughout the trunk and pelvis. Specific techniques of sensory stimulation such as approximation, tapping, and vibration can be incorporated into treatment, but need to be applied with good judgment. (Scherzer & Tscharnuter, 1982). The unique demands of the client coupled with the skills of the therapist will determine the precise use of intervention.

PRECAUTIONS: The prone position can cause dizziness in some clients due to the strong vestibular stimulation while the horse is walking. This position should only be used as a preparation for function at a

* Horses are drawn without tack and riders without clothes and helmets only to show positions. A rider should never be on a horse without proper attire and a horse is never used without tack.

higher level (moving from developmental sequential position to one requiring more maturity). Be aware of a rider with a shunt, with stomach tubes or ileostomies, and use experienced side-aides as the client has a tendency to slip in this position. A properly fitted helmet is a must.

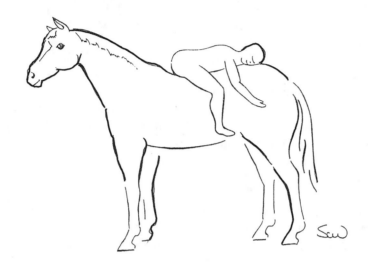

FIGURE 2.
**PRONE ON THE HORSE'S BACK: POSITION TO INCREASE MUSCLE
RELAXATION AND TO DECREASE SPASTICITY**

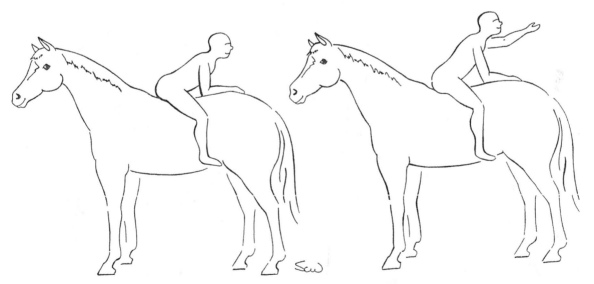

A. SYMMETRICAL BILATERAL WEIGHT ON ELBOWS

**B. UNILATERAL WEIGHT BEARING ON ELBOW
REACHING WITH NON-WEIGHT BEARING ARM**

FIGURE 3.
**FACING BACKWARD: PRONE ON ELBOWS: POSITION TO DEVELOP HEAD,
SHOULDER, AND UPPER TRUNK CONTROL**

II. CLIENT LYING PRONE OVER THE HORSE'S BACK AND SITTING BACKWARD ON THE HORSE

This position is usually more comfortable for the client and provides greater opportunity to incorporate relaxation techniques to reduce spasticity (Figure 2). This position can also be used to improve symmetry and upper extremity weight-bearing in bilateral and unilateral prone propped (Figure 3 A & B) positions. Improved trunk control and abdominal/extensor strength may be achieved by facilitating control of upper body flexion/extension, lateral righting, and rotation through the body axis (Figure 4 A&B). The position of the client's legs around the horse's barrel promotes abduction and external rotation; also, a strong hamstring stretch frequently occurs in this position. When the client can transition to an upright sitting position (Figure 4B) while facing backwards on the horse, trunk extension and a neutral pelvis can be facilitated. By regulating the speed, length of stride, transitions, and direction of the horse, this dynamic treatment surface provides the opportunity to facilitate weight shift, proximal co-contraction (Figure 4A) equilibrium reactions. As in all therapy sessions, emphasis is placed on good bio-mechanical alignment of the client, symmetry, and the reduction of compensatory movements or postures. Occasionally, therapists prefer to ride with the client to achieve greater facilitation of normal movement.

PRECAUTIONS: Some horses impart a very strong anterior/posterior movement which is transmitted to the client while facing backward. Constant vigilance of head and neck control of the client is required. Some clients fatigue rapidly in this position and some complain of disorientation due to decreased visual input.

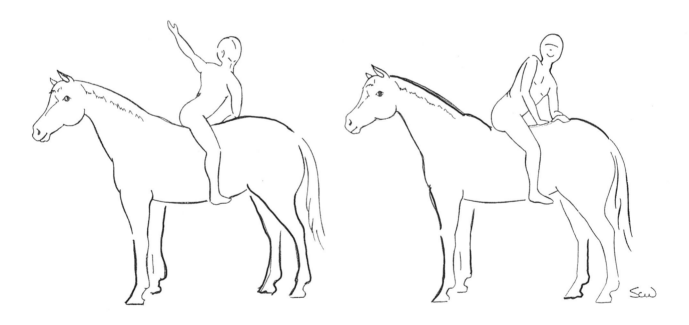

A. ASYMMETRICAL   B. ASYMMETRICAL

FIGURE 4A.
SITTING BACKWARD--THESE POSITIONS NATURALLY FACILITATE TRUNK EXTENSION AND A NEUTRAL PELVIS - VERY USEFUL FOR RIDER WITH POSTERIOR TILT AND A ROUND BACK.

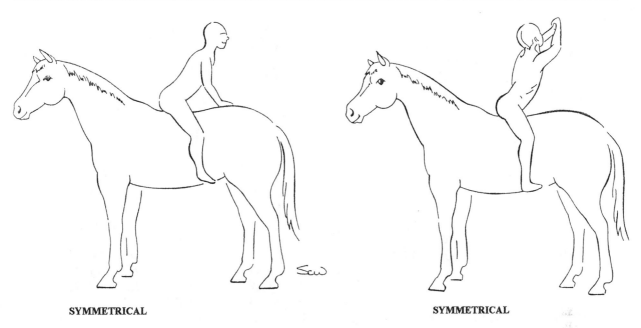

SYMMETRICAL   SYMMETRICAL

FIGURE 4B.
**SITTING BACKWARD--MORE POSITIONS THAT FACILITATE TRUNK EXTENSION AND A
NEUTRAL PELVIS**

III. CLIENT LYING SUPINE ON HORSE'S BACK

This position may also cause discomfort to the client (Figure 5) and proper handling/positioning is extremely important, particularly in the client's low back region. (A pillow under the head may help to reduce the strain on the back in this position). The selection of the best modality (horse) is also crucial in this position. When lying in the supine position is used effectively, the therapist can focus on elongation techniques of the neck and trunk, active-passive stretching of upper and lower extremities, shoulder/pelvis dissociation and abdominal strengthening activities. In preparation for riding astride, the client can lie supine over the horse's back with legs straddling the horse.

Activities to promote neck elongation and head control may be used in this position, with extreme care. Many therapists prefer to assess the effect of this position on the client while the horse is standing still and gradually incorporate movement. A scrutinizing eye and keen observation skills are paramount to discern when the client is becoming over-stressed or when the position is not therapeutic.

PRECAUTIONS: Occasionally, the client becomes fearful in this position due to feelings of vulnerability and the strong effect of gravity on the client in the supine position. Specific treatment goals may be more readily achieved in other positions. A small pillow can be used under the head to decrease the hyperextension of the head/neck region. Monitor the helmet fit carefully when in this position for the helmet has a tendency to slip. The legs of the client should be supported and the lower back of the client should be monitored to avoid strain.

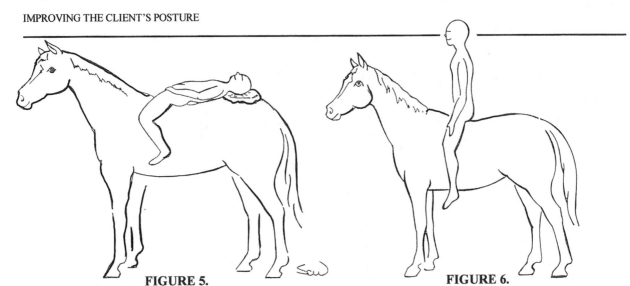

FIGURE 5.
SUPINE POSITION ON THE HORSE'S BACK

FIGURE 6.
SITTING FORWARD--MORE DIFFICULT AS RIDER IS SITTING ON NARROWER BASE AND THE HORSE'S NECK IS A NARROW BASE TO WEIGHT-BEAR ON.

IV. CLIENT SITTING FACING FORWARD

This position is more difficult for many clients as the base of support and weight bearing surface is more narrow (yet more "normal" and easier to integrate for vestibular/visual input) (Figure 6). As with all positions, it is the therapist's role to analyze the client's response to the horse and direct the movement of the horse. (Heipertz, 1981). Treatment goals of improving the client's posture, balance, mobility, and function are continually stressed in this position. Direct intervention by the therapist through "backriding techniques" is most readily used with this position (Glasow, 1984). This position is also used in "classic hippotherapy" to emphasize the influences of the horse on the client. A well-trained dressage horse and a knowledgeable horse trainer with expertise in long-reining will provide the client with a variety of tactile, proprioceptive, and vestibular inputs by performing school figures on one or two tracks.

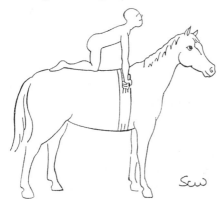

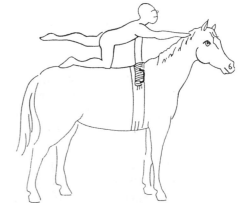

A. SYMMETRICAL WEIGHT BEARING ON ALL FOUR EXTREMI-TIES

B. ASYMMETRICAL WEIGHT BEARING PROGRESSING FROM THREE EXTREMITIES TO TWO EXTREMITIES

FIGURE 7. QUADRUPED POSITION (HANDS AND KNEES) DEVELOPS PELVIC AND LEG STABILITY

V. HIGH LEVEL DEVELOPMENTAL SEQUENCES (VARIATIONS OF QUADRUPED, KNEELING, STANDING)

The use of these positions (Figures 7,8,9) in therapeutic riding are similar to some of the exercises used in sports vaulting (flag, free kneel, stand) (Feiedlaender, 1970). Due to the extreme demands on the client's balance, postural control, proximal stability, and motor planning; these developmental positions are more suitable for clients with mild movement disorders, sensorimotor disorders, sensory-integrative dysfunction, perceptual-motor disorders, cognitive disorders, behavioral disorders, or language impairments. The emphasis of treatment is usually placed on <u>movement transitions</u> versus postural control within a position. (Tebay & Rowley, HIPPOTHERAPY PROJECT, 1990)

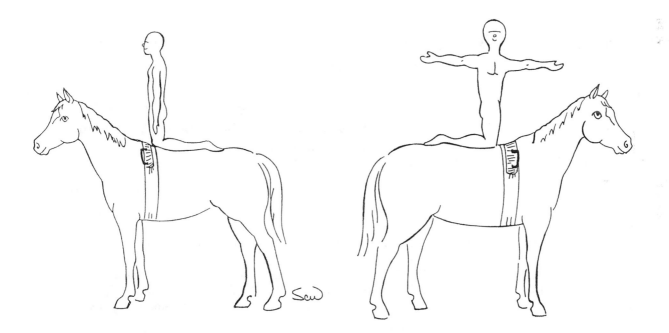

A. SYMMETRICAL WEIGHT BEARING ON BOTH KNEES

B. ASYMMETRICAL WEIGHT BEARING ON BOTH KNEES, ROTATING AND FLEXING TRUNK AS IN REACHING FOR AN OBJECT

FIGURE 8
KNEELING: REQUIRES GREATER PELVIC AND TRUNK CONTROL

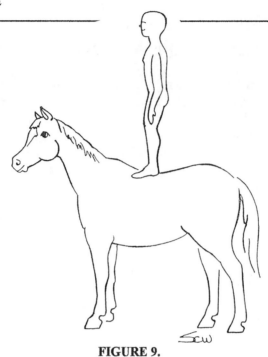

FIGURE 9.
STANDING: REQUIRES INTEGRATION OF TOTAL BODY MOBILITY AND STABILITY
COMPONENTS OF MOVEMENT

SUMMARY AND CONCLUSIONS

This article provides the reader with a historical perspective and rationale for the use of developmental sequences in therapeutic riding. It is strongly recommended that a therapist receive additional education through seminars on this precise use of the horse for improving the client's posture and balance before experimenting with this dynamic treatment tool.

References
Banus, B.S., Kent, C.A., Norton, Y.S., Sukiennicki, D.R. (1979). *The Developmental Therapist*. 2nd ed. Thorofare: Charles B. Slack, Inc. 1-163.
Bertoti, D. (1988). Effect of Therapeutic Horseback Riding on Posture in Children with Cerebral Palsy *Physical Therapy*, 68, 10. 1505-1512.
Bobath, B. (1978). *Adult Hemiplegia Evaluation and Treatment*. London: William Clowes & Sons Limited.
Conolly, B., Montgomery. P. (1987). *Therapeutic Exercise in Developmental*. Chattanooga: Chattanooga Corp.
Friedlaender, E. (1970). *Vaulting: The Art of Gymnastics on the Moving Horse*. Brattleboro: The Stephen Greene Press: I-44.
Glasow, B. (1984). *Hippotherapy - The Horse As a Therapeutic Modality*.
Glasow. B. (1985). *Abnormal Movement Blocks In Cerebral Palsy and Their Correction in Hippotherapy*.
Glasow, B. (1985). *Principals of NDT and Normal Development Applied to Progressions in Hippotherapy*. Published in the proceedings of the Fifth International Riding Congress. Milan, Italy.
Heipertz, W., et al (1981). *Therapeutic Riding: Medicine Education and Sports*. Translated by M. Takeukichi. Available from Canadian Equestrian Federation, 1600 James Anismith Drive Glouchester, Ontario, Canada.
Scherzer, A. L., Tscharnuter, I. (1982). *Early Diagnosis and Therapy in Cerebral Palsy*. New York: Marcel Dekker.
Tebay, J., Rowley, L., (1990). *National Hippotherapy Curriculum Committee*. (1990). Box 41, Riderwood, MD.

CHAPTER 14

TECHNIQUES USED IN HIPPOTHERAPY AND EQUINE-ASSISTED THERAPY

THE FELDENKRAIS METHOD AND HIPPOTHERAPY*

Dr. med. Ingrid Strauss

INTRODUCTION

Moshe Feldenkrais was born in Russia in 1904 and died in Tel Aviv in 1984. He was a physicist, who also conducted research and experiments in neurophysiology, the physiology of behavior, and neuropsychology. In 1949, he published ground-breaking studies. As the result of research, over a period of decades, into human learning processes, he developed his concept of "awareness through movement" (the book appeared in 1967 in Hebrew and in 1968 in German, published in Germany by Insel) [in English: Awareness Through Movement. New York: Harper and Row, 1977 *tr.*] and "the discovery of the obvious" (1981)[in English: The Elusive Obvious. Cupertino, CA: [Meta Publications, 1981 *tr.*]. From his experiences, Feldenkrais gathered together a large body of exercises that has, in the intervening time, also, and repeatedly, influenced hippotherapy.

FUNDAMENTAL CONCEPT

The fundamental concept of Feldenkrais' movement treatment is that a person be mentally involved in his or her movement activity. By developing a sense of feeling their body and controlling it, a person becomes significantly involved in their exercise activity and achieves an intensification of the effects of the treatment it provides. A growing sensitivity to bodily processes - *i.e.* their visualization runs parallel to increased capabilities. Feldenkrais recognized and researched this functional interrelationship [the English term that he used is "functional integration" *tr.*]: that movements mirror the state of the nervous system. In learning a movement, a person completes the exercise successfully when they perceive the movement in their muscles and joints. To think movements, to repeat them mentally and be able to notice their qualities in your mind is better than repeating the movements only mechanically [physically]. Sensory, perceptive, and conscious processes are always connected and involve the whole person. This "functional integration" leads to optimal sensorimotor functioning, which in turn reflects back on psyche and spirit ["Geist"]. "What interests me are not movable bodies but movable brains" [no reference *tr.*]- long experience with his treatment methods over a period of decades brought Feldenkrais to the insight that [human] consciousness meant entering into a new phase of evolution. "We need a more imaginative scientific orientation in order to understand the reciprocally interconnected functions of all aspects of the whole self, and understood as a whole instead of satisfying ourselves with inaccurately imagining local functions." [no reference *tr.*] At the end of his life, Feldenkrais said, all too prophetically, "I believe that we are living in a short transitional period which announces the coming of homo humanus, the truly whole person."[no reference *tr.*]

---

* *Eberhard W. Teichmann translated this article from German to English.*

His observations and perceptions are acknowledged in many forms of therapy that have developed during the last years. I can name, for instance, the extensive field of sensory integration pioneered by Jean **Ayres** and Jean **Piaget**, **Perfetti**'s treatment ideas, and the latest results of research on functions of the central nervous system by A.R. **Luria** and his book, <u>Working Brain: An Introduction to Neuropsychology</u>, published in 1992. Feldenkrais published his first book - <u>Autosuggestion</u> - in 1930, at the age of twenty six. Even at that time he intuited the mental forces that he would later experience and reconfirm, during the vicissitudes of his work over a period of decades, in ever renewed ways, as the central force for all activity. Today it is known that there is a measurable difference in the central nervous system between motor exercises that are done purely mechanically and those that are done with the participation of the mental processes of perception, observation, and attention. Mental integration while doing an exercise brings more success than without it. This was reported on long before it was confirmed scientifically, especially as experienced by musical virtuosos. Feldenkrais developed his exercises for developing general human capabilities, limited as they are, of course, by physiological facts. That these exercises would be helpful as well in different, pathological, circumstances is an obvious consequence - the "elusive obvious" - and thus arose, over decades, an inexhaustible fund of experience useful for treating patients. Had Feldenkrais known about hippotherapy, his creative genius would have been tirelessly at work on it.

A GUIDE TO EXERCISES THAT FIT INTO THE FRAMEWORK OF HIPPOTHERAPY

Feldenkrais conceived of thousands of exercises to develop awareness through movement; he was convinced "that the latent abilities of each of us are substantially greater than those with which we [actually] live. The fact that they have remained latent arises from our lack of consciousness...My students have difficulty imagining how I can improvise thousands of movements year in and year out and for each theme, provide ten or more variations." It is said of him that he was uniquely and unusually creative. In relating this, I want to say that my selection of exercises for our purposes can be no more than a minute stimulus; it is meant to be an invitation to choose from the huge abundance of Feldenkrais exercises appropriate for patients.

<u>Carriage of the head:</u> All the muscles of the body are dependent on the functioning of the neck and head muscles. The easier and more freely the head moves, the easier it is to carry out movements in the entire body, especially those involving turning or twisting. His instructions for achieving this goal involve repeated diagonal movements of the head in relation to the trunk, also using the arms and hands, and coordinated with movement of the eyes.

The large muscles of the <u>middle of the body</u> accomplish the main work of movement: exercises for this area involve turning movements of the trunk and pelvis, coordinated with movements of the arms, legs, head and eyes, mostly in a diagonal pattern.

<u>Looking,</u> control of the eyes and closing the eyes lead to many exercises.

<u>Working with one side of the body</u> and noticing differences between the two halves of the body constitutes a substantial portion of the exercise plan.

<u>Thinking the movements,</u> imagining the feelings of the movements in the muscles and the system of bones and joints and differentiating between successful and unsuccessful movements is essential.

Perceiving and developing the <u>breathing function</u> is a separate theme on the one hand; on the other hand it is a red thread that runs through all the exercises. The exercises always begin from a carefully set up initial position.

In the next section, I will try to convey, from my own experience, how hippotherapy can be made more intensive by including Feldenkrais exercises.

PRACTICAL SUGGESTIONS FOR USING FELDENKRAIS EXERCISES IN HIPPOTHERAPY

It is essential to differentiate two spheres of influence in therapy: a <u>verbal</u> sphere that uses words and language to develop "awareness through movement;" and a <u>nonverbal</u> sphere in which movement sequences are coordinated or corrected by manipulations [of the therapist] and exercises in the sense of "functional integration." If possible, the work should be done on the horse without a saddle.

"Awareness through movement" is always the first phase of the treatment; [and] it is carried out in every stage of hippotherapy. The patient should learn to perceive his or her body processes. The therapist directs the patient's attention by asking questions about the process of movement; the patient is to notice the answers without verbalizing them. By following a number of such questions in practice, they can be tailored to the mental capacities and physical problems of the patient. These [following questions] are to be thought of only as suggestions:

- Do you notice the connection between your seat bones and the back of the horse? Are both sides of your seat bones pressured in an equal way? Is it [the pressure] heavy? Is the pressure of your body on the horse's back equal on both sides [of your seat]? Do you notice the movement of the horse's back under your seat bones? Do your seat bones always take on the same position? Are your seat bones moved or do you move them yourself?

- Is your pelvis straight? Is one side of it higher or lower than the other?

- Can you notice the transition from your sacrum to your lumbar vertebrae? Is this transition area free to move or is it rigid? Notice the direction of movement in your lumbar vertebrae.

- Are your legs equally long? Is the distance on your legs between your knee and your hip joint equally long on both legs? Are both of your feet the same distance from the ground?

- Do your dorsal vertebrae form a straight line or are they curved? Does your sternum change position when you breathe? Does your sternum rise when you inhale?

- What do your shoulder blades do when you inhale? Where do your shoulder blades move to when you bend your back? Are your shoulders at the same height? Is the distance between your shoulder and your ear lobe equal on both sides of you? Can you drop both shoulders equally or does one drop more or less than the other?

- Do your arms swing when you move? Do both arms swing equally wide? Do your arms swing without any effort on your part?

- Is the crown of your head the highest part of your body? Does it lie perpendicular to the extension of your backbone? Where does it move to when you move your head to the side?

The point of such exercises is to develop a feeling for movement as a whole and at the same time center [attention] on movement sequences in a particular locality.

"Functional integration" can be seen as the second phase of the learning process; to carry it out in an active program of exercises on a moving horse requires that the patient has learned to sit [on the horse] in a relaxed way and that he or she is not bothered by exercises or manipulations [of the therapist]. That means that the harmony of movement that the patient and his or her horse have achieved must be preserved during the corrective movements. Under these conditions, and starting from the initial position of "balanced seat," the following program of exercises, appropriately chosen, of course, may be undertaken. Dividing them by sections of the body is proper in the sense that they address crucial areas to exercise but improper in the sense that each exercise addresses the entire body and that this is indeed the essential idea behind the work.

Head:
The position of the head influences the entire musculature of the body. One's capacity for balance and the extent to which one can turn [the head] can be [improved] by exercises in which the head and shoulders are turned in opposite directions; by turning the head and the pelvis in opposite directions; by turning the trunk to the left and then nodding the head to the left and to the right and noticing at the same time how that movement affects the ischia. The patient practices his capacity for balance by placing the crown of his head in its highest position (which he determines). Then he takes a tuft of hair at that point, pulls lightly and balances the head as if it were suspended by a silken thread. The turning movements of the head are coordinated with the eyes - the direction of gaze; also practice rotating the direction of the gaze opposite to movement of the shoulders or the trunk; experience all of the movements also with the eyes closed.

Rib cage:
Turning and twisting movements as described above; noting the position and function of the vertebrae by rounding, straightening, extending backward and moving the back side to side; by drawing the shoulder blades together, by raising the sternum and correlating all these movements to the breath; expanding the rib cage while straightening the trunk by turning the thumbs outward; noticing the rising of the sternum by lightly touching it with the second to fourth fingers of both hands; lifting the crown of the head and allowing the seat bones to sink by pushing down with the feet.

Pelvic region:
Engagement of the large muscles of the middle of the body by turning the trunk and pelvis in opposite directions; rotating the pelvis dorsally during the in breath while relaxing the abdominal muscles; and rotating it ventrally while tightening the abdominal muscles on the out breath; developing pelvic rocking movements (be careful of the horse's reaction to this!) in coordination with the gait of the horse; alternately pushing the left and then the right seat bone forward while moving the corresponding shoulder in the same direction; then, to increase the effect, doing the same movement with the seat bones but moving the opposite shoulder. Rounding the lower back in a pronounced way while rotating the pelvis to the back and then reversing the movement, rotating the pelvis forward while making the lower back a hollow curve; practice achieving an exaggerated lordosis of the spine during the forward pelvic rock. Combine the movements of the pelvis with light bending and stretching of the hip joints.

Extremities:
Arm exercises can facilitate increasing coordination, support achieving stability in the trunk, and improve the capacity of the vertebrae to rotate. Interlace the fingers and fold the arms in unaccustomed positions and practice changing positions with increasing speed; fold the arms by putting the palms of the hands on the armpits, allowing the fingers to touch the shoulder blades at the same time, if possible; alternate this exercise to the right and to the left; develop arm swings with the shoulder at the lowest possible point, while observing the effects of different hand positions. Move the lower extremities minimally, both together and alternately, in the direction of their joint axes, while coordinating corresponding or opposite arm movements. Move the feet by flexing the ankles, both together and opposing; notice each toe by pressing it against the shoe, or better yet, against the therapist's hand; have the therapist stimulate the various zones of contact of the sole: the individual toe pads, the outside edge of the sole, its inside edge, the extent of the heel, done with a flat hand and light pressure. (Feldenkrais called this "work with an artificial floor" and he carried out the manipulations using a board while the patient was lying down in a relaxed position).

Effects of diagonal movement:
The effect of the aforementioned frequently used diagonal exercises can be intensified by stretching one arm out at eye level while looking at the back of the hand and while twisting the trunk in first one and then the other direction. The extent of rotation can be increased by bending the elbow; head to the left while placing the palm of the left hand on the back of the right hand, and then reverse the movements.

Effects of moving one half of the body:
Carry our exercises with one side of the body only, noticing the differences in both sides of the body. Notice if working on one side of the body has an effect on the other side: each side of the body moves differently and is perceived differently. In working with patients who have neurological symptoms on one side of their body, practice the exercises with the healthy side while asking the patient to imagine doing the same exercises with the disabled side. In a subsequent series of exercises, the patient will be asked to notice or perceive the lack of volitional reaction of the disabled side.

Eye - direction of gaze:
The aforementioned exercises have the following goal: movement of the eyes organizes the movement of the body. Further mental training involves perceiving movements with the eyes closed: think through the position, direction and extent of each movement several times and then do the movements and notice if the results change.

Breath:
Many of the aforementioned exercises are accompanied by changes in the breathing spaces of the body; these should be noticed. For example, increase the volume of the lower abdomen by simulated yawning, move the diaphragm by doing little coughs. Include [conscious] breathing in and out in all the exercises.

Mental exercises:

Repeat the exercises in the mind, practice the capacity for imagining, think the movements, imagine the feelings of the movements in the muscles and bones. All these activities bring real success in the exercises.

Prerequisites for the effectiveness of all the exercises are the following:
- quiet
- carrying out the exercises slowly and gradually
- rhythmic repetitions
- no exertion
- periodic long rest pauses
- alertly attending to the proceedings

Only under these conditions can sensitivity to the processes of the body become established and grow. The inner reality of a movement determines its quality and its value. The principles of the Feldenkrais method are equally helpful for working with children, modified, of course, in age appropriate ways.

Dr. med Ingrid Strauss
Kreuth [Germany]
Leonhardiweg 14
83708 KREUTH
Germany
March 19, 1997.

THE EFFECT OF HIPPOTHERAPY ON ATTENTION AND AROUSAL

Craig Nettleton Ph.D.

Many of the beneficial effects of hippotherapy are mediated through the achievement of optimal arousal in the central nervous system. Traditionally, the effects of hippotherapy have been explained as occurring through the imitative process created by the motion of the human pelvis astride the moving horse. More recently, dynamical systems and motor learning theories have been invoked to better describe the complex interactions of multiple systems in learning new motor skills through hippotherapy. Additionally, sensory integration approaches to hippotherapy have emphasized the role of central processing to bring together kinesthetic, visual, and vestibular inputs to create the self organization of new motor plans. The integration of sensory and motor systems requires a level of brain activation that is sufficiently aroused to perform those functions but not so hyper aroused as to become disorganized. The purpose of this paper is to describe the structures and functions of the brain which are impacted by the movement of the horse and how to use that knowledge in the practice of hippotherapy.

We developed this approach to the use of the horse as a therapeutic tool at Skyline Therapy Services by observing our patients at the two ends of the arousal continuum. Our most involved brain injury patients were more activated after riding supine with wedges. Our most hyperactive and distractable patients were more focused after trotting. In order to grasp how patients at the extremes of the spectrum became "normalized" by hippotherapy input, we must understand optimal levels of arousal. Performance is determined by the level of arousal. Too little arousal and the response is poorly established, too much arousal and the response becomes chaotic. Additionally, different tasks require different levels of arousal. Reading this text requires an alert mind and a calm body. Learning to post at the trot requires an alert mind and an activated body. Each task makes its demands on multiple arousal systems.

Arousal systems have three primary functions:
1) Attention - preparedness for sensory input,
2) Activation - motor readiness and performance
3) Self monitoring - observation of the interaction of sensory, motor, and central processing systems.
Each function has several contributing subsystems.

In order to pay attention, we must first have sufficient arousal or alertness. Normal wake-sleep cycles contain variable levels of cortical activity. Abnormal states such as coma or stupor are characterized by arousal levels which are too low for normal perceptions or actions. Hyper-arousal, such as the confused agitated state of some brain injured patients, and the excessive emotional reaction of mania or anxiety, interferes with the organization of both sensory and motor systems. At the normal level of alertness, signal detection occurs. We must orient to the input (where), categorize it (what), and determine its meaning to us at the moment (when and why). The latter functions require comparisons to short and long term memory and current plans. Signal detection, like religion, has both errors of omission (failure to detect the target) and commission (misidentifying the non-target). Distractibility draws attention away from the task to irrelevant stimuli. Double tracking requires shifting attention back and forth between tasks. In addition, we must know how long to maintain attention, i.e. when we need to be vigilant and when to relax.

Activation is the process of preparing for and executing motor responses. One must first initiate the response, then sustain the action through to its completion. In order to stay on task, we must control impulsivity and hyperactivity which lead to irrelevant actions. Feedback helps modify the performance of some actions; others are based on past performance and are preprogrammed in a feed forward fashion. One must also know when to stop performing the activity and switch sets to an alternate activity. Failure to do this constitutes perseverative error.

Self monitoring is the observation of the consequences of one's actions. It involves higher order cognitive processing, the comparison of behavior with plans and goals and/or with social expectations. This is one of the executive functions of the brain - to monitor whether or not the attentional focus is on the appropriate stimuli and whether the appropriate actions are being successfully carried out.

Many brain structures are involved in attentional processes. Sub-cortical systems are necessary in maintaining normal alertness. Lesions in the brain stem, whether caused by head injury, stroke, or viral infections such as polio, effect the reticular activating system and create lower levels of arousal and increased fatigability. Midbrain structures such as the thalamus constitute the switchboard for both sensory and motor networks, and are necessary for efficient information processing. The hypothalamus interacts with the endocrine system and regulates responses to stress. Other midbrain structures are involved in the perception of pain and pleasure and are critical in understanding motivation. The limbic system regulates emotional reactions and thus stimulates cortical tone.

Several cortical structures are necessary for attentional control. Anterior to the limbic system is the cingulate gyrus which is involved in initiation and motivation. The frontal lobes are most important to self regulation. The effects of damage to this area are apparent in head injured patients who have difficulty in establishing plans, organizing the steps to carry them out, maintaining task focus through to completion, and evaluating the results. Metabolic and EEG studies of patients with attention deficit disorder also show abnormalities in frontal lobe functioning. Another cortical region which is involved in attention is the right parietal lobe. Patients with cerebrovascular accidents in this region show the phenomenon of neglect, lack of sensory perception or motor activity on the left side. Not only do right CVA patients show this unilateral finding, but they exhibit a global lack of awareness of their own deficits.

All brain structures have connections which form neural networks. These networks combine to form functional systems. Functional systems incorporate the reciprocal interactions of sensory and motor systems. Subcortical activation is necessary for cortical processing. Cortical structures in turn impact subcortical systems. The intricacy of attentional processes is but one example of the complexity of brain functions.

The previous discussion makes it apparent that many patients have disruptions in their systems of attention. Pharmacological interventions are often implemented to attempt to normalize brain chemistry. For example, Ritalin is commonly prescribed to patients with attention deficit hyperactivity disorder. It may seem counter intuitive to use a stimulant in children who are hyperactive. However, hyperactivity is a symptom of brain under arousal. Hyperactive children are attempting to use motor activity to stimulate themselves and increase brain activity. Patients taking Ritalin often report that they are calmer. This is not because it has a paradoxical effect, but rather that it brings the brain to an optimal level of functioning, making processing more efficient. In turn, the patient does not have to use motor activity to achieve this level, thereby allowing a calmer body. The movement of the horse can be used in a similar fashion.

Just as stimulant medication must be titrated to find the optimal dose, the movement of the horse must be used strategically as well. A careful physician starts with a low dose of psychoactive medications and gradually raises it until maximum benefit with minimum side effects is achieved. The effect of the movement of the horse on arousal systems needs to be conscientiously observed as well. Too little movement can mean a less efficient system and a less effective session. Too much movement and the patient may be agitated or overloaded to a glazed state. The quality of the movement of the horse is as important in this area as in traditional applications of hippotherapy. Long slow strides at the walk may have a calming effect. The concussive impact of a horse with straight pasterns and a choppy trot may have an arousing effect. It is difficult to predict the effect of a particular horse and gait on a particular patient at a specific moment in time. Careful observation of the impact of horse's movement on attentional systems is essential to achieving optimal levels.

The horse's movement is not the only variable in hippotherapy which affects arousal. The level of activity in the clinic is an important factor. Simultaneous sessions, loud music, or schooling horses may be overstimulating for some autistic or early recovery head injury patients. The patients level of participation is a variable which can be manipulated to therapeutic advantage. Active participation, such as steering through an obstacle course or vaulting, engages the patient more fully.

Working with the patient at optimal levels of arousal improves therapeutic response across disciplines. Whether the patient is being seen by a physical therapist, occupational therapist, speech therapist, or a psychologist, the quality of responses improves if the patient can attend adequately. Although many therapists may begin with warm up activities off the horse, sometimes immediate exposure to the horse's movement may facilitate therapeutic progress. If the patient is under or over aroused, addressing that issue immediately will allow other goals to be achieved later in the session. If arousal issues are not addressed, other activities will not be accomplished as well.

Attention span can be increased through learning. The hippotherapy setting provides many opportunities to work on these issues. Patients who are distracted by stimuli such as other horses entering the arena can be taught to return to task with cuing. Vigilance can be maintained for increasing time spans by creating longer strings of directions to be followed. Double tracking can be strengthened by having the patient engaged in a demanding horsemanship skill while being simultaneously required to perform a cognitive task. Tacking the horse up provides opportunities to observe initiation, accuracy, and bringing a task to completion. Self monitoring can be facilitated by pointing out the horse's reaction to the rider.

In summary, the patient's level of arousal is crucial to their ability to adequately perform a task. Both extremes of the arousal continuum have disruptive effects on performance. Many different structures in the brain regulate aspects of attention, and lesions affect the entire system. Attention and arousal issues should be observed as a routine part of therapeutic interactions. Hippotherapy provides an opportunity to manipulate arousal through the movement of the horse. Training attentional skills in the hippotherapy setting is limited only by the imagination of the therapist.

STABLE MANAGEMENT PROGRAM: AN ADJUNCT TO EQUESTRIAN THERAPY

Ellen Adolphson, PT & Gillian Forth, PT

The concept of therapeutic stable management used at Bryn Mawr Rehabilitation Hospital by the therapists was originally developed to make good use of the time the clients spent while waiting for their therapeutic riding sessions. As the clientele is comprised primarily of young adults with head injuries, the program quickly expanded to address the range of cognitive and physical impairments found in this population.

The primary goals are to improve a client's:

- Attention span.
- Recognition and recall.
- Sequencing skills.
- Right/left discrimination.
- Laterality.
- Ability to follow directions.
- Eye/hand coordination.
- Visual-spatial awareness.
- Motor planning skills.
- Fine and gross motor skills.
- Appropriate social interaction/communication skills.

The first lesson is a tour of the barn. This allows the clients to acclimate to this novel environment and appease some of their curiosity. As they become familiarized with the setting and where the tack room, the feed room, where the helmets are kept, etc. Safety is emphasized as the primary concern. Care and time is spent demonstrating and reinforcing safe movement around a horse, proper and safe handling of equipment, and the attention to and understanding of horse "body language." These basic skills are then incorporated into all horse-related activities. Clients are encouraged to move around the horses, touching and interacting with them. This interaction reduces the anxiety level of clients and provides them with multi-sensory stimulation. At the same time, it allows the staff to become familiar with the behaviors of clients in this environment. Ground rules and expectations are communicated.

Subsequent lessons can include, but are not limited to: horse safety, feeding, grooming, knowledge of tack, tacking/untacking the horse, parts of the horse, and colors and markings. Throughout these sessions, the therapist is constantly evaluating and cuing the client as needed, tailoring these one to one "treatment" times to address individual needs. Is the client attending to the task? Is he incorporating prior knowledge? Is body awareness (both of horse and client) demonstrated? If an answer is "no," the problem must be identified and dealt with accordingly.

The therapist can increase or decrease the challenge of a situation for the client by controlling the environment, but the number of available choices can be limited. Visual, verbal, or written cues can be provided as needed. A task can be made less difficult by decreasing the number or complexity of choices involved. On the other hand, for example, balance can be challenged by increasing the range of motion or rotation involved in a task. Grooming and tacking are excellent high level balance activities!

Do not let yourself fall into the rut of limiting clients in wheelchairs to interaction with a book. From grooming to tacking to feeding, the properly and well-trained horse in the correct situation with an attentive therapist will allow full participation of just about anyone, not the least of whom are those in wheelchairs. Get all clients actively involved!

Stable management can be a successful experience for all. However, keep a few things in mind as the program evolves.

- ◘ This aspect is an adjunct to riding. Do not encourage a "You must learn; you will be tested," environment. Clients are here to ride.

- ◘ If you do not know the client's cognitive abilities, start simply, stay on the subject, and gradually increase the complexity of the task.

- ◘ Always allow for success but without insulting the client's intelligence.

- ◘ Have a basic plan for each session, but be flexible.

- ◘ Health, attention span, and mood of both client and therapist, as well as unexpected happenings seem to play a role in the mechanics of a session. Allow the clients to assist in these problem-solving tasks.

Finally, make it fun. We owe it to our clients, ourselves, and our horses.

Reference:
Bryn Mawr Rehabilitation Hospital, 414 Paoli Pike, Malvern, Pennsylvania 19355 USA.

RHYTHMIC FACILITATION - A METHOD OF TREATING NEUROMOTOR DISORDERS USING THE RHYTHM AND MOVEMENT OF THE WALKING HORSE

Jill Wham, Dip OT/NZ, OTR

DEFINING RHYTHMIC FACILITATION

Rhythmic facilitation is a neuromotor facilitation technique which is synchronized with the movement and rhythm of a walking horse. The horse provides the mobility and the rhythm, the occupational therapist organizes the client into an optimum posture and augments and mobilizes action with rhythmic facilitation (Wham, 1990). The rhythmical movement of the horse needs to be carefully analyzed in order to use this technique.

THE RHYTHM AND MOVEMENT OF THE WALKING HORSE

The horse has been described as a walking simulator machine (Riede, 1988). The movement is not like that of riding in a car or wheelchair but is three-dimensional and rhythmical. The horse produces a pulse through its back which works against the client's forward, upward and lateral movements (Figure 1) (Riede, 1988). A posterior view of a client who is wearing reflective markers down the spine and across the buttocks (level with the hip joints) was video taped. This shows that as the horse walks, an upward pulse is transmitted rhythmically and alternately through the client's left and right side of the pelvic girdle. The movement is absorbed through lateral flexion of the lumbar spine and elevation of the pelvis alternately on the left and then right. The markers above the waist remain in a neutral position (Figure 2).

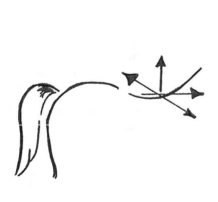

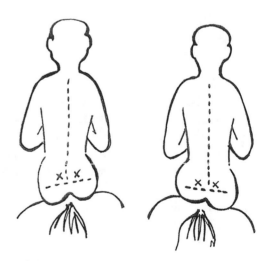

Figure 1.

Figure 2

When analyzed further, it was observed that the elevation of the pelvis coincides with the stance phase of the horse's hind leg on the same side, i.e., during the stance phase of the left hind leg, the horse's rump elevates on the left side, the client experiences pelvic elevation on the left and the lumbar spine's left side flexes accordingly to absorb the movement. The same movement can be observed from a posterior view when the person walks. During the stance phase of each leg the pelvis is elevated and the lumbar spine flexes to absorb the movement. Videos comparing the posterior views of the client with those of the walker show that the same quality and dimensions of movement are experienced. A lateral view of the client shows that with each step there is a corresponding opening and closing (flexion/extension) of the hip joint (Figure 3). The client's hip is thrust forward and the lumbar vertebrae "ripple" to absorb the forward impulsion through the horse's back. This occurs alternately at each hip during the stance phase of the horse's hind leg. It is this action which brings in a rotational movement into the client's trunk, invaluable for inhibiting spasticity and reducing abnormally high muscle tone in cerebral palsy.

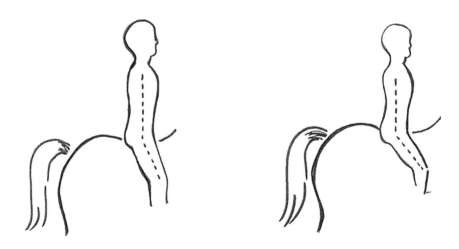

Figure 3.

Thus as the horse walks, the rider's lumbar spine, hips, thighs and associated musculature of the pelvic girdle and abdominal muscles act as "shock absorbers" while the upper body remains still. The implications are exciting in the field of rehabilitation related to neuromotor disorders such as cerebral palsy and head injuries. The ability to experience and learn the normal movement patterns and balance reactions necessary to sit, stand and walk is dependent on stability and freedom of movement in the pelvic girdle and trunk.

As in hippotherapy the client can be placed in a variety of other positions. These may include: supine lying along the length of the horse, sitting backwards, propping on extended arms or forearms, and lying prone across the horse. The emphasis can be upon developing stability in these positions or using a rhythmic technique to facilitate movement, for example, rolling along the horse's back. Rhythmic facilitation techniques may also be used by the therapist while backriding. **In this case the therapist needs to be very well seated and able to feel the left, right, upward and forward pulses of the horse's walk.** A simple numnah (saddle pad) and surcingle are favored as providing the optimal benefit in terms of using the horse's shape, warmth, and movement.

SPECIFIC RHYTHMIC FACILITATION TECHNIQUES

The therapist must first be able to assess the client and analyze the aspects of the posture to be targeted for work. The most suitable position or positions to be used on the horse are selected, and after the mounting procedure the therapist helps the client settle into a relaxed and comfortable position. Warm-up procedures may be used initially, such as breathing, upper body exercises, or creative visualization techniques, such as those used by Sally Swift (1985). The therapist directs the horse's pace and shape via the leader. For example, a slower pace may often be required but the horse will be expected to make itself into a rounded outline and track up so that the movement through its back is fluid and rhythmical.

The horse leader is required to keep the horse's steps uniform and to encourage the horse's concentration upon his work. It is important that the horse's rhythm and movement is not broken or that he does not become distracted and turn his head or alter his shape. A leading technique similar to "long reining" can be used where the leader stands just behind the horse's ear, placing one hand over the horse's neck to make contact with the reins onto the bit. The leader then "rides" the horse from the ground using the reins and voice commands instead of leg aids. The horse is trained to an advanced level of obedience and is capable of producing the rounded outline, fluidity of movement, and concentration expected in good dressage.

The therapist walks beside the horse and firmly attaches one hand <u>over the client's thigh onto the surcingle or numnah.</u> Often a second sidewalker works on the other side of the horse, opposite the therapist. The purpose for holding onto the numnah or surcingle as opposed to the client's leg or waist is two-fold: 1) safety and 2) as an "anchoring point" for using rhythmic facilitation techniques. Although the horses are highly trained and the leaders are skilled and competent, the therapist and sidewalker must always be aware of the horse's instinctive potential to shy. Any environment has its surprises to which a horse may react. The client with disabilities often does not have necessary protective reactions and is likely to sustain a more severe injury than other people if he or she falls. Being firmly attached to the horse means that if the horse shies, the client will remain anchored by the two sidewalkers. If the situation continues to be dangerous, the sidewalkers will be in a position to take the client off safely.

As an anchoring point for a rhythmic facilitation technique, the attachment to the horse itself allows the therapist to be sensitive to and work in harmony with the horse's pace and rhythm. The support given to the client can be varied. The sidewalker's arm may rest lightly on the rider's leg or it may be used to anchor the client firmly onto the horse. Placing the arm closer to the hips gives greater proximal support and helps the client with poor pelvic and trunk stability. Supporting closer to the knee is a more distal contact and the client will need to work harder to stay balanced.

When using rhythmic facilitation techniques, the therapist times his or her own stride length and has to synchronize exactly with the horse's hind legs. When backriding, the therapist feels the horse's rhythmic pulse and will be able to identify exactly when each of the horse's hind legs are striking the ground. Using this rhythmical pattern (left... right... left... right... /one... two ... one... two...) the therapist can time the use of his or her hands to augment the horse's mobilizing action.

Three examples of this technique are outlined as followed:
   A. <u>To improve pelvic mobility,</u> the therapist uses the forward pulse of the horse and during the stance phase of the hind leg, he or she augments the forward movement of the client's hip. The heel of the hand and the flat

of the fingers are applied just below the ischial spine (Figure 4), and pressure is used to alternately push the client's hips forward with the horse's movements. The client needs to be seated with good alignment of the body. This is observed as recommended in classical riding books. The client is encouraged to sit tall with the ear, shoulder and hip all being in the same vertical plane. This classical position may be modified to further augment the forward impulse through the client's hips by the rider leaning back slightly. This moves the ear-shoulder-hip line behind the vertical and the movement is exaggerated through the client's hip.

This rhythmic facilitation technique is effective with clients who have restricted mobility in the hips, e.g., spastic diplegia, spastic quadriplegia. It may also be used to challenge the client with low muscle tone and/ or poor pelvic stability. It should be noted that if the therapist's timing does not coincide with the horse's rhythm, the desired mobilizing action will be blocked.

B. <u>To improve symmetry, particular emphasis is on even weight-bearing through both seat bones</u>. Most clients with a neuromotor problem show asymmetry in their sitting position. There is often more weight distributed through one side than the other. When asked to transfer some of this weight to sit evenly, they are not able to maintain this symmetry for long. Their body schema (i.e., the perception of themselves in space) has altered so that sitting asymmetrically feels correct and sitting evenly may feel strange and insecure. The asymmetry is easily identified by walking behind the horse and observing the rider. Sometimes they may be placing so much weight on one side that they have slipped off the midline of the horse's back. The horse must be halted and the client brought back to the centre before the rhythmic facilitation technique can be used. Once the client is re-centered, the horse walks on and the therapist can now facilitate for symmetry. The client is "asked" to shift his or her weight distribution with rhythmic pressure being applied upward and into the client's hip on the 'heaviest' side (Figure 5 - point **X**).

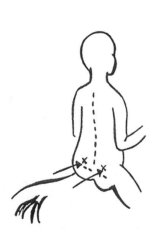

Figure 4.
Points of pressure applied below
the ischial spine

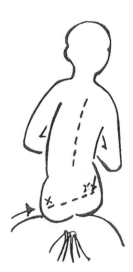

Figure 5.
Point Y and X

Compression downward may also be used to "ask" the client to sit into the horse's movement on their `lightest' side (figure 5--point **Y**). The stance phase of the hind leg on the 'lightest' side of the client is used in this case to encourage him or her to sit into the upward pulse of the horse's walk. As the client practices, the therapist can be lighter with his or her hands and can gradually replace the facilitation with verbal prompts or visualization techniques. A horse walks comfortably at 75 steps per minute, which translates into over 2000 steps per half hour. This gives over 1000 opportunities to practice the skill. In this case the skill is weight-bearing on the right side in sitting (Figure 5). In this way the client can accept and learn to tolerate the new sensation of symmetry.

C. <u>To decrease scoliosis</u> , the client is positioned supine along the length of the horse's back. The therapist places one hand over the client's thigh and onto the numnah at the withers. The other hand is placed under the client's axilla. As the horse walks, a rhythmic stretch is applied to match the elongating action of the horse's side, i.e., during the stance phase of the hind leg on the same side. For example, a client who needs elongation on his or her left side will be stretched rhythmically on the left during the horse's elongation or stance phase of the horse's left hind leg. The assistant sidewalker can help by bracing against the client's thoracic region to assist the elongation (Figure 6). This uses similar key points to the three point bracing systems used in modular seating systems for children with scoliosis. Walking the horse in straight lines or various circles can vary the amount of elongation used. As the client becomes more "pliable" a smaller circle can be tolerated (the elongation is on the outer edge of the circle) and a greater stretch achieved. The results of this method of stretching for clients with scoliosis have been promising in many cases at Ambury Park Riding Center*.

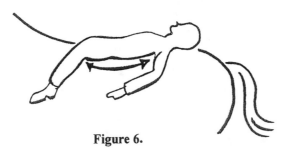

Figure 6.

The above examples illustrate some of the many ways rhythmic facilitation can be used in hippotherapy. As the therapist becomes more attuned to the horse itself and its rhythm, facilitation techniques can be worked in harmony with the horse. The therapist may work on foot, walking in time with the horse's hind legs, or on top of the horse as in back riding. The rhythm is the key to the client's learning with the repetition and expectation provided by the horse. The mental application is supplied by the client and the therapist. A well-trained horse and leader ensure that each step is identical to the last, giving the client a chance to practice the postural skill over and over until it is mastered. A positive expectation is generated with the rhythm. The client knows what to expect and when. He or she is able to anticipate, prepare him or herself posturally and respond adaptively. The expectation is one of success and there is no time to be bored or complacent as the horse keeps moving. The rhythm does not wait for the client, but *"asks"* him or her to *"do it now" .... now ...now"*.

* In a research study by Dr. Jill Calveley, children with this problem showed improved sitting balance following a course of therapy using this method.

When neuromuscular facilitation techniques are used in harmony with the horse's rhythmic movement, specific therapeutic goals can be targeted. Rhythmic facilitation can be used to develop improved muscle tone, head control, trunk righting reactions, pelvic stability, hip mobility, postural extension against gravity, symmetry and other functional goals. These, along with the cognitive and social aspects of development achieved by clients are the basis for major accomplishments such as independent sitting, standing, and walking needed for occupational roles.

CONCLUSION:

RHYTHMIC FACILITATION - A THREE POINT MODEL

Rhythmic facilitation is a method of treating neuromotor disorders using the rhythmic action of a walking horse. The <u>horse</u> provides the mobility and rhythm, and the <u>therapist</u> organizes the client into a desirable position to benefit and augment the mobilizing action with <u>rhythmic facilitation</u>.

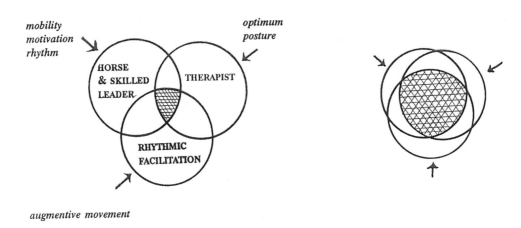

Figure 7.

The three interlinking elements merge so that all work simultaneously and harmoniously to become one operation. The client, the most important person, is the nucleus of the operation and the more these circles merge, the greater the benefit to him or her.

References:
Bertolli, D. (1988). "Effect of Therapeutic Horse Riding on Posture in Children with Cerebral Palsy." *Proceedings of the 6th International Therapeutic Riding Congress*. Toronto, Canada.
Calveley, J. (1988). The Effect of the Horse Riding upon Sitting Balance in People with Cerebral Palsy. *Proceedings from the 6th International Congress of Therapeutic Riding*. Toronto, Canada.
Dacum Hippotherapy Curriculum Committee. (1988), October. *National Hippotherapy Project 3/91*. Warwick: New York
Glasow, B. *Division of Vaulting for Disabled*. Warwick: New York.
    North American Riding for the Handicapped Medical Subcommittee. (1988). Therapeutic Riding Classifications.
Reide, D. (1988). *Physiotherapy on the Horse*. Therapeutic Riding Services, MD
Swift, S. (1985). *Centered Riding*. North Pomfret: David and Charles.
Tebay, J.M., Rowley, L.L., Copeland, J.C., Glasow, B.L. (1988). Training Physical and Occupational Therapists as Hippotherapy Specialists.
Wham, J. (1990). Abstract, paper presented at the New Zealand Association of Occupational Therapists Jubilee Conference. Christchurch, New Zealand.

DEFINING STRATEGIES FOR REMEDIATION IN REHABILITATION

Barbara T. Engel, M.Ed, OTR

Practitioners using the horse in therapies can use many different techniques with equine-assisted therapy and/or hippotherapy. Some strategies and remediation techniques are listed here to give the reader a brief understanding of the terms and their use in equine-assisted therapies.

Affolter Method
Dr. Felicie Affolter, a Swiss language pathologist, has developed a treatment approach involving *Guiding as a Perceptual Cognitive Approach* to functional development of persons with motor disorders. This approach is based on Piagetian theories of development. It assumes that perception is a prerequisite for interaction, tactile-kinesthetic information is necessary for interaction to occur and interaction is always goal-directed. The technique, as described by Affolter, requires a hands-on approach in which the therapist assists the client in performing a task. The therapist (her) puts her arms and hands over the client's (his) arms and hands and guides the client through the performance of a task. The client learns to register sensation of touch and movement while performing the task. The client learns to register information regarding his environment. He gains the ability to interact on a tactile-kinesthetic basis with his environment as he becomes aware of himself and his actions within the surroundings (Affolter, 1991). The Affolter technique can effectively be applied with occupational therapy in the equine setting both on and off the horse. For example: the therapist, Judy, backrides an eight-year-old Mary who has a moderate motor planning problem. Judy places her arms and hands over Mary's as Mary holds the reins. Judy guide Mary's arms and hands with light contact as Mary guides the horse around a series of cones.

Alexander Method
F. Matthias Alexander deals with the concept that physical and mental processes work together in any form of human activity. All training, despite method must be based on the mind-body awareness or the indivisible unity of the human organism. The Alexander Technique is referred to and used by Sally Swift.

Brummstrom Approach
Brummstrom sought to facilitate motor recovery by the development of primitive reflexes and active movement in synergy patterns.

Centered Riding
Centered Riding is an approach developed by Sally Swift of Brattleboro, Vermont. It asks the rider to use mental and physical images resulting in perfect body balance and an increased inner awareness of both oneself and one's horse. It is not necessarily a method used to teach riding. Centered riding teaches one how to breathe, balance, and how to move the body and limbs. The approach is clearly based on classic dressage dating back to the early 1600's. By using the centered riding approach, any person may improve his or her ability to control his or her body while learning to ride a horse or while accommodating the movement of the horse. It teaches one NOT to interfere with the moves of the horse. This is an important element in becoming one with the horse and in providing the appropriate stimulation from the horse to the client during hippotherapy. The technique is used by instructors with their students and by therapists with their clients to improve functions. If a therapist is not trained in dressage, this is an excellent book to gain an understanding of the principles of

riding and communication with the horse. In addition it helps the therapist understand the steps needed to treat clients with sensory processing deficits.

Conductive Education System

Also known as the Peto System, Dr. Andras Peto from Budapest developed conductive education in the 1950's. This is a method of learning called "rhythmic intention." In it each task to be learned is broken down into component parts; each part is practiced separately until success is reached. This aspect is the intent. Meanwhile, the client counts while practicing the tasks, providing the rhythmic component and stimulus that guides the movement. Rhythmic intent is a method of learning that involve the client's motor, linguistic, perceptual and cognitive abilities. When several clients are working together, the group provides further motivation (E.Cotton) This technique can clearly be used with equine-assisted therapy.

Craniosacral Therapy

John Upledger, an osteopathic physician, developed *Craniosacral Therapy* (Upledger, Vredevoogd, 1983). The technique involves the understanding of the craniosacral system. It uses gentle and non-invasive palpatory skills to detect subtle biological movements, and to perform fascial and soft-tissue releases. This modality is used with persons with a neuromuscular dysfunction. It helps to identify and reduce accumulated pain and stress. It calms down the autonomic system, lowers the blood pressure and reduces fevers. Additionally, it removes transient and minor restrictions, relaxes muscles, improves fluid exchange and blood flow. With tissue manipulation, it lengthens the spine, and promotes general relaxation and a balancing of the body system. It can be used effectively with backriding by those who are highly skilled in backriding techniques and those trained in Craniosacral therapy. It is especially effective in developing centering in the client and developing the "feel" of being centered, a primary skill in sitting in a balanced position on the horse.

Developmental Stimulation

Developmental stimulation includes all types of facilitation and stimulation techniques based upon the normal growth process. Techniques arise from different theories as they are developed by various professionals. The new research of the late 1990's has explained the developmental process more clearly. Many of the techniques such as the one which claims to teach infants to read, are unfounded. For example, the techniques used by early childhood specialists to encourage movement and play will vary from techniques used by pediatric occupational, and pediatric physical therapists treating children with cerebral palsy. Techniques that have been found to be currently accurate can be incorporated into the therapeutic riding program by many specialists.

Eutony

Greta Alexander, a German, calls her method *Eutony*. "Eu" in Greek means good, well, harmonious, and "tonus" means tension. This method involves focusing on the unity of the total person. This "feeling of unity and integrity liberates the creative forces and develops the capacity of contact with others without losing one's own individuality." Her method increases one's awareness of own's bodily systems and influences the way one functions (Alexander, 1985).

Feldenkrais Method

The Feldenkrais method is an educational, neuromuscular approach to improve function. It strives toward ease of movement and improved coordination. This is accomplished through increased awareness, sensitivity and coordination (Feldenkrais, 1981). The entire sensory-motor system is involved to unravel habitual patterns and replace them with better motor function through changing the person's perception of movement. Dr. Moshe Feldenkrais developed the techniques of *functional integration* and *awareness through movement*.

Functional Integration uses touch, the feelings of pressure and pull, and the warmth of the hands and their caressing stroke. This technique is based on neurological milestones in development. Feldenkrais felt that a "crucial point of learning was the arrival of the impulses sent by the nervous system in patterns such that all the intricate movements can be performed" (Feldenkrais, 1981). When the nervous system is damaged, *Functional Integration* techniques help the nervous system to respond and establish impulses that facilitate normal movements.

Feldenkrais's *Awareness through Movement* technique is based on several concepts: that one needs to learn at one's own rate, that movement is the vehicle for learning, and that one needs to have alternative ways of moving. Learning must be pleasurable and it must be easy. These two elements increase relaxed breathing. He felt that emphasis should be on the action of learning the movement, not the goal to be obtained; one needs to be aware of the learning process. Feldenkrais's technique has been used with hippotherapy in Germany. See page 189 for Feldenkrais and hippotherapy.

Handling Techniques

Any hands-on technique that can be used to manipulate the posture or limbs of a client for therapeutic reasons is called a "handling technique." Bobath's methods involve many techniques for handling children and adults with spastic disorders. Facilitation techniques are special handling techniques used by the therapist to increase the ease in carrying out a functional action or to inhibit neural responses. They help the client by enhancing function. Handling techniques are used by care givers and therapists to handle a person at key points in a way that maintains *normal* or *near normal* posture and are used when moving a person from one position to another (Finnie, 1975). Inhibitory techniques are also handling techniques that inhibit - or restrains or interfere with - an action or a process. Therapists use inhibitory techniques to reduce spasticity, or to relax or slow undesirable actions.

Holistic Treatment

Holistic refers to treatment of the whole or consideration of all functional aspects of a person. Holistic treatment deals with all aspects of a person's function and dysfunction and usually encompasses many different approaches. A holistic occupational therapy approach to learning disorders was developed by Barbara Knickerbocker, OTR (Knickerbocker, 1980) which incorporates sensory integration theory but uses a different treatment approach. (Jean Ayres and Barbara Knickerbocker were close friends and shared their theories.) Occupational therapy has historically been a holistic treatment since "work" skills involve mind, awareness, cognition, motivation, physical mobility and skills.

Motor Behavior Theories

The dynamic systems theory places the responsibility for motor control among most the central nervous system. The brain prepares and tunes the motor system to respond to the changing environment and to the tasks given tasks. Skilled motor performance is the ability to perform a task in several different number of ways according to the variation in the environment. The maintenance of posture control is understood to be controlled by a feed-forward mechanism. Balance control varies by position of the person, by the tasks being performed, the context in which the activity occurs, and the individual's perception of their most stable body part.

Myofasial Release

This technique was developed by John F. Barnes, a physical therapist. Myofascial release is designed to be used with appropriate modalities, mobilization, exercise and flexibility programs, neurodevelopmental treatment (NDT), sensory integration, and movement therapy. Myofascial release relates to the fascia of the body. The fasia is three-dimensional connective tissue that runs from the head to the foot throughout the body. Its purpose is to support structures by holding tissues together and separating structures so that they can move without friction (Barnes, 1989). Myofascial Release is the lengthening of superficial and deep body tissue through a gentle and sustained stretch (Boehme, 1988)(Barnes, 1991).

Neuro-developmental Treatment (NDT)

NDT, also called the Bobath technique, was developed by Berta Bobath, a British physiotherapist, and her husband, physician Karel Bobath. This method is based on the recognition of the interference of normal maturation of the brain leading to arrest of motor development and the presence of abnormal postural reflex activity (Bobath, 1970). The aim of this handling technique is to inhibit abnormal movement patterns while facilitating normal reactions and movement. NDT has been traditionally used with hippotherapy.

Perceptual-Motor-Stimulation

Perception refers to the interpretation in the brain of sensations one takes in. Movement is a motor response. Perceptual-motor stimulation refers to physical activities that increase when the brain interprets, responds to feeling, or senses changes in the environment, and a motor response is the result. All therapeutic horseback riding involves perceptual-motor-stimulation.

Proprioceptive Neuromuscular Facilitation (PNF)

Herman Kabat, MD, and two physical therapists, Margaret Knott and Dorothy Voss, developed *Proprioceptive Neuromuscular Facilitation* techniques for the treatment of neuromuscular problems. PNF is "a method of promoting or hastening the response of the neuromuscular mechanism through stimulation of the proprioceptors" (Hopkins & Smith, 1978). The PNF patterns and techniques are used both independently and with exercises, gait training, and self-care activities to develop strength, balance, and motor learning. The technique applies itself well to hippotherapy.

Rood: Neurophysiological Approach

Margaret Rood, an occupational and physical therapist, developed a treatment approach that involves activation, facilitation, and inhibition of muscle actions, voluntary and involuntary, through the reflex arc. This approach assumes that an exercise is a treatment only when the response is correct and the feedback results in enhanced learning of that response (Hopkins, Smith, 1978).

Sensorimotor Stimulation

There are many therapeutic treatment applications of sensorimotor stimulation that have developed during the last 50 years. They are based largely on the work of Sherrington and others, and include approaches of the Bobaths, Fay, Doman-Delacato, Rood, Kabat, Pavlov, Brunnstrom, Fuchs, Ayres, Cratty, Kephart and others. Most have emerged as current knowledge of the nervous system has progressed. Sensorimotor stimulation

techniques are applied according to the theoretical base of the professional using them -, i.e., physical, occupational, and speech therapists; physical educators, movement therapists, child development specialists and so on. There is a great deal of change occurring in the approaches being used in treatment because of the growth in the knowledge of how the central nervous system functions. Many "old" techniques are outmoded since the reasoning behind their development has been inaccurate and the techniques have been either "revised" or discarded in order to apply to the current base of knowledge about function. Sensorimotor stimulation is very rich upon the moving horse.

Sensory Integration or (SI)

Sensory Integration is a system of treatment techniques based on theories of evaluation and treatment developed by A.J. Ayres, an occupational therapist. It involves active participation by the client in purposeful activities that are always initiated and directed by him or her. It requires the client to make an adaptive response to his or her environment. In this process, activities that are rich in proprioceptive, vestibular and tactile stimulations are not repeated but are done as a continuous series of events. After careful evaluation using Ayres's tests, the therapist manipulates the environment to obtain the desired results for the dysfunction and to facilitate or inhibit neurological functions for the stated goal of improving the processing and organization of sensation. Sensory integration does not include the teaching of skills or the arousal of specific sensations such as applying tactile stimulation to a client or placing the client in an activity that gives him or her vestibular stimulation. Sensory integration methods must be administered by an occupational or physical therapist who is specifically trained in the techniques. (Sensory Integration International, 1990). A Sensory integration-certified therapist (occupational or a physical therapist) is recognized by SII (Sensory Integration International) as qualified for testing purposes only. Sensory integration techniques can be used in riding and with equine activities.

Tactile Stimulation

Tactile refers to the sense of touch. Tactile stimulation can include any type of arousal of the touch system; it may include direct excitation to the skin or having the client engage in tactilely arousing activities. (Sensory Integration International, 1990). Tactile stimulation by it self is not sensory integration. Tactile stimulation is involved in all aspects of horsemanship. In siting astride the horse provides sensation that is passed through the back of the horse to the seat of the rider.

Vestibular Stimulation

Vestibular refers to the vestibular apparatus of the inner ear that includes those parts enervated by the eighth cranial nerve: the saccule, utricle, semicircular canals, vestibular nerve and vestibular nuclei, and those parts of the brain that are directly affected by this system. The vestibular system responds to type, direction, angle, speed of movement, and the head position, movement percieved by the eyes, enabling a person to orient in space and time and maintain a sense of equilibrium or balance (Dunn, 1991). Vestibular stimulation can include any excitation that arouses the vestibular system (Sensory Integration International, 1990). Vestibular stimulation by it self is not sensory integration. Vestibular stimulation is involved in all aspects of horsemanship and riding skills.

References:

Affolter, F.D. (1991). *Perception, Interaction, and Language*. Berlin: Springer-Verlag.

Alexander, G. (1985). *Eutony*. Great Neck: Felix Morrow

Barnes, J.F. (1991) Myofascial Release Techniques. *Occupational Therapy Forum*. July 19, 1991.

Blakiston's Gould Medical Dictionary 4th Ed. (1979). New York: McGraw-Hill Book & Co.

Bobath, B. (1972). *The Concept of Neuro-developmental Treatment*. Lecture notes Western Cerebral Palsy Centre, London Cermak, S. (1989).

Boehme, R. (1988). *Improving Upper Body Control*. Tucson: Therapy Skill Builders.

The Efficacy of Sensory Integration Procedures in *Sensory Integration Quarterly*. Torrance: Sensory Integration International.

Cotton, E. (no date given). *The Hand as a Guide to Learning*. London: The Spastics Society.

Dunn, W. (1991). In Christiansen-Baum (ed) *Occupational Therapy, Overcoming Human Performance Deficits*. Thorofare: Slack Inc.

Feldenkrais, M. (1981) *The Elusive Obvious*. Cupertino: Meta Publications.

Finnie, N.R. (1975). New York: E.P.Dutton & Co., Inc.

Hopkins, H., Smith, H. *Willard & Spackman's Occupational Therapy*, 5th Ed. New York: Lippincott Co. p 127-28

Knickerbocker, B.M. (1980). *A Holistic Approach to the Treatment of Learning Disorders*. Thorofare, Charles B. Slack,Inc.

Sensory Integration International (1990). Course notes.

Swift, S. (1985). *Centered Riding*. North Pomfret: David & Charles Inc.

CHAPTER 15

BACKRIDING

KEY WORDS
TREATMENT
HANDLING TECHNIQUES

BACKRIDING TECHNIQUE IN THERAPY

Elizabeth A. Baker, PT

Within the past decade and a half, backriding has attracted a level of acclaim shared by few other teaching or therapy techniques in the field of therapeutic horseback riding. A simplistic description of backriding is riding double on horseback. Backriding is used in therapeutic riding to improve the quality of the individual riding session. The acclaim that backriding has received, and deservedly so, results from observations of the rapid progress made by riders with whom this technique has been successful. In these instances, backriding has provided the initial physical facilitation and/or emotional support needed to allow the development of skills for more independent riding and for improved balance and movement skills off the horse. Presumably, the same support or facilitation could not be adequately provided from staff on the ground. However, some areas of concern have also surfaced. These have included safety practices; the use of appropriate equipment; horse size, conformation, maintenance and training; and other ethical concerns related to both horse and client. It appears that while backriding can be a tremendously effective technique, it must be carefully and judiciously used.

Backriding is a technique in which two people sit astride a horse. One is the client, who is physically, emotionally or mentally disabled, and who cannot be adequately supported or assisted from the ground by sidewalkers or the therapist. The other is a specially trained individual, usually a therapist or riding instructor (the backrider may also be a designee of the instructor or therapist, under that person's direct supervision). For the physically disabled client, the backrider should be an experienced physical or occupational therapist; for a client with an emotional or mental impairment, the backrider should be a therapeutic riding instructor. When the backrider is a physical or occupational therapist, the choice of backriding as a therapeutic technique has been made because the therapist can skillfully provide the physical handling and facilitation required to maximize the physically disabled rider's balance and posture during the therapy session. If the backrider is a riding instructor, backriding has been chosen as the best possible means to further the development of riding skills in that person. For example, the close physical contact of the backrider may alleviate the initial fear of riding found in the student with mental or emotional disabilities. In any instance, the choice of backriding should be a timely one; that is, backriding is used as a therapy or teaching technique at the appropriate time in the development of the client's skills, when it will do the most good, and with the expectation of progressing beyond backriding toward his or her optimal level of independence.

Whatever his or her educational background, the backrider must be a skilled rider and knowledgeable "horse person." The backrider must be able to ride independently at a walk, trot, and canter; and to ride by being longed on a longe line siting on a pad without "holding on" to the surcingle at the walk and trot. Good riding skills are extremely important, because the backrider is responsible for maintaining the safety of the client should the horse shy or stumble. However, the backrider is seated behind--rather than over--the center of gravity of the horse, Figure 1. In this position it is more difficult to remain balanced and to follow the movement of the horse. Thus, the backrider with inadequate riding skills will have difficulty maintaining his or her own balance, impairing his or her ability to provide skilled assistance to the client.

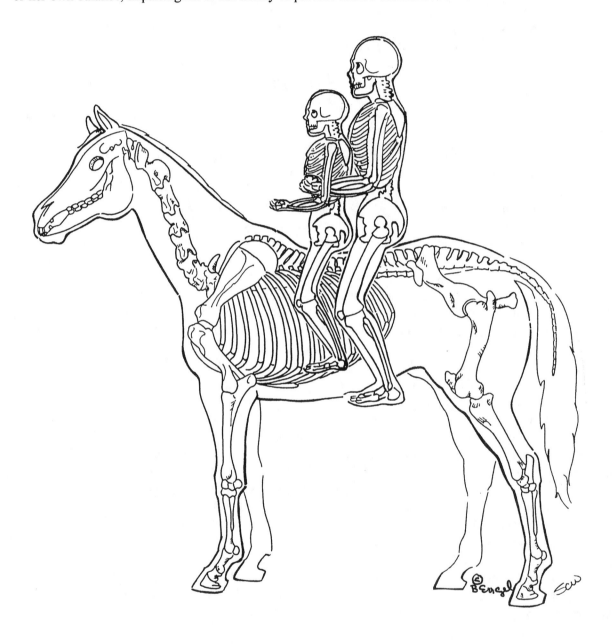

FIGURE 1.
BACKRIDER IS SEATED BEHIND RATHER THAN OVER THE CENTER OF GRAVITY OF THE HORSE

The backrider should be able to correctly groom and prepare the horse for a backriding session, as well as recognize and anticipate signs of emotional and physical stress in the horse which would indicate that backriding may be inappropriate. The backrider should be familiar with effective equine training methods which improve the horse's suppleness, strength, and overall mental health. While the backrider may not be capable of providing the training, he or she should be knowledgeable enough about such methods to recognize their necessity and advocate for them. Other considerations are weight and height. Previous unpublished writings have indicated that the backrider's weight should not exceed 150 pounds, and that this is also true for the client. The combined weight of the client and backrider should be a factor in selecting a horse of suitable size and conformation.

Backriding may be chosen by a physical or occupational therapist as an equine-assisted therapy technique. The client who will benefit from this therapy technique usually manifests a movement dysfunction, and as noted cannot be adequately supported or facilitated from the ground. This may include a variety of diagnoses, such as cerebral palsy, multiple sclerosis, spina bifida, spinal cord injury, and others. Backriding is never prescribed on the basis of the diagnosis alone; it is the accompanying deficits in muscle tone, strength, balance, postural stability and symmetry which provide the indicators for the use of this technique. These indicators include the following: poor head/trunk control, poor balance, significantly asymmetric position and movement patterns, increased tone as a result of the position of horse's movement, severe tone and movement abnormalities, rapid fatigue, and lack of progress due to the effort required to ride. All these problems, in certain instances, can be effectively treated without backriding. Backriding thus should be the chosen approach because the therapist on the ground cannot provide the client with the input needed to allow progression in treatment.

Backriding allows the therapist to provide facilitation and support in a symmetrical, precise manner because the backrider is at the same level as the client. This in turn allows the motorically impaired client to relax, to achieve a balanced and symmetrical position, and to follow the movement of the horse without excessive effort, spasticity and fear. What input the therapist provides depends on the specific needs of the client at that point in the treatment program. Very often, the client for whom backriding is utilized is one whose head and body postural control is so impaired that sitting balance is poor or virtually nonexistent. The therapist's hands can provide assistance to maintain the correct spine and pelvic alignment until the horse's movement facilitates control there; they may gently emphasize the pelvic rotation caused by the horse's movement to enhance normalization of muscle tone and postural control. Manual facilitation of oblique abdominal flexor musculature or hip extensors, and approximation through the shoulders or pelvis, may also be used. This input facilitates the development of proximal stability needed to support upper extremity use such as bearing weight on the hands, patting the horse, and reaching for objects. When very small adults or children are treated, the therapist may also choose to utilize developmental positions and movement transitions during the backriding session. This might include positioning the client in prone inversion, in front of the backrider. The backrider may also sit facing backwards on the horse, positioning the client in supine or prone, or in upper or lower extremity weight-bearing positions to develop proximal stability, midline control, and weight-shifting skills. Experience in neurodevelopmental treatment and handling techniques off the horse is necessary for their correct application when using the horse in treatment. Also necessary is practice in the use of these techniques while backriding a normal adult or child. Although it is preferable for the therapist to be the backrider in a therapy session, the riding instructor or knowledgeable horse person may assume this role under the direct supervision of the therapist. As in all therapy sessions, independent function is a goal; thus the therapist gradually withdraws support and facilitation as the client's independent postural control improves. This includes progressing from backriding the client to treatment from the ground.

Therapeutic riding instructors may also choose to use backriding as a teaching technique. A client with emotional, psychological, or mental impairment may be very fearful of riding yet fascinated by the horse. The reassuring presence of the backrider may enable such a client to begin a riding program. The withdrawal of the backrider when appropriate to a position on the ground will also provide a very concrete measure of success and a source of pride to the client, who can now ride "all by myself." (It may be said that with certain clients with physical disabilities, the therapist may backride initially for the same reason--to alleviate fear). Clients who have no overt physical disability but have mild postural insecurity and sensory processing problems may also seem fearful and overwhelmed by the horse's movement, clinging to the surcingle or sidewalkers. In such situations the additional tactile and proprioceptive input provided by the close physical contact of a backrider may help. It is also true, however, that children with such problems will show greater ability to integrate and organize the input they receive from the horse with greater success--e.g., less fear, improved postural security and confidence--while the horse is moving. Thus it should not be assumed that a backrider is necessary; the vestibular input provided through the horse's movement may be of equal value. There may be other client-specific reasons an instructor would choose to backride. The determining factor in that choice, as always, is whether or not the client can be effectively managed and taught from the ground; or is backriding, at this specific point in the individualized riding program, a necessary teaching tool or part of a progression.

Helping the client to progress beyond backriding is always preferable. If necessary, it can be done gradually. For example, backriding can be used in the beginning of a therapy session until postural control improves; the therapist may be able to dismount and complete the session from the ground. This reinforces the need for a very safe, reliable, well- trained horse, since dismounting from behind the client can be difficult.

The horse is the critical component of the backriding session. It must have a safe, quiet, reliable disposition, and be completely comfortable with all situations and equipment used in the therapeutic riding program. This includes the ability to stand quietly at the mounting ramp during a slow, difficult mounting procedure, as well as to tolerate the presence of several side-aides if needed. The horse should be trained to quietly carry two people before being used for backriding in the program.

The horse's conformation will also dictate whether or not it is appropriate for backriding. The horse should have good basic conformation and be sound, because backriding will impose additional weight and stress on any structural abnormality present. This stress is compounded by placing a good deal of that weight over the horse's loin area, the weakest part of the back. Thus, an older horse that has a mild unsoundness or structural problem, suitable for light work (a common description of the donated program horse) may become unsound and unusable if backriding is attempted. The horse's back should be muscular, strong and supple, with a "level topline," for example, without high withers, high rump, swayback deformity, or prominent backbone. The length of the back should be short to average; a horse with a long back is inappropriate for, and likely to be injured by, backriding since a long back is bio-mechanically weak before the addition of the backrider's weight. A short back with the withers sloping evenly into the back and a short loin area are ideal. In assessing the horse's back, looking down at it from a high point such as the mounting ramp can help identify weakness. If the loin area is weak, the spine will be prominent and the muscling will slope downward; if it is strong, the area will appear round and full. The ideal height has been described as 14.2 to 15.2 hands, but a safe larger horse with well-trained taller side-aides may be appropriate. If a smaller horse is used, the previously mentioned weight limits for the backrider and client may begin to seem excessive (unless one uses a Haflinger, though small and stocky, can carry the weight of a big horse). A smaller horse may also be inappropriate for use in therapy when backriding is needed. Its stride may be too short, quick, and choppy (as is that of most ponies); the combined weight of the client and backrider may additionally shorten the stride and decrease the movement imparted to the client, negating any therapeutic benefit. The horse's width can vary, but if the client's hip and pelvic mobility is adequate, a wider base of support is preferable.

The horse's quality of movement and flexibility is extremely important, particularly in therapy. The horse should be balanced, symmetrical, and able to "track up" (at the walk, the hind foot steps forward and past the hoofprint of the same side forefoot) even with the weight of two riders. It should be able to bend with equal flexibility to either side. The horse should be able to vary his stride length in response to cues from the leader or when on long reins, without losing rhythm. This requires careful initial training and a maintenance training regimen maintained by a skilled rider who is knowledgeable in training methods. Activities such as classic longing, cavalletti work, and training in the classic dressage method will help strengthen the horse's back and abdominal muscles.

The backriding horse should receive a gradual introduction to its task. Since backriding requires the horse to carry additional weight in an area of the back unused to it, the horse should be allowed to strengthen its back by practicing backriding with gradually increasing weight in the backrider's position. The length of the practice sessions should also gradually increase. It is very reasonable to assume that a horse unaccustomed to backriding will suffer at least muscle soreness and soft tissue trauma in the loin area. To help prevent this, a several week introduction to backriding could occur. During the first week, the horse could carry up to a 150 pound person in the normal riding position, with a small child of 50 pounds or less in the backriding position, for five minutes per session, at two or three sessions per week. Over the next few weeks the backrider's weight and the session duration could progressively increase, dependent on the needs of the therapeutic riding program, and the anticipated weight of the clients who may utilize that horse. A slow introduction to backriding in this manner may also clearly indicate what the horse's ability and weight tolerance will comfortably be, before an injury occurs.

There are other ways to minimize trauma to the horse's back. One is to limit backriding sessions with an individual horse to twice per week, and no more than one half-hour per session, coupled with a good maintenance training regimen. During a backriding session, the horse should be kept to an engaged medium or working walk when possible. It should be constantly monitored for signs of distress which may be related to backriding. These can include a change of mood or reluctance to work; flinching or uneasiness during grooming, saddling, or mounting; decreased hind leg stride length; pain and muscle spasm in the back, and also at the poll, and unsoundness. When backriding, heavy pads that allow the horse's sweat to evaporate, or that wick it away, should be used. A very high density closed cell foam pad which does not "bottom out" under the riders will distribute pressure; such foam does not have to be particularly thick to be effective. Often a combination of pads provides the best result.

It is inappropriate to use a saddle for backriding. One would be sitting behind the saddle and behind the client. This places the backrider to far on the back of the horse and severely limits handling the client appropriately. Easing onto the horse during the mounting process enables the animal to accommodate to the weight more easily. Warming the horse up prior to the backriding session and cooling down afterward helps; in both instances, activities which encourage the horse to elongate and round the back, use the abdominal muscles, and stretch its legs forward and under itself are appropriate. After a session, particularly in cold weather, a pad or blanket over the back for a short time will prevent rapid loss of body heat and resultant cramping along with walking him till he has cooled down. It is interesting to think that all these concepts--warm-up, cool-down, muscle strengthening, and so on--are very familiar subjects to not only therapists, but all those who appreciate personal physical fitness. If these same concepts are applied to horses used for backriding, the animals will retain their usefulness and health longer in all aspects of the program.

The riding program staff, volunteers and environment require careful consideration when backriding is utilized. The leader must be an experienced, knowledgeable horse handler who can recognize the signs of the horse's moods, and who can react appropriately to its behavior. The leader should be attentive to the instruction, needs and safety of the backrider and/or therapist. A minimum of one side-aide is required; two are strongly recommended, and more may be needed. While the backrider ensures the client's safety, the side-aides are responsible for assisting the backrider to maintain his or her balance. The side-aides may need to stabilize the backrider at his/her hips, thighs, knees or feet during the session; this may also be helpful during the client's dismount. The side-aides should only provide physical contact to the backrider for stability when and where needed, as indicated by the backrider. If the client is a larger adult, additional side-aides may be needed to help the backrider maintain the client's position. The side-aides should be of a height and strength appropriate to the needs of that particular session. They should be trained specifically for their responsibilities during backriding, as these differ from other types of sessions. The need for a sufficient number of well-trained side-aides during a backriding session should never be underestimated, as the result may be injury to both backrider and client.

The physical environment used for backriding should be considered prior to its use. It is preferable that the environment be quiet, clear of obstacles, reasonably distraction free, and enclosed by a fence with the gate closed. The footing should be even and soft, without rocks or significant debris. An indoor arena may best provide these components as well as further limiting the sometimes overwhelming array of sensory stimuli of the program site. Appropriate music can enhance an indoor session by providing a regular rhythm to which the horse can walk and by alleviating boredom for the staff and client. The site should also be safe because it is predictable--that is, reasonably free from unexpected, noisy events which might frighten the horse.

The equipment used in backriding is specific to both this technique and to the needs of the client. As noted, a saddle is not used due to its negative impact on the position of the backrider. The horse should be well-padded to protect its back and for the comfort of the client and backrider. The type of pad chosen to be directly under the client will be determined by the client's stability, weight, and balance. A pad which provides less friction, and allows the client to slide a little easier, might be chosen to facilitate improving the client's sense of midline and balance. A sheepskin often provides great comfort and may be less aversive to touch for the client with tactile hypersensitivity. The pads are held in place by a surcingle, which is also chosen for specific reasons. Considerations in the choice of a surcingle include the number and position of the handles, and its overall width. A vaulting surcingle may provide security and handles for upper extremity weight-bearing. A vaulting surcingle which is narrow and with the handles placed well toward the withers of the horse is preferable because it takes up less space, is better accommodated by clients with decreased range of motion at the hips and more easily reached. An anti-cast roller, with its centered handle, is easily accessible by client and backrider, should it be needed, and again, usually accommodates clients with decreased hip range of motion, but it does take up space, and can make weight-bearing through the hands on the horse's withers impossible. A surcingle without handles may be the least in the way but leaves the client or backrider without a handhold. While it is hoped that the session is safe enough that the backrider will not need a handhold, he or she may prefer one. Finally, the use of a helmet by both the backrider and client is usually considered an essential safety feature in most countries. The helmet should have an attached harness and no brim. If the client's head control or posture is impaired by a regular riding helmet, a lightweight helmet may be chosen.

For this client, the "North American Riding for the Handicapped Association, Inc.'s Guidelines for the use of a Lightweight Helmet" should be consulted.

The use of backriding as a therapy or teaching technique can be very effective. However, for the many reasons discussed herein, the choice of backriding should not be lightly made. It is a safe technique for therapeutic riding clients only when all safety concerns have been successfully addressed. The selection, training, and maintenance of the backriding horse will always truly show if or whether or not the use of the horse is humane and ethical, because the potential for harm to the animal through the use of this technique is both known and preventable. Clearly, the credo, "Do No Harm," is one to be adhered to where backriding is concerned. Yet when correctly and safely done, backriding can provide a tremendously effective technique for improvement-- and enjoyment--in therapeutic riding.

References
North American Riding for the Handicapped Association. (1990). *Backriding Guidelines*. Denver, CO.
Barnes, T. (1990). Houston, TX
Stanford, E. (1983). *Guidelines for Backriding*. unpublished educational seminar.
Glasow, B. (1983). *Putting Backriding into Proper Perspective*. NAHRA News, Denver, CO

Editor's note: The two articles in this chapter on backriding may present you with variances. These are not intended to confuse you. They present points of views from two very experienced backriding therapists. The material should make you **think** what they are saying and make decisions based on your specific situation. Backriding is a very specific, complex treatment technique. It is because of its importance and the skill required that is covered by two therapists in this book. Additionally, a third article will be found in the *Therapeutic Riding I Strategies for Instructors* by a third therapist with extensive experience.

WHY BACKRIDING IS USED

Beth Standford Werkheiser, PT

This technique is an extremely valuable adjunct to a therapeutic riding program allowing the program to meet the needs of a wider variety of clients. Clients with more serious physical disabilities can be served as the therapist is able to provide effective proximal facilitation techniques. In many cases, backriding fosters a client's ability to function more independently on the horse and allows the staff to meet the physical, educational, psycho-social, and recreational needs of the client more effectively.

Backriding offers many advantages when working with clients with physical disabilities. The therapist has a much broader range of handling techniques available when seated behind the client. If the therapist is experienced with working with horse's, he or she is able to use more subtle handling techniques which facilitate the clients trunk to move with dynamic dissociation in rhythm with the horses movement. The therapist is able to utilize bilateral symmetrical and asymmetrical handling techniques much more effectively from behind the client than from the ground. It is very difficult to utilize handling techniques through the client's shoulder girdle and lateral trunk when handling from the ground, while these techniques are simple when riding behind the client. It is easier for the therapist to grade the amount of therapeutic input and the location of this input. This allows the client to receive only as much input as is needed for them to utilize their own muscle activation optimally. Particularly when backriding adults or children with significant head control problems, the therapist is able to use his or her other body to assist with positioning the client's trunk behind the vertical and becoming aligned over his or her pelvis.

Because the therapist is able to utilize more effective handling techniques, the client will be able to ride a horse which facilitates more dissociation in the pelvis and lower extremities. Taller horses with better movement qualities can be used as the therapist will not be trying to reach the client's body from the ground. Effective handling techniques and better movement qualities will change the client's dynamic postural control faster, resulting in improved functional skills and quality of motor control.

Backriding may also be utilized to improve the client's riding skills. The backrider can assist the client with his alignment and balance leaving the client free to focus on learning skills to control the horse. This type of backriding is most frequently used for teenagers and adults. Backriding can be used for a limited number of sessions to quickly assist a client in developing his or her ability to ride with quality alignment and move his or her pelvis freely with the horse's movement.

STAFFING REQUIREMENTS
Backriding is a highly skilled therapeutic technique which requires ongoing problem solving utilizing a team approach between the therapist, therapeutic riding instructor, and volunteers. When backriding, skilled professionals and experienced volunteers should be involved, allowing a quality session without injury to the client.

Volunteers and staff should receive training about the appropriate safety and handling techniques needed for backriding prior to working with a client. Roles and responsibilities should be clearly defined. For example, the leader is responsible for control of the horse and sidewalkers are responsible for keeping the backrider and client on the horse or safely dismounting them. During an emergency volunteers should attempt to communicate what they are doing. Emergency dismounting must be practiced, particularly with the volunteers who will be responsible for this during a session.

The Leader

Whenever a backrider is on the horse with a client, there must be an experienced horse person leading the horse. The leader is responsible for controlling the horse during a backriding session. The leader must be able to:

1. Control a horse effectively at the walk and trot.
2. Regulate the amount of impulsion and speed of the horse
3. Grade the speed of transitions from the halt, walk, trot.
4. Complete various figures while leading such as: circle, cross the diagonal, and serpentine.
5. Recognize the behavioral characteristics and signals indicating the mood of the horse
6. Calm and reassure a horse when it is nervous
7. Remain calm during an emergency situation
8. Utilize effective leading techniques while a horse is spooking, backing up quickly, or otherwise misbehaving.

Sidewalkers

Sidewalkers are primarily responsible for assisting with the safety of the client. They may be asked to assist with the client's position on the horse, such as helping to maintain the client's leg position. During a backriding session, there must be at least one sidewalker next to the client at all times. Usually two sidewalkers are present, one on either side of the horse. Sidewalkers should always be in physical contact with equipment on the horse, usually using a thigh hold on the client which may extend over the backrider's leg to give them extra stability. If the sidewalker holds only the client and the horse jumps forward suddenly, the sidewalker could pull the client or backrider off the horse. By holding the pad or surcingle and resting their arm over the client's thigh they are likely to follow the horse if it moves suddenly.

It is important to consider the sidewalkers' height and strength for they need to be able keep the backrider/client on the horse when it is spooking. Generally, in an emergency, the sidewalker keeps the backrider on the horse and the backrider maintains the client safely on the horse. However, if backrider and client are going to fall off the horse, the sidewalker is primarily responsible for the client's safety. Sidewalkers should practice the special safety techniques used during backriding prior to assisting in the session. During the dismounting procedure, the sidewalkers are responsible for the safety of the client.

The Backrider

The selection of a backrider should be considered carefully. There is always an added risk when two people are on the horse at one time. The backrider must be a skilled rider in order to be able to comfortably ride the horse. When the therapist in your program is not a rider, he or she must achieve certain riding skills prior to backriding a client. He or she should backride a normal child before backriding a client. If a horse moves suddenly or spooks, it is unsafe to be dependent on the volunteers to keep the backrider and client on the horse. It is important that the backrider have the necessary riding skills to assist with the safety of the client in an emergency situation.

The backrider should be able to complete the following tasks:

1. Ride at the walk and trot without any loss of balance or holding on using the equipment that will be using during backriding (a pad and strap or vaulting surcingle).
2. Be able to control a horse well at the walk, trot, and canter. (Be a rider not a passenger.)
3. Be comfortable caring for the horse including grooming, leading, and tacking-up.
4. Recognize basic behavioral characteristics and signs indicating the mood of the horse. For example, recognize the difference between a comfortable and frightened horse from its head and ear position.
5. Recognize signs of back strain in the horse, both on and off the horse. This includes being able to feel a sore back when on the horse, feeling the horse's back sink when mounting, or feeling the horse's back arch when walking. All of these skills are necessary for the backrider to provide quality therapy, to attempt to prevent an accident, and to allow an appropriate response during an emergency situation.

Backriding for Therapy

A team approach involving a therapist working with the therapeutic riding instructor is necessary to provide a holistic therapy session addressing the client's physical, psychological, and educational needs. The backrider must be a physical or occupational therapist who is able to utilize dynamic handling techniques to enhance the sensorimotor skills of the client. The team approach allows the therapist to focus on the neuromuscular goals while the instructor addresses the psychosocial and educational needs of the client. The instructor is usually responsible for monitoring safety considerations during the treatment. The therapist generally communicates with the leader about the gait, stride figures, and direction of the horse. If the client uses voice control, the therapist communicates the desired change, and the instructor talks to the client so a consistent flow is established. If the client is an adult, the therapist may choose to communicate directly with him or her.

Backriding the Physically Involved Client

Backriding a client with a physical disability should be done by or under the direct supervision of a physical or occupational therapist. The handling techniques of a therapist are more effective than that of a therapeutic riding instructor; therefore, the therapist will be able to respond to the client's postural needs more appropriately. The therapeutic riding instructor may be walking near the horse, may be a sidewalker, or a leader, depending on his or her role in the session and the availability of qualified volunteers. The therapeutic riding instructor is usually responsible for the educational and recreational aspects of the session. The therapist and therapeutic riding instructor should discuss who is primarily responsible for telling the leader where to go and for the safety aspects of the session.

There may be situations where it is not possible for the backrider to be a therapist. For example, if the therapist is not able to ride. If the therapist and instructor decide it is safe for the client to ride with the instructor backriding, the therapist should train the instructor to use basic support handling techniques with the client. The therapist should directly supervise the backriding session. Often the client's medical background indicates that only a therapist with skilled handling techniques should act as the backrider. An example would be a client with cerebral palsy who has a hip subluxation. Skilled handling techniques are necessary to prevent further subluxation of the hip. Under these circumstances the client should not be on the horse until the therapist can perform the backriding. When backriding is utilized as a therapeutic technique by a therapeutic riding program, the goal should be for the therapist to be the backrider.

Backriding for Emotional Support

Staffing needs are quite different when backriding a client with mentally or emotionally disabilities for the purpose of emotional support. A therapeutic riding instructor rides behind the client on the horse. Unless the client is physically disabled there is no need for a physical or occupational therapist to be involved in the session. If the client has sensory integration difficulties, an occupational or physical therapist may be needed to provide direct or consultative intervention.

THE BACKRIDING HORSE

The horse is a critical team member. The degree of risk involved in backriding is closely associated with the horse selected. The quality of therapeutic input from the horse relates to its conformation, movement characteristics (flexibility, impulsion, stride length, movement pattern), type of training, and level of training. The movement characteristics of the backriding horse are extremely important and directly influence the quality of the backriding session. An experienced therapeutic riding horse is best as it has been exposed to the unique stimuli in a therapeutic riding program, such as adaptive equipment, unusual client behavior, sidewalkers, and varied mounting procedures. Because the program staff have worked with the horse for a while, its behavior will be more predictable. The horse must be trained to carry two people on its back prior to a client with a disability being placed on the horse with a backrider.

The horse must:

1. Have a calm temperament.
2. Stand still for prolonged periods of time.
3. Not spook easily even when startling stimuli occur (obviously no horse is spook proof, but your backriding horse should be as close to this as possible).
4. Be accustomed to therapy equipment such as walkers, wheelchairs crutches.
5. Be familiar with teaching equipment used in the session (balls, rings and educational materials).
6. Stand quietly at the mounting ramp even during slow difficult mounting procedures.
7. Tolerate various methods for the backrider to dismount such as off the rump.
8. Comfortably carry weight of a backrider behind its center of gravity.

Conformation of the backriding horse will influence its durability, movement characteristics, and the client's posture. The height of a backriding horse should be between 14 to 15.3 hands. Some smaller horses work for children and petite backriders while some larger horses worth their weight in gold necessitate tall sidewalkers. A horse with a strong back is essential. Usually, if the horse has a medium length back they will last longest. If the back is too short the backrider may be sitting too far back on the horse. Long backed horses rarely last as they usually hyper-extend their spines with two riders. The withers should be low with a gradual slope down each side. Well shaped withers assist with midline positioning. A gentle widening of the withers into the horse's barrel allows the client's legs to be well-supported and encouraged to move gently into abduction/external rotation. A horse with high withers is uncomfortable for the client while a horse with no withers is very difficult to stay on if it spooks. For narrow-withered horses with an upward dip below the withers a double padding system can be used to fill this space and decrease the client's tendency to internally rotate his or her hips. Generally, a horse of moderate width is desirable. If the horse is narrow, it decreases the base of support resulting in decreased postural stability and increased compensatory hypertonus in the pelvis and lower extremities.

Do not waste a good backriding horse. The work is physically strenuous and emotionally stressful for many horses. Give them regular vacations and make sure they are ridden by an experienced rider who can let them have a little fun as well as keeping them fit and well-balanced. Monitor the horse's back for soreness and take appropriate action immediately if soreness develops. Do not use your backriding horse for all of your difficult clients or it will burn out quickly.

EQUIPMENT
When selecting the equipment to be used, the therapy team should consider protection of the horse's back, conformation of the horse, desired alignment of the client's lower extremities, tactile tolerance, and comfort of the client. The basic equipment includes a pad with a surcingle to hold the pad on the horse. Never backride a client with a saddle on the horse. Saddles are dangerous, interfere with effective handling techniques, and are uncomfortable for horse and client when used during backriding.

Pads
The padding must be long enough to allow both the client and the backrider to sit on the pad. If a thin foam backsaver can be found that will meet the client's needs, more effective protection of the horse's back is possible. A Western saddle pad, vaulting pad, or a fleece pad is placed on top of the backsaver. If the horse is broad, or less thickness is desired, a square quilted dressage saddle pad may be adequate. Clients who are have problems with tactile defensiveness will need a tactile neutral pad. Fleece pads assist with developing tonal adaptability to the weight-bearing surface.

If stirrups are desired, some bareback pads may be effective, though they tend to be too short. For children, a felt saddle which is extremely thin can be placed on top of the protective pads for the horse. Felt saddles do not cause the problems regular saddles do because they are flexible and about 1 inch thick. Stirrups can be attached to a strap surcingle if rings are added, or they may be attached to vaulting surcingles.

Generally, stirrups are not appropriate for clients who require backriding as they frequently elicit extensor tonus in the lower extremities. If weight bearing is desired through the client's legs, sidewalkers can use their hands for a weight-bearing surface. Handling techniques are more responsive to changes in the client's tonus than stirrups.

Surcingles
Three kinds of surcingles are available. The strap surcingles, the vaulting surcingle, and the anticast surcingle. The strap surcingle is thin and will not interfere with the client's leg position. Vaulting surcingles allow the client to hold handles if desired and the therapist can hold them during an emergency. The anticast surcingle has a midline handle, therefore requiring less abduction of the legs. Frequently, handles interfere with the positioning of the client's lower extremities. More effective trunk activation can often be elicited if the client is not holding a handle.

Other Equipment
Side-reins may improve the quality of the horse's movement but should be used only on a reliable horse who is trained to be ridden safely with side reins. Some horses will panic when ridden in side reins, particularly in situations when they are frightened. This type of horse should never be backridden with side reins.

The horse can be lead from a bridle with a therapy lead or from a halter. It is very important for the therapist to have reins within reach. If the leader is separated from the horse, the backrider must have some way to control the horse. Some backriders have a neck strap or breast plate on the horse to be used as a handle in an emergency.

SELECTION OF THE CLIENT FOR BACKRIDING

Determination of whether backriding is appropriate for a client, must be made on an individual basis by the physical or occupational therapist and the therapeutic riding instructor.

Physically Involved Client

The following are examples of situations which might indicate backriding would be beneficial:

1. A client who is unable to sit on the floor independently unless he or she W-sits, has a moderate to severe posterior tilt in ring sitting, or uses one or two hands to assist with sitting balance.
2. A client who has difficulty maintaining head and neck alignment in sitting, indicating significant trunk and pelvic instability.
3. Client with an asymmetrical postural pattern which is difficult to correct.
4. Moderate to severe hemiplegic client who sits with an asymmetrical sitting posture that is difficult to change with facilitation. The therapist is unable to facilitate a neutral pelvis and straight spine within 5-10 minutes with the client receiving therapeutic handing from the ground.
6. Sidewalkers or therapist become fatigued when attempting to assist a client from the ground.
7. When trotting is indicated for a client with low postural tonus to facilitate trunk activation, but when trotting, the client's head moves forward and back on the neck in a whiplash fashion. A skilled backrider can provide adequate facilitation and support unwanted movement of the head and the neck.

Backriding can be beneficial for a wide variety of clients. It may be used for a short period of time or it may be necessary for all of the riding sessions. Typically, clients who lack independent sitting balance on the floor need to be back ridden. Some clients who are ambulatory would benefit from backriding particularly if they have significant alignment problems in sitting. If the therapist suspects a client may need to be backridden, it is best to start with a backrider as the initial riding experience. It will be a more positive experience.

As the therapist gains experience working in therapeutic riding, it will become much easier to appropriately assess which clients must be backridden and which clients could ride without a backrider, but would benefit from backriding as part of their therapeutic riding experience. Backriding is useful for clients with a progressive disease as it may prolong the amount of time riding is possible. The backrider can decrease the physical effort of riding for the client and therefore prevent excessive fatigue. This may be particularly beneficial for clients with muscular dystrophy or multiple sclerosis.

Emotionaly Involved Clients

A variety of clients have emotional needs that may indicate backriding is necessary. The backrider is able to use touch to promote a client's emotional independence and security. When a child is extremely fearful of riding, a few sessions with a backrider may help them to gain the confidence needed to ride with sidewalkers. This is commonly observed when working with young children. Backriding may also help with young children having separation problems from their parents, as the backrider can use physical contact to enhance the child's emotional security at the same time he or she is being encouraged to enjoy the experience of riding. Using a parent as a backrider is not appropriate and may not be covered by your insurance.

Occasionally, emotionally disturbed children or children with sensory integration deficits may benefit from having a backrider on the horse. The horse may help the client to enjoy touch and proprioceptive input from another person. The following is an example of backriding for emotional purposes with a client having severe sensory integration difficulties. Initially, the client rode with two sidewalkers and a leader. The client enjoyed the proprioceptive and vestibular input from the horse. In the course of her treatment, she became emotionally dependent on people and needed to be held most of the time. Change from one situation to the next was threatening to her. The combination of these problems made it very difficult for her to tolerate the transition from being held by her parents to riding with the therapist and instructor on the ground. When placed on the horse alone, she would try to get off or cry for long periods of time. Backriding was the solution for her. After approximately 15 minutes of backriding, she was confident and absorbed in the input from the horse allowing the therapist to dismount and continue the session from the ground. When backriding, the therapist was able to provide input similar to what she felt when held by her parents. As she became more organized and confident, the therapist began to enhance the input from the horse, utilizing handling techniques to provide deep proprioceptive input through the client's trunk. This further developed the client's physical and emotional security. As the client became more secure, the therapist decreased body contact and handling techniques. Eventually, the therapist was able to dismount and enhance the tactile, proprioceptive and vestibular input of the horse from the ground.

When backriding for emotional purposes, it is often not necessary for the entire session. The therapist or instructor will dismount when the client no longer needs the support of a rider behind them. The client should be assessed on a continuous basis to determine if backriding is still appropriate. It is common for backriding to be reinstated after it has not been needed for awhile, particularly if the client experiences a traumatic event when not at the riding program.

TREATMENT TECHNIQUES

When backriding, the therapist combines neurodevelopmental and sensory integration handling techniques with hippotherapy treatment concepts. Individualized treatment programs are designed to address the client's physical, psychosocial, and emotional needs. Ongoing reassessment is necessary to determine which techniques are effective allowing program modification to be made. To provide effective intervention, the therapist must coordinate hand placement, direction of input from her hands, and trunk alignment in relation to vertical gradations of the horse's movement and the figures the horse completes.

Backriding allows the therapist to utilize a variety of handling techniques to facilitate improved dynamic postural alignment and postural control. The therapist can use her hands to facilitate postural alignment while movement impulses from the horse facilitate automatic postural reactions; or the therapist can enhance the movement of the horse using subtle weight shifting techniques in rhythm with the horse's movement. It is crucial for the handling techniques to be subtle and in coordination with the postural responses elicited by the horse's movement. If the horse causes a weight shift to the right and the therapist facilitates a weight shift to the left, the input will be extremely disorganizing for the client. Enhancing the horse's movement through facilitation is an advanced technique and should only be used by an experienced therapist. This technique is usually not introduced until the client has achieved adequate alignment, and a stable bases of support during facilitation, A therapist with experience utilizing the horse as a treatment modality can usually accomplish this within each treatment session.

The therapist's goal during a treatment session is to enhance the client's ability to respond appropriately to the horse's movement with dynamic energy-efficient postural alignment and control. As the treatment session progresses, the client will need less input from the therapist. The following suggestions will assist the new therapist to develop a successful treatment progression for his or her clients. During treatment, always respond to the client's individual needs and modify the treatment approach as needed.

Symmetrical or asymmetrical handling techniques are possible when backriding. Hand placement is determined by the client's alignment, postural activation, and response to the combined facilitation from therapist and horse. The therapist's hands can be parallel or perpendicular to the ground depending on the desired direction of input. Modification of the therapeutic input will be needed as the client's postural control changes. During handling, the therapist can easily align the client's trunk in front of, on, or behind the vertical. The following is a list of typical hand placements:

1. Symmetrical
   A. Top of shoulder
   B. Lateral trunk (upper, middle, lower)
   C. Lateral pelvis
   D. Lateral thighs
   E. Upper extremities

2. Asymmetrical
   A. Shoulder girdle/lateral trunk
   B. Shoulder girdle/pelvis
   C. Trunk pelvis
   D. Upper extremity/trunk

Upper extremities may be used as a point of control to elicit postural responses. Depending on the alignment of the arms, increased trunk extension or flexion can be facilitated. After the pelvis is established as a base of support, the upper extremities can be used to facilitate subtle elongation of the trunk on the weight-bearing side in response to the lateral weight shift of the horse.

Side sitting may be used for the client who has moderate to severe hypertonus in his or her pelvis and lower extremities. Both of the client's legs are on one side of the horse with the top leg in more flexion than the bottom. Sidewalkers should be instructed to prevent internal rotation of the lower leg while the therapist supports the client's trunk behind the vertical. As the client's pelvis relaxes, it can be repositioned in a more upright position. When the lower extremity hypertonus has been reduced, the horse is halted and the client is repositioned sitting astride the horse. Side sitting is not appropriate for all clients and is rarely used when backriding teenage or adult clients due to their size and body weight.

Initially, most hypertonic clients are unable to achieve a neutral pelvis and erect spine even with maximal facilitation techniques. Allow the client's legs to be aligned with excess hip flexion. As the tonus changes, and the pelvis is able to be aligned in an upright position, more hip extension can be achieved. The first priority is the development of pelvic flexibility allowing vertical alignment of the pelvis and a stable base of support. Attempt to position the client's pelvis in an upright position. Bring the client's trunk behind the vertical and align it with a straight spine over the pelvis. Positioning the trunk behind the vertical elongates flexor muscle groups which will prepare them for activation in response to movement impulses generated by the horse. Often, combining this position with an active walk will encourage pelvic mobility and trunk activation. As hypertonus is decreased, the therapist will be able to shift the client's pelvis forward until an upright pelvis and erect spine are achieved.

At the halt, the client can be encouraged to lean forward and hug the horse. The therapist handles the client from his or her pelvis and spine to facilitate a forward weight shift initiated at the pelvis. In the hug position, the client's hamstrings and hip extensors are elongated while spinal extensors are activated. For many clients it is beneficial to utilize this technique periodically during the treatment session to gain further mobility in the pelvic area and activation of trunk musculature. For clients with more advanced trunk control, it may be effective to have the horse walk with a less active pattern while the client uses his or her upper extremities to weight bear on the horse's shoulders. This is a difficult task and can easily elicit a hypertonic response if the client does not have adequate proximal stability and trunk control. Any time the client sits up from a forward position, care must be taken to prevent initiation of the weight shift with cervical hyperextension.

When backriding, it is possible to use trotting to facilitate improved trunk activation and pelvic mobility. However, this is a highly skilled technique and requires the therapist to be a competent rider. If the backrider's balance is not well established on the horse when it is trotting, the situation is dangerous and the backrider will not be able to use effective handling techniques to assist the rider. It is extremely important to monitor the client's head and neck alignment during trotting to ensure that a whiplash effect is not occurring. Usually, trotting is done for short distances on a horse with a smooth trot.

PROGRESSION TO RIDING WITHOUT BACKRIDER

Transitioning a client from backriding to riding without a backrider should be planned carefully. It is best to slowly progress the client towards more independent riding. Typically, treating from the ground is considered when a client requires minimal facilitation techniques through the lower trunk and pelvis during most of the session. Often, these clients are able to sit on a walking horse in good alignment for short periods of time without facilitation. The client's alignment should be basically symmetric as asymmetric alignment is difficult to correct from the ground.

Usually, the session begins with backriding. When the client sits with appropriate alignment when given minimal to light touch facilitation, the therapist dismounts, continuing the treatment session from the ground. If the horse is too large to allow handling from the ground, then the client may be transferred to a smaller one. As the client's postural skills improve, the amount of time the backrider is needed on the horse will decrease.

When backriding is no longer indicated, several treatment options are helpful to decrease hypertonus, facilitate proximal stability, and lessen the need for handling techniques to the upper trunk. Many clients benefit from riding prone on the horse. This can be done over the barrel of the horse or with the client's head near the tail and his or her legs on either side of the withers. Prone facing the back of the horse is usually more effective as the client's body is well supported by the horse's body facilitating improved tonal adaptability. The horse's movement encourages cephalo-caudal weight shifting and lateral weight shifting. As the horse walks in a rhythmical fashion with minimal impulsion, distal hypertonus is reduced and proximal tonus is facilitated.

When the preparation for sitting is completed, it is often beneficial to have the client sit facing the back of the horse. This position allows for comfortable weight bearing on extended arms facilitating trunk and shoulder girdle stability and pelvic mobility. If a client has significant hip flexor tonus with tendency for trunk flexion due to flexor hypertonus, riding backwards is usually more difficult then riding forwards. With these clients, it is more effective to transition from riding prone to sitting facing the front of the horse. The pelvic belt technique can be very useful when transitioning a client from backriding to riding without a backrider. A description of the pelvic belt technique can be found in the NARHA Guide in the special equipment section.

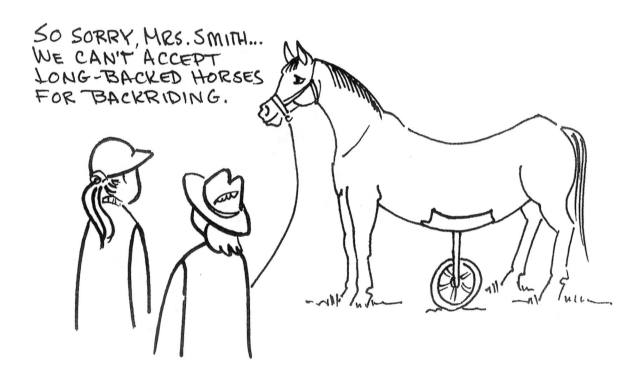

BACKRIDING STANDARDS AS PROPOSED BY NARHA

As you have read in the two previous papers, backriding is a highly skilled treatment technique. Not only does it require a therapist with highly developed skills in neurodevelopmental treatment but it requires the back rider to be a skilled rider, able to maintain ones self on the horse without holding on by saddle, reins, or stirrups at the walk and trot. Though backriding is performed at the walk, one must be able to remain balanced in case the horse is spooked and jumps forward or sideways. Not only balanced but balance while holding a client securely on the horse.

Backriding is a therapeutic technique used by licensed health care professionals. The technique is an integral part of a prescribed treatment by the licensed credentialed health care professional and must be in compliance with their professional practice act and standards of their profession. The health care professional is most typically an occupational, physical or speech therapist. He or she must be a skilled rider. Backriding is provided or directly supervised (on a one-on-one basis)by the licensed credentialed health care professional. The licensed credentialed health care professional has been trained in and has a strong treatment background in movement dysfunction.

"In backriding, the client is provided with neuromuscular facilitation or guidance with motor control by a specially trained individual who rides behind the client, on the client's same horse. As backriding is a highly skilled therapeutic technique, it requires constant problem solving using a team approach. The backrider may be the licensed credentialed health care professional, or a person designated and directed by the health professional; in either case, the backrider must meet the standards for backriding" as written in the backriding NARHA standards for all approved programs in the US. The backriding team consists of a licensed credentialed health care professional, two side helpers to monitor the safety of the backrider, a therapeutic riding instructor and or qualified horse handling expert to lead or longline the horse. And a backrider (with a secure and balance seat) if that person is not the health care professional

CHAPTER 16

ASSESSMENT AND EVALUATION PRIOR TO THERAPY WITH THE HORSE

ASSESSMENT AND EVALUATION OF THE CLIENT IN A THERAPEUTIC RIDING PROGRAM BY A PHYSICAL OR OCCUPATIONAL THERAPIST

Gertrude Freeman, MA, PT

During recent years a holistic approach both to life and to the study of the human body has found wide acceptance. In most cases attention is concentrated on one system; however the influence on an individual of all systems should be considered. A therapeutic riding session may offer an example of input from the sensory, musculoskeletal and perceptual-motor systems combining for function. For example, a riding session is aimed at the overall goal of trunk control while specific work is being directed to the development of the musculo-skeletal system. However, this session would also include the creation of an intensive contact between the horse and rider, setting up a sensory relationship. In addition, having the client pronounce the order to walk not only encourages speech, but when the horse responds, the rider has realized a cooperative behavior (Hauser, 1988).

Whatever the goal for the riding program, one is evaluating the ability of the student to perform a motor act which requires planning (feeding information forward) and preparation (predictive set). Having an explanation of the theories which attempt to describe the mechanism that allows the central nervous system (CNS) to control movement will enhance the instructor's ability to identify problems and develop treatment strategies.

When discussing control of movement, great emphasis used to be placed on how the CNS produces movement. Currently there is a shift in emphasis from studying how the brain produces movement to how it controls movement or behaviors in order to achieve specific tasks, thus the term **motor control**. Motor control stresses the importance of all the body's systems interacting in a balanced way to enable an individual to perform an act. This is explained by the systems model of motor control. Examples of systems which are important to establishing motor control are the perceptual-motor and musculo-skeletal systems.

EVALUATION PROCESS
A thorough evaluation based upon the systems model of motor control is of critical importance in order to select the most appropriate therapeutic riding program for the rider. The evaluation should be divided into two parts: measurement and assessment. **Measurement** is a process of reducing behaviors to numbers; these numbers provide objective data of change. **Assessment** combines these measurements with judgment, considers all systems influencing the client, and arrives at decisions regarding the needs to be addressed in the client's riding program. It is of the utmost importance that specific, standardized, and normative based measurements be employed when evaluating clients for therapeutic riding (Krebs, 1980).

Evaluation is a continuing process involving a series of interrelated steps which enable the evaluator to design and continually alter the riding program. During each step of the process the evaluator must employ effective decision-making as well as knowledge of and skill in therapeutic riding. Also critical to an evaluation process are change and effective communication with the client and other members of the riding team. The therapy program chosen should be compatible with the goals of the client and interrelated with the client's other therapy programs.

The first step of the evaluation process is the preliminary measurement which includes measurement of the client's present level of function and dysfunction, organization, analysis and interpretation of the assessment data, and establishment of long term and short term goals. The evaluation is ongoing during riding sessions. The instructor must constantly assess what is occurring and know how to alter the program to accomplish the established goals. Immediately following each individual session it is important to assess the outcome. Lastly, a long term reassessment of the treatment outcome is necessary to determine which goals have been met and what will be transferred to other activities in order to provide long term results.

The preliminary evaluation includes the gathering of both subjective and objective information. The medical or school record can be an important source of objective information regarding history, precautions, and present status. An interview with the client or parents is a subjective measure which can reveal information regarding the client's lifestyle, personal goals, and expectations. It can assist the evaluator in determining goals and the appropriate means of motivation for this individual. In some instances, therapeutic riding can serve as an extension of physical, occupational, speech therapy, psychotherapy, or of programs in special education centers. It is not expected that the therapeutic riding instructor will obtain nor analyze the objective data. It is the task of the therapists/psychologist/teachers to formally assess the rider and to clearly transmit relevant information for riding instructors to incorporate into treatment plans (Longden, 1988).

A client is first assessed by the therapist in terms of program offerings and the tabulated limitations of his particular disability. Record such things as sight, hearing, communication, comprehension, intelligence, confidence, balance (in sitting, standing, and walking), coordination, skin sensation, attention span, behavior and social skills, mobility, deformities, aids and appliances, and gait. Such an assessment reveals the potential client's capabilities on the ground, reveals any area of potential danger and highlights areas of particular need (McNab, Poplawski, 1988). **Together** the therapist and instructor should analyze the data to develop a problem list. Identify which of the problems can be addressed effectively through the riding program; those which cannot be helped but must be accommodated; and those which do not have an impact on the program and can be ignored. Based upon these decisions, goals for that particular client and the barriers to achieving the goals will be identified and incorporated into a plan for therapeutic riding. The determination may be made at this time as to whether or not the client can participate in therapeutic riding or if he may need to be involved with the therapist in treatment sessions.

Long term goals should integrate functional outcomes into an interdisciplinary treatment plan. They should describe a functional outcome of riding in terms of activities of daily living, mobility within the environment, and communication or interaction within the environment. Once long-term goals have been established, the next step is to determine the component skills that will be needed to attain these goals. Each component skill then becomes the objective of a short-term goal. The short term goal should identify a task in which the rider is actively able to participate and is difficult enough to be a challenge. The final step of evaluation is ongoing and involves continuous reassessment of the rider and the efficacy of the program. Compare the effectiveness of the session to the established goals and modify the plan as needed. Long-term goals may be revised if the client progresses more rapidly or more slowly than expected. The lesson plan therefore becomes a fluid statement of progress.

EXAMPLES OF AREAS TO EVALUATE

An evaluation based on the systems approach will **assume** that many systems interact to produce the outcome of intervention. To design an effective riding program one needs to evaluate all of the systems or subsystems that participate in or should participate in the riding session. It is important to know which of the client's systems are intact and how one can best stimulate those which are faulty. Examples of areas to evaluate are the environment, the perceptual-motor system, the musculoskeletal system and other functional systems which may be affected by riding, and learning (Barnes, el al 1990).

Environment

Consider the physical environment: is it motivating, appropriately challenging? What spatial and temporal demands does it make on the rider? For example, what effect do the level of noise, lighting and the presence of other riders in the arena have. Is the rider distracted by this external input, or is it appropriate to add external input to the session in order that he may be prepared to ride in varied environments?

Perceptual-Motor System

In evaluating the perceptual-motor system, one is determining how the rider sees him or herself and his or her environment. Perception is a process which integrates past experiences, memory and judgment with the sensations one is currently experiencing preparatory to movement. Think of perception as programming from the inside out as compared to sensation as programming from the outside in (Montgomery, 1990). The rider's ability to extract information from the stimuli present in the environment must be measured, as well as his or her capacity to develop an appropriate motor response. Examples of subsystems of the perceptual-motor system to be evaluated include visual-motor coordination, auditory-motor responses, cognition, body image, gross and fine coordination and motor planning. During an interview, try to perceive the attitude of the client and his family toward the riding program. What is their motivation for riding? What do they hope to accomplish? Evaluate how these characteristics (e.g., fear) may affect the goals of the riding program. To determine **cognitive** impairment, evaluate such areas as attention to task, memory, and sequencing and organization of information. Is the rider able to organize the sensory input and perceive the requirements of the activity he or she is being asking to perform? Can he or she remember the parts of the horse? The process of mounting may be a means of assessing sequence. Examine how the rider learns. Is immediate feedback appropriate? If someone with poor short-term memory, for example, is provided some delay between tasks so he or she can process what he or she has accomplished, will he or she be more successful with the riding program (Barnes, el al 1990) (Riolo-Quinn, 1989)? **Body image** refers to the client's perception of his or her body, its parts, movement abilities, and the limitations. Evaluation of **motor planning** involves determining the rider's perception of the need to move, and initiating or modifying movement as needed in response to environmental demands. Determine the perceptual areas of need and the guidance required in order for him to successfully carry out the riding program. As the client progresses, the program should be modified to maintain a challenge.

Musculoskeletal System

Examples of subsystems of the musculoskeletal system include joint motion, muscle strength and sensation. If the joints required for riding are restricted due to limitation of joint motion, alterations in muscle length or strength, the client will have limited ability to assume certain postures and respond correctly to the movements of the horse. Pain will also affect the riding program since normal movement cannot occur in the presence of pain. A thorough history should detect the level of pain and indicate its effect upon the quality of movement, and therefore the potential success of the riding program (Barnes, et al, 1990).

Functional Skills

The horse represents a multisensory medium for the improvement of antigravity trunk control. This improvement is often reflected through gains in functional skills. Therefore it is important to evaluate those skills which may be affected by the program. Examples of skills to measure include sitting balance, reach, and gait.

Riding is an excellent method for treating balance disorders. Effective means of measuring balance that are available to most therapeutic riding programs are cameras, timed video-cameras and posture grids. A camera and posture grid can evaluate the rider's ability to maintain a stable trunk both on and off the horse. Employing a timed video camera, one can evaluate how far the rider is able to move in each direction in response to the horse's movement and still maintain balance (boundaries of stability). Another important component of balance which can be evaluated is the appropriateness of the strategies employed by the rider to regain the sitting position following displacement, including his perception of this control. Weight shifts are automatically imposed upon the rider in response to the movements of the horse; assess how well the disabled rider responds in comparison to normal riders. Does the weight shift come in automatically as anticipatory postural adjustment? If so it is incorporated as part of the predictive set (Barnes, 1990; Calveley, 1988; Donahue, 1988; O'Sullivan, 1988). The rider has incorporated preparation for weight shift into his predictive set.

Improved reach is often an indirect result of improved sitting balance. One may also observe improvement in gait resulting from improved trunk control. Gait may be evaluated by measuring foot prints or by video recordings. Measured footprints can evaluate changes in step width or length; base of support or the degree of toeing out can also be determined. With the addition of a stop watch, measurements of velocity and cadence can be included (Nelson, 1974; Shores, 1974).

Learning Medium

Riding is an ideal learning medium for children with disabilities. In order to progress with academic learning a child must first master the abilities of language, cognition and perception. Realizing the value of horseback riding as a learning medium reinforces the necessity of including in the evaluation process activities which occur both during and outside of the riding or treatment session; i.e., concentration and retention in the classroom (Krebs, 1980).

Conclusion

According to recent rehabilitation literature, an individual needs to perform activities which are functional, challenging and related to the real environment in order for lasting improvement in motor capabilities to occur (Barton, 1989). Therapeutic riding is an activity which meets these requirements. To improve the credibility of therapeutic riding in the United States, further research to document its value is of critical importance (McGibbon, 1990). Many claims are made concerning the benefits of the rhythmic movement of the horse in respect to the physiological improvement of the client's balance and coordination. In addition the rider's friendship with and understanding of the animal and the horse's acceptance of the rider are said to improve self esteem. The social occasion is thought to be beneficial in modifying behavior. However, very little empirical research is available in this country which can adequately substantiate the benefits of therapeutic riding (Armstrong-Esther, 1985). Well-structured, carefully documented evaluations of clients and their individual programs can form the basis for this much-needed research. These evaluations need to be as objective as possible; simple descriptions are not reliable for base line measures or as the basis for treatment progression.

Development of a quantitative research methodology requires that scientific principles be applied to therapeutic riding including basing results on normal values and applying standardized tests for measuring outcome. There is a need to develop methods of systematic observation and devices for measuring the effect of riding programs. The instruments currently accepted by the individual disciplines involved in therapeutic riding need to be applied. Reports of studies which may serve as guides for further research are published in the proceedings of the 5th and 6th Congresses on Therapeutic Riding.

Only by performing quantitative studies will we realize the value of the horse. Through systematic evaluation and planning, members of therapeutic riding teams together should strive to apply stricter standards and methods in order to develop a concrete data base through which the validity of therapeutic riding can be substantiated. Only when this data base has been achieved will the barriers which currently exist in the areas of recognition and financial support be overcome.

References

Armstrong-Esther, C.A.. Myco. F., Sandelands, M.L. (1985). An Examination of the Therapeutic Benefits of the Horseback Riding Technique Used by the Lethbridge Handicapped Riding Association. *Proceedings of the 5th International Congress on Therapeutic Riding.*

Barnes, M., Crutchfield, C., Heriza, C., Hardman, S. (1990). *Reflex and Vestibular Aspects of Motor Control, Motor Developmentand Motor Learning.* Atlanta: Shakesville Publishing Co.

Barton, L., Black, K. (1989). Setting Functional Outcomes for Inpatient Rehabilitation. Measurement and Assessment Problems in Physical Therapy. *Proceedings from the Forum on Neurological Physical Therapy Assessment.* Neurological Section of the American Physical Therapy Association.

Calveley, J. (1988). The Effect of Horse Riding Upon Sitting Balance in People with Cerebral Palsy. *Proceedings of the 6th International Therapeutic Congress.* Toronto, Canada.

Donahue, K. (1988). The Use of Hippotherapy as an Adjunct Treatment for Traumatic Brain Injured Clients. *Proceedings of the6th International Therapeutic Congress.* Toronto, Canada

Hauser, G. (1988). Hippotherapy Under the Aspect of Therapeutic Pedagogics. *Proceedings of the 6th International Therapeutic Congress.* Toronto, Canada.

Krebs, D. (1980). Measurement and Assessment Problems in Physical Therapy. *Proceedings of the Forum on Neurological Physical Therapy Assessment:Neurology Section of the American Physical Therapy Association.*

Longden, M., Lane, B. (1988) Riding Instructors: the Vital Link. *Proceedings of the 6th International Therapeutic Congress.* Toronto, Canada.

McGibbon, N. (1990). Theories of Motor Control, A Historical Perspective. Presented at the *National Meeting of the Delta Society.* Renton, WA

McNab, J.R., Poplawski, V. (1988). Sharing the Experience of the World if the Horse. *Proceedings of the 6th International Therapeutic Congress.* Toronto, Canada.

Montgomery, P. (1990). *Presentation II Step Conference,* Norman, OK. July.

Nelson, A. J. (1974). Functional Ambulation Profile. *Physical Therapy.* 54:1059.

O'Sullivan, S. (1988). Chapter 1 Clinical Decision Making in *Physical Rehabilitation Assessment and Treatment.* O'Sullivan & Schmitz ed. 2nd ed. Philadelphia: F.A. Davis & Co.

Riolo-Quinn, L. (1989). Motor Learning Considerations in Treatment Neurologically Impaired Patients.*Proceedings of the Forum on Neurological Physical Therapy Assessment: Neurology Section of the American Physical Therapy Association.*

Shores, M. (1974). Footprint Analysis in Gait Documentation. *Physical Therapy.* 60:1163-1167.

RAFFERTY THERAPEUTIC RIDING PROGRAM EVALUATION FORM

This form maybe copied for use in a riding program only.
Copies can be obtained from The publisher of this book.
Sandra L. Rafferty MA OTR ©

Date _____

STUDENT _____

Initial Report _____

End of Year Report _____

Period Covered _____

STUDENT REPORT

Student: _____   DOB: _____

Instructor: _____   Lesson type: _____

No. Years Riding: _____   Diagnosis: _____

Ambulatory [ ] Non-ambulatory [ ]: Appliances used: _____

Verbal [ ] Non-verbal [ ] Attentive [ ] Inattentive [ ] _____

Comments:

_____

_____

A. BEHAVIOR	INITIAL (I)	YEAR END (YE)
1. How does rider come to lessons? (happy, resentful, apathetic, ecstatic)		
2. Is the Rider Cooperative?		
3. Does rider follow directions? How (spontaneously, quickly, with encouragement, detailed explanation, periodically, infrequently, slowly) ?		
4. Rider's behavior toward: horse/instructor/volunteer: (cooperative, over-affectionate, aggressive, inappropriate, spitting, ignoring, no interaction, distractibility eye contact, touching, defensive)		
5. Does rider exhibit inappropriate behaviors while riding? (Spitting, screaming, biting self, moving arms or legs, hyperactive, distractable)		
6. Does rider show allergic response to environment and how?		
7. Medications		
8. Allergies to Medications?		
9. What is rider's general Affect? (Happy, lethargic, cool, over excited, distractable, dull, in & out of reality, appropriately content)		
10. Does rider enjoy lessons?		

ASSESSMENT AND EVALUATION

B. SENSORY SYSTEM	INITIAL (I)	YEAR END (YE)
1. Can rider hear? (Distractable to sounds, deaf-uses sign language, hearing aids, lip reads)		
2. Can rider see? (blind, partially sighted, visually distractable, aids)		
3. Can rider tolerate being touched & touching? (Tactilely defensive, seeking, giggles)		
4. Is rider aware of position in space? (Follows imitation of postures, positions body without eyes)		
5. Rider's vestibular system function (balance, seeks movement, rigid-won't leave midline)		
6. Can rider remember previuos movements? (kinesthetic/synaptic memory, exercises, reining, 2-point, games)		
7. Can rider keep balance against movement & how? (walk, trot, halt, falls forward, backward, sideways)		

C. LESSON SKILLS	INITIAL (I)	YEAR END (YE)
1.Mounting Procedure: all mounting occurs with a leader steadying the horse and an offside person holding down the stirrup leather on the offside to prevent the saddle from slipping (ground, block, ramp, assist, independent, extend left leg, pull with arm, support with arms)		
2. Behavior once astride (cautious, comfortable, aggressive, non-reactive)		
3. Manner of **communicating** to horse (gesturing, facial movements, vocalizations, verbalization, appropriate, inappropriate, body movements.)		
4. Volunteer assistance needed (leader, side-walkers, full, partial, stand-by, at halt, walk, trot, back rider)		
5. Equipment used (English/Western, pad, hand hold, neck strap, reins)		
6. Can rider **move** horse forward & how ? (squeezes legs, kicks, moves seat, verbalizes, whip, spurs, gives with hands)		
7. Can rider halt horse & how? (says "whoa", closes hands on reins, closes legs, half-halts)		
8. After first step, rider (loses balance, holds on, moves with horse, smiles, cries, screams, no affective reaction, posture changes)		
9.Rider holds reins (incorrectly, correctly, consistently, inconsistently)		
10. Manner of steering (direct unilateral, crosses over withers, over hands)		
11. Equestrian/ postures (astride, at walk)		
a. Heels (down parallel to ground, up)		
b. Knees (softly hugging saddle, too tight, clinching saddle, winged outward, floppy)		
c. Pelvis (tilted toward ground, held parallel to ground, tilted upward)		
d. Lower back (arched, flat, rounded)		

240

C. LESSON SKILLS	INITIAL (I)	YEAR END (YE)
e. Upper back (straight, rounded, scoliosis)		
f. Shoulders (level and even, one shoulder higher than other, one more forward than other, which one)		
g. Upper arms (too close, squeezed to sides, held too far away from body/chicken winged)		
h. Elbows & forearm (forearm pointing to sky/upward, forearm in direct line from bit to elbow, forearm pointing downward)		
i. Wrists (cocked backwards/hyperextended, flexed, neutral, correct,)		
j. Hands (palms downward, palms facing each other, palms upward, fists too close)		
k. Thumb & fingers (thumb squeezing rein too hard, thumb correctly holding rein, thumb softly holding rein between thumb & index, thumb sticking upwards)		
l. Fingers (loosely holding reins, correctly holding reins, too tightly, hold rein between baby finger & ring finger)		
m. Neck & head (head too far back with chin up in air, in neutral position with chin parallel to ground, tilted forward chin to chest		
n. Eyes (looking forward in direction of movement, looking downward, looking upward, looking everyplace except in direction of movement)		
12. Can rider assume 2-point position & how (neck strap, mane, hips stabilized in mid-position, too weak, arm drop, trunk too forward, too upright), competency over cavaletti, trotting jumps		
13. Manner of trotting & how (holding neck strap, mane, saddle, volunteers, arm prop, balance, arms, legs, heels, position)		
14. Manner of cantering		
15. Manner of jumping		
16. Exercises (yes, no, assistance & comments)		
a. Toe touches same side		
b. Toe touches cross over		
c Touching horse's ears		
d. Touching horse's rump		
e. Trunk rotation		
☺ Putting ring on horse's (cross lateral) ear.		
☺ Putting ring on own toes (cross over)		
☺ Putting ring on horse's rump		
☺ Catches ball from front		
a. 45 degrees - side		

C. LESSON SKILLS	INITIAL (I)	YEAR END (YE)
b. 90 degrees - side		
c. 75 degrees - rotation to rear		
f. Knows right & left		
g. Throws ball using 2 hands		
h. Throws ball using l hand		
i. Takes feet out of stirrups		
j. Puts feet in stirrups		
k. Sits sideways on horse		
l. Sits backwards on horse		
m. Sits frontward		
n. Arm swings/airplane wings		
o. Swimmer's motion		
Can the rider do exercises at walk, which ones?		
17. Games (yes, no assistance, comments, N/A=non-applicable)		
a. Can rider play red flag, green flag ?		
b. One-step simple relay race (rider goes around barrel or end cone and comes back)		
c. Can rider play 2-step relay race? (weave cones, go around barrel and come back)		
d. Can rider play 3-step relay race? (weave cones, pick up an object or place object on barrel and come back)		
e. Can rider pass object to another rider ?		
f. Can rider slap hand of teammate ?		
g. Can rider do obstacle course?		
h. Play musical cones?		
i. Balance nerf balls on tennis racket ?		
j. Cone polo (knocking nerf ball off cone with stick)		
k. Nerf basketball		
l. Throwing & catching between teammates		
m. Egg & spoon		
n. Ride a buck		
Ride, run, lead relay race		

C. LESSON SKILLS	INITIAL (I)	YEAR END (YE)
o. Ride, run, lead relay race		
p. Do a drill team ride		
q. Ride a dressage test		
r. Ride blind-folded		
s. Ride a Caprilli test		
t. Ride a course of jumps		
u. Trail-rides		
v. Ride cross country/up & down hills		
w. Does rider ride in special events Horse Shows for the disabled Horse shows for the non-disabled Horse-a-thons Program Demos		

SUMMARY

Date initial: _____   Riding instructor _____   Head instructor _____

Date year end: _____   Riding instructor _____   Head instructor _____

Rafferty Therapeutic Riding Program Evaluation provides a method to determine eligibility and progress.

This form may be duplicated for center use only. Permission must be granted by Sandra Rafferty for reproduction for any publication. Sandra L. Rafferty, MA, OTR, RR 1, Box 369, Troy MO 63379.

The G.R.E.A.T. Postural Scale
(Gainesville Riding through Equine Assisted Therapy)

Linda Frease, MOT, OTR/L

BACKGROUND

Those involved with the therapeutic use of the horse are confident that this technique contributes to positive changes for the rider. Unfortunately much of the literature is anecdotal. Attempts to design *scientifically* sound studies to measure improvement have been frustrated by a lack of reliable instruments to document expected changes (Fox, Lawler & Luttges, 1984, Brock, 1986, Bertoti, 1988, Biery & Kauffman, 1989, MacKinnon, Nob, Lariviere, MacPhail, Allan, Laliberte, 1995). The G.R.E.A..T. (Gainesville Riding through Equine Assisted Therapy) Postural Scale for Therapeutic Riding is a new assessment tool designed in partial fulfillment of the requirements for the Master of Health Science degree in Occupational Therapy at The University of Florida. While the original plan was to document rider improvement in postural alignment, it was first necessary to design a tool that would provide structure for observational assessment of the characteristics of postural alignment. The preliminary results indicate that the tool has good to excellent interrater reliability. As with any new tool, there are areas that will need to be reevaluated and refined. It is anticipated that several years could be required for that process so the G.R.E.A.T. postural scale is presented here in the initial stage of development.

DESIGN OF THE GREAT SCALE

Texts on riding instruction often define the correct rider position as one in which an imaginary straight vertical line could be drawn through the ear (head), shoulder, hip, and heel of the rider. Instructors of riding may use verbal cues to correct the position of the rider by referencing the rider's position in relation to the imaginary vertical line, i.e., behind or in front of the vertical. Bases on this practice, the vertical line became the structure upon which the scale was based. The correct position of the head, shoulder, pelvis, hip and heel are located at the center of the scale. Postures that would place the rider's body in front of the vertical line are located on one side of the center and those that place the rider's body behind the vertical are on the opposite side. Two variations of the seat (pelvis) and upper body positions, arbitrarily defined as mildly and moderately off center, are located on each side of the center. Limited by the circumference of the horse, there are fewer possible positions for the leg. Therefore, only one variation is shown.

INSTRUCTIONS FOR SCORING POSITION WITH THE SCALE

The exact procedures for use of the scale will be refined as the scale itself is modified and refined. Consideration is being given to the addition of "between" ratings. For example, a rider may be leaning back only slightly. As the scale is currently designed, the rating would be a 1. Scoring a 1+ to indicate a position closer to the center may be more meaningful. Should users elect to use this technique, defining the criteria sufficiently to insure consistency, would be important for the "in-between" ratings.

At this writing, it is recommended that the user begin with a global assessment of position in relation to the center or vertical alignment of the rider. For example, is the rider in front of or behind the vertical line?

The seat (pelvis and lumbar spine) should be the initial area rated. The rider is behind the vertical, which drawing on the scale most accurately reflects the rider's position? A score of **2**, described on the scale as "moderate posterior pelvic tilt with lumber curve reversed" might also be described as a "chair seat" or a rider

The seat (pelvis and lumbar spine) should be the initial area rated. The rider is behind the vertical, which drawing on the scale most accurately reflects the rider's position? A score of **2**, described on the scale as "moderate posterior pelvic tilt with lumber curve reversed" might also be described as a "chair seat" or a rider "sitting on his/her pockets." A score of 1 is described on the scale as mild posterior pelvic tilt with decreased lumbar lordosis. This is a less extreme chair seat, but the rider's seat is still leaning back. The same logic applies to riders who are positioned in front of the vertical. For a score of **2**, defined on the scale as a moderate anterior pelvic tilt with increased lordosis, the rider may appear to be sway backed. Again, a score of 1, mild anterior tilt with normal to mild increase in lumbar lordosis, would be less extreme, but the curve of the lower back is more exaggerated than normal. The anterior pelvic tilt would be described by some as a "crotch seat." For riders who demonstrate the correct seat position (neutral pelvic alignment with normal lumbar lordosis), deviation may be noted in other areas.

The shoulders and thoracic spine would be assigned a rating after the seat (pelvic) position is determined. During the design of the scale, it was theorized that the position of the seat (pelvis) would frequently determine the position of the trunk area. If a rider is rated a **4** on the pelvis, the forward tilt of the pelvis would imply that the rider's shoulders must be drawn back to the upper body and over the base of support. This posture is defined on the scale as a flattened thoracic curve with shoulders adducted and elevated. This type of positioning might be called "stacking" and may be observed in riders with various neuromuscular disorders. Again the rating of **3** is a less extreme version of a forward leaning position in which the shoulders may be drawn back to balance the upper body. A very rounded back (kyphosis) superimposed on a pelvis tilted forward could result in the inability to maintain an upright posture. Located on the same side of the scale as chair seat, the rounded back positions would most likely be seen in combination with the backward leaning seat.

The head and neck position would logically be the next area rated. Again, an attempt was made to group the most likely combinations of body positions, but there are always exceptions. How often do riders with a correct position look down? Having every part of the body except the head in "correct" alignment is entirely possible. The reader is here warned that the head positions represented on the scale had the lowest ratings for reliability during the initial study and is the most likely element to be modified in future versions.

Next one will look at the hip angle. This will, of course, be influenced by equipment. If a rider is seated in a saddle with short stirrups, the hip angle may be affected. The "correct" positions shown on the scale anticipated a rider without stirrups and legs hanging naturally or a rider with stirrups adjusted to permit the heel to be aligned with the hip. Riders with very tight hip flexors are those most likely to have a closed hip angle. Riders sitting in front of the center, (this position is sometimes referred to as a "crotch" seat) may be able to open their hip angle more than they could if they were sitting correctly.

Finally, the knee and heel are rated based on the amount of bend in the knee and the position of the heel in relation to that of the pelvis. Sometimes a rider will extend the lower leg from the knee and push the foot forward in an attempt to get heels down. This position would be rated a **1**. If the knee is bent so much that it is unlikely that the rider would stand if the horse were removed, the rating would be a **3**.

SCALE FOR A SERIES OF EVALUATIONS

Some riders may exhibit relatively static postural alignment throughout the riding session, but the very nature of the intervention is to encourage dynamic postural accommodation. There will be movement in the rider's pelvis, when the alignment deviates from neutral. The observer must record the prevailing alignment at the time of assessment. The rider may make observable changes at one or two alignment points, the entire alignment may change, or there could be multiple changes in a single session. Demonstrating trends during a single session is also possible for a rider. For example, a rider with spastic muscles may exhibit one alignment pattern early in the riding session. As the rider's muscles relax, a different postural alignment may be observed. For the instrument to be an effective means of recording the variation of alignment patterns demonstrated by a rider in a single session, the assessment must be quickly completed. Because the scores for each alignment point are similar and cluster on one side of the vertical or another, it is hoped that those familiar with the scale can assess a rider's postural alignment in seconds. A field trial was completed in which the scale was used to assess rider postural alignment at five minute intervals during a thirty minute session.

It was possible to observe and record the initial and interval postural alignment of the rider in less than one minute per observation.

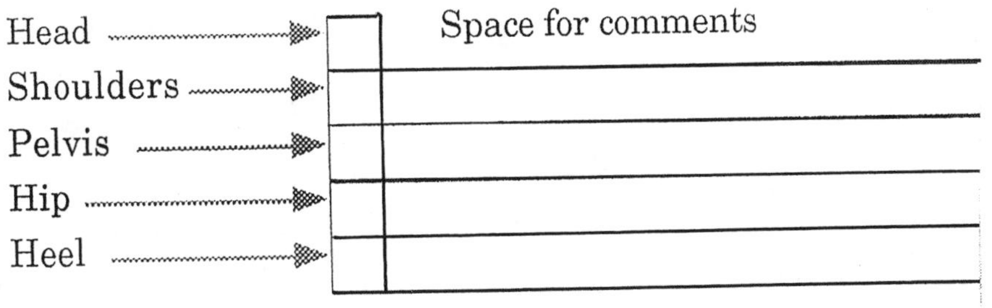

Head ⟶
Shoulders ⟶
Pelvis ⟶
Hip ⟶
Heel ⟶

Space for comments

Figure 1.
Explanation of grid for trial ratings using the G.R.E.A.T. Scale

1	3:43 pm Mounting
0	posture fairly erect
0	horse at halt - equipment adjusted
0	transition to walk w/verbal cue
1	

1	3:50 Continue at natural walk
1	Upper body and pelvis posture
1	"collapse"
0	Appears inattentive to posture
0	may be tired

0	3:46 pm Proceeded at natural walk
0	Position correction follow verbal
0	cue and maintained except while
0	responding to conversation
0	

1	3:52 Introduce forward walk
1	Rider spontaneously corrected
0	pelvis alignment with gait
0	change and sustained for 60 seconds
1	

Figure 2.
Rider observation of April 24, 1996 using the G.R.E.A.T. Postural Scale for assessment of postural alignment

	3:55 Continue at forward walk
	Begin upper body exercise
	Rider hands on shoulder during
	transitions between walk/halt and
	between natural and forward walk

1	3:58 Work on rider transitions
1	between t-point and sitting
1	positions
0	
0	

	4:02 Practice posing at walk
	Halt to adjust stirrups

1	4:05 Riding complains of being too
1	tired to respond to verbal cues
1	to sit up straight
0	
0	

Figure 2. Continued
Rider observation of April 24, 1996 using the G.R.E.A.T. Postural Scale for assessment of postural alignment

1	4:03 Mounting
1	Rider appears "floppy"
1	Adjust equipment and walk on
0	Warm up with no demands
1	allow rider to accommodate

1	4:20 Continue natural walk
1	Increase demand on rider through
1	exercise-no change in alignment
0	Note increased pelvic mobility
1	anterior/posterior

1	4:25 Continue natural walk
1	Introduce exercises to encourage
1	mobilization of trunk muscles
0	
1	

0	4:30 Continue natural walk
0	Provide verbal cues for corrected
0	posture-maintained for 45 seconds
0	
0	Rider complains of being tired

Figure 3.
Rider observation of October 14, 1996 using the G.R.E.A.T. Postural Scale for assessment of postural alignment

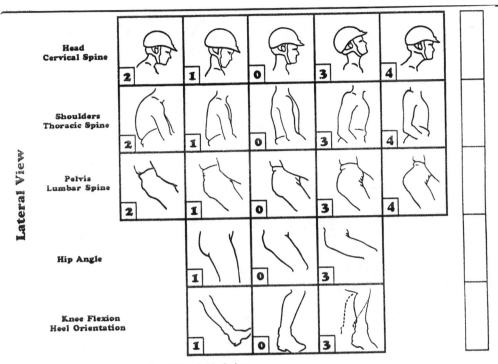

Head/Cervical Spine

Score 2   if head extended in front of shoulder and cervical spine flexed
Score 1   if head erect and balanced over trunk but cervical spine flexed - looking down
Score 0   if head is erect and balanced over trunk with ear aligned over center of shoulder
Score 3   if head extended in front of shoulder and cervical spine extended
Score 4   if head balanced on extended cervical spine - looking up

Shoulders/Thoracic Spine

Score 2   Moderate kyphosis with shoulder ahead of hip - continuous curve "C"
Score 1   Mild kyphosis with shoulder ahead of hip - slumped
Score 0   Normal thoracic curve with shoulders aligned over hip
Score 3   Flattened thoracic curve with shoulders adducted
Score 4   Flattened thoracic curve with shoulders adducted and elevated

Pelvis/Lumbar Spine

Score 2   Moderate posterior tilt with lumbar curve reversed
Score 1   Mild posterior pelvic tilt with decreased lumbar lordosis
Score 0   Neutral pelvis with normal lumbar lordosis
Score 3   Mild anterior pelvic tilt with normal lordosis to mild increase in lumbar lordosis
Score 4   Moderate anterior pelvic tilt with increased lordosis

Knee Flexion/Heel Orientation

Score 1   Knee extended with heel down - may be in front of or behind pelvis
Score 0   Knee flexed with foot perpendicular to ground - with stirrup, heel aligned with pelvis
Score 3   Knee angle closed with heel "drawn up" - may be in front of or behind pelvis

Hip Angle

Score 1   Hip angle open
Score 0   Hip angle approximately 135°
Score 3   Hip angle closed or "drawn up"

Figure 4.
Guide for Scoring

The author would be interested in comments and observations from anyone using the scale and will assist as much as possible, should someone wish to use the scale in a research project.

References:

Bertoti, DB. (1988). Effect of therapeutic horseback riding on posture in children with cerebral palsy. *The Journal of American Physical Therapy Association.*

Biery, MJ., Kauffinan, N. (1989). The effects of therapeutic horseback riding on balance. *Adapted Physical Activity Quarterly.* (6)221-229.

Fox, VM., Lawlor, VA., Luttges, MW. (1984). Pilot study of novel test

Frease, LA. (1996). Interrater reliability of the GREAT postural scale for therapeutic riding. Unpublished master's thesis, University of Florida, Gainesville, Florida -

MacKinnon, JR., Noh, S.,Lariviere, J., MacPhail, A., Allan, DE., Laliberte, D. (1995). A study of therapeutic effects of horseback riding for children with cerebral palsy. *Physical & Occupational Therapy in Pediatrics.* 15(1):I7-31.

CHAPTER 17

PROCESSING CONSIDERATIONS DURING EQUINE-ASSISTED THERAPY AND HIPPOTHERAPY

THE LEARNING PROCESS: COGNITION AND PERFORMANCE

Barbara T. Engel, MEd, OTR

The human being is endowed with the process of thinking, and the ability to acquire knowledge, and use it to perform functional tasks. Human cognition, as this is called, involves all of the processes necessary to take in information, reconstruct it, embellish it, interpret it, store and recover it, and use it to solve simple or complex problems. We use this process in our daily lives either in work or play in the performance of life skills. How successful one is in carrying out these skills is dependent on the ability to fully develop each component of the learning process. It has now been established that many of these processes develop very early in life - between 0 to 36 months. "People deprived of language as children rarely master it as adults, no matter how smart they
are or how intensively they're trained". (Newsweek's Special Your Child Edition, Spring/Summer 1997.)

Most of us have learned this material while in college - so much has changed for those who have been out of college for a while. Since it is so critical to the rehabilitation process, we will review some of the basic material here. When working with children and adults with processing problems, it is important to keep up with the current research that is developing. This article does not attempt to complete these topics but to present a simple overview of current knowledge.

Probably one of the most important elements in (re)habilitation is to be keenly observant of the client's behaviors and to know what to look for. Without critical observations, the problems the client is having will be missed and can not be addressed.

In classic hippotherapy where the client is a passenger on the moving horse, the sensory systems must be aroused, must perceive, and respond to the stimulation. This is a basic learning process without which no progress can occur.

In therapeutic riding programs, therapists, instructors, and educators are confronted with individuals who have deficits in one or more areas of this process. In order to assist our clientele in overcoming some of these deficits so they are able to carry out basic balance, good posture, riding and horsemanship skills to their maximum abilities, the staff must have a basic concept of the **normal process** in order to deal with the **abnormal mechanisms**. When the therapist can break down a task into increments, he or she will be able to assist a client by stimulating aspects of the learning and performance process. This stimulation will hopefully aid the rider in improving a deficit or a weak area. This process is complex. Not only does the therapist need to be able to identify problem areas but must also know the stimulation needed to assist in the reduction of dysfunction without **over stimulating the client**. Because of this complexity, the instructor will seek the assistance from the consultant therapists. In so doing, the instructor will be taking on a truly professional role in **therapeutic** riding.

LEARNING

Learning is defined by Webster (1966) as "knowledge of a subject or skill in, by study of, experience in, or by instruction" and defined by Lawther (1968), as "a change due to training and experience. One must learn: to survive and be happy, to progress, and to be socially acceptable." In order to effectively introduce new skills one must have an understanding of the *learning process*. This is especially true when dealing with a population in which many have difficulty learning. *"Learning is something that goes on inside a person and one cannot watch it as it happens. The therapist can only see the results, not the process of learning"* (Ross, 1977). If one cannot see how a child learns, how can he or she be taught? First one must understand how the learning process develops in clients. Then one can better understand how to teach them. De Quiros & Schrager (1978) divide learning into four processes:

- *Primary learning* allows adaptation to the environment. This process deals with survival and the adaptation of a species to changes in its environment. Animals and infants have primary learning mechanisms. They are alert or **attend** to something in their environment; they **perceive** the smell of food; since they are hungry they are **motivated** to make **adaptations** to receive the food. If they do not receive food, they may be under **stress and anxious** because of their hunger.

- The *second process* allows the use of generational (knowledge from other species' members) knowledge. Customs, cultural expectations, and social behaviors are involved in the second process. We perceive through our senses and learn from experience. We interact with others of our species. This process can be seen in young children and some animals. For example: the child attends to his or her environment; he or she perceives his or her mother's voice; he or she is **motivated** to gain attention; he or she adapts his or her behavior with a social smile and chuckle (since he or she has learned this behavior gains a favorable response).

- The *third process* implies the use of symbols which allow for the transmission and reception of knowledge through language such as writing and speech. This is a process only humans have. One must be able to attend, perceive, adapt, be motivated and use conceptual thinking in this process. Bonding has been identified as an early communication process. Riding involves all these processes. The client is said to bond with the horse. The client must be aroused, then **attend** and must be **motivated** in order to listen to directions and must **perceive** what is said. The client must then understand the therapist's **concepts** and **adapt** their behavior to carry out the directions.

- The *fourth process* implies the ability to think with verbal symbols and to formulate diverse, different and new patterns of creative communication. This last process is what can be called scholastic learning or cognition and is also restricted to humans. This process involves all aspects of learning and functioning with increasingly difficult demands to solve complex tasks and problems.

ROLE OF MOTIVATION

Lawther (1968) defines motivation "as a state of *being aroused* to action - aroused from passivity or calmness to restlessness, to a degree of dissatisfaction or disturbance, and then to directed purposeful acts." A person can be motivated to act for reasons of survival, maintenance of basic needs, pleasure, security, social status, praise, achievement, approval, or for exploration. Motivational needs can be divided into physical needs and emotional needs. Scott (1978) questions what can appeal to a person enough to induce him or her to organize his or her experiences into concepts and to think out and try solutions. Feldenkrais (1981) and Skinner (1971) feel that choice allows freedom. "When there is no option of choices, a person feels that he or she cannot change even though he or she knows that he or she engenders his or her own misery" (Feldenkrais, 1981). Choice entails self-knowledge, self-control, self-direction and allows one to manipulate his or her environment. This freedom enhances the person's sense of competence and self-worth. Therapeutic riding literature frequently mentions how much riders gain in self-esteem. Here the motivating element is the horse who provides the rider freedom in movement and, therefore, choice.

Other motivating factors include positive and negative reinforcements. Positive reinforcement includes food, praise, hugs, gaining self-worth, fulfilling values, and being given a reward (Lewin, 1935). Skinner (1971) mentions that positive reinforcements can include doing something one is told to do in order to get away from the nagging that occurs when one is not doing it. In this way one is free from attack, the attack of being nagged. This technique is used when training horses. The horse learns "trot" when asked. If he does not trot he learns he will be tapped (nagged) with the sound of the whip or the whip itself.

Operant conditioning can also be a motivating factor. One learns that he or she gets hot in the sun but becomes cool in the shade. One therefore seeks the shade for comfort and pleasure. When our actions are followed by a certain kind of positive consequence, it is more likely that we will repeat that action. The therapist or an instructor uses those methods of motivation which work well for a specific situation and in which the individual feels comfortable. The therapist or instructor must believe in the methods he or she uses with students as well as with the horses. Horses respond well to this method of training - a pat after a good job or a carrot or apple after a good session.

ROLE OF ATTENTION AND FOCUS

Webster (1966) states that "attention is the ability to give heed, carefully observe, notice; give thoughtful consideration to others; or the readiness to respond to stimuli". Attention is an important process for all instructors, for without attention, learning cannot occur. Marsh (1983) states that attention involves:

- Arousal- a positive change in behavior when a stimulus is presented
- The ability to perceive a stimulus and respond to it
- Paying attention that includes watching and/or listening to what is happening or to a task
- Attending to an appropriate or a specific stimuli
- Finding a specific stimulus among many
- Sustaining attention in order to complete a task

An infant begins to attend to speech sounds at birth or in utero. A child may attend to a stimulus but may find it too unrewarding to warrant a response (Tjossem, 1976). Children or adults with central nervous system (CNS) impairment may not be able to "tune in" or "tune out" multi-visual, auditory, vestibular and sensory stimuli. Receiving massive input may prevent the individual from attending appropriately to a selected task or to instructions. In some of our clients, each process may take more time then usual. A child is asked to lay back on the horse. He is aroused and shows good attention - nothing happens. After waiting two minutes the therapist does not expect any action from the child and continues to lead the horse - four minutes later the child lays back on the horse as requested. His arousal and sustaining attention were there, but the child had difficulty processing the command to carry out the action. Before attention occurs the individual must first be *aroused* to orient or to perceive a stimulus. Arousal, referred to as alertness, occurs on a physical and mental level. It prepares a person for some form of action. The stimulus can be perceived through any of the sense organs such as hearing, touch, vestibular/proprioception, sight, taste, or smell. The CNS provides a sensory-filtering mechanism that focuses attention by eliminating irrelevant, trivial input (Heiniger & Randolph, 1981). The information is processed through the CNS and is transmitted to the input-output centers where integration occurs. The next step involves interpretation regarding the relevance and importance of the stimulus. When the CNS has identified a pertinent stimulus, the individual must then have the ability to respond to the information in a meaningful or appropriate way. If there is a time lag in the transmission and reception of a stimulus that needs to be integrated in order for a response to occur, the individual may lose the meaning of the original information and be unable to find it meaning. Therefore, the reason to respond is lost.

Duchek (1991) describes four elements of attention:
- **Alertness**

Alertness refers to both the physical and mental levels of arousal that are needed at a given time to respond to a stimulus.

- **Selection of attention**

Stimuli bombard each of us through any one or all of the sense organs. Once attention has been focused on the selected stimulus, it must be maintained at the exclusion of other information in order for a task to be completed. In a complex task, **selective attention** may need to be maintained while shifting from one area to another. In riding instruction, selective attention will shift from the instructor to the riding aids.

- **Allocation of attention.**

When performing a task such as bridling the horse, we must allocate enough attention in order to complete this task. This is referred to as *attentional capacity*. More capacity is needed to bridle the horse than would be needed to return the brush to the basket. A complex task such as controlling and bridling a horse may require the total capacity of attention the person has available. A simple task such as putting the brush back into the basket requires less attention and may allow a reservoir to be carried into another activity such as talking with a friend.

- **Automaticity**

More attention is required when a task is unfamiliar. A task that has been learned and performed many times requires less attention, since it becomes automatic. When this process occurs a reservoir of attention is created which is then available for additional tasks.

There are a number of theories on the sequential development of the CNS pathways which influence attention and which of these pathways must first be stimulated. Scientists now have methods to study the CNS; future findings will shed light on all areas of human and animal function. **What is of concern is the complexity of a person's ability to attend. It is also important to know that attention can be facilitated by either increasing or decreasing certain stimuli.** Learning how to manipulate stimuli to increase attention is a process that takes both knowledge of and ability to analyze subtle effects on behavior and experience. But, with sensitivity and close observation of what responses are caused by which stimuli, one can get a good feel for the situation and how to handle it. For example:

Jimmy does not attend when other activities are carried out in surrounding areas. He becomes hyperactive after ten minutes; within fifteen minutes, he becomes very distracting and cannot function. Jimmy is able to attend to two-step directions when he is in a quiet area on a one-on-one basis. Jimmy's attention is better and he can remain calm when his session is in the indoor arena. There he is able to attend and organize himself to perform a requested task.

The observation of Jimmy's reactions suggests that Jimmy cannot filter out irrelevant information. He attends to all stimuli in his environment--stable noises, other clients, instructor and helpers--all this information overloads him and he reacts with hyperactivity. Jimmy can focus better and stay calmer when he is with the therapist and in the indoor arena. When most of the environmental stimuli are removed (indoor arena) Jimmy can attend. He can attend even better when visual stimuli supports oral instruction. The therapist asks Jimmy to walk his horse between the parallel poles. Jimmy could attend to part of the instruction but not all. It may be that Jimmy not only has difficulty attending but also has a problem with recall from the memory bank. The therapist cues him on the task and helps him to remember to complete the task.

Attention can be affected by: the level of development, alertness, selective attention, motivation, attractiveness of a stimulus or how it is presented, ability to perceive information, dichotic listening, stimuli from internal organs, stress, pain, or fatigue (Ross, 1977). In addition to these common influences, attention is affected by abnormal development, prescribed and illegal drugs, trauma, seizures, inherited deficits, emotional stress, physiological, psychological and metabolic deficiencies (Thomas, 1968). These multiple influences may cause an individual to be very alert and responsive one day and function poorly the next, thus affecting attention. These phenomena are especially observable in learning disabled individuals and in related disorders such as hyperactivity and attention-deficit disorders.

The following description of terms (Cruickshank, 1967) may help one understand the variables which enter into the complexity of attention:
- Distractibility or hyperactivity--inability to refrain from responding to all stimuli
- Motor hyperactivity or hyperkinetic behavior--the inability to refrain from reacting to any stimulus without a motor response (wiggling, poking, twirling, pulling, pushing, talking)
- Perseveration--inability to move from one action to another--fixation or getting "stuck" in any act (repeating a phrase or motor act over and over)
- Disassociation--the condition of seeing parts, not the whole (the head but not the body--the letter but not the word), inability to integrate
- Figure-ground--the inability to separate visually an object from its environment (the tree-barn- horse are all attached) aural figure-ground--to separate a sound from the total environmental sounds (the sound of a word/horse's neigh/airplane are all one sound)

There are other aspects of attention that must be considered. What may appear to the therapist an inability to attend, may not be a problem of "attention" but rather a problem of responding (Grandin, 1986) which can be seen in people having autistic or learning disability disorders. The author remembers as a child of five, being asked by strangers, "Does she not talk?" The problem was not the "attention" to the question being asked or the ability to talk but the slowness in the ability to retrieving the answer. By the time Barbara could respond to the stranger, the stranger had already gotten involved in something else and was no longer paying attention to her. One quickly learns to avoid certain social situations where questions might be asked or to pretend not to "attend" if one cannot **perform as expected**.

Grandin (1986) points out that autistic individuals have difficulty putting order to their world and therefore must be provided an organized and predictable environment. In a predictable and familiar environment, the individual may be able to focus and attend more readily. Grandin also points out that both in autism and in learning disabilities, a person can do only one thing at a time. This may literally mean listening, or thinking, or doing. If pressured to combine these processes, the simplest reaction may be to "phase out" and avoid the stimulation or situation. Affolter (1991) states that the search for information requires a capacity for the amount of information that can be processed (or attended to) in a given time span. We are all familiar with responses such as: "That is enough," "That is too much noise," "I can hardly think any more", "I'm too tired to go on" (Affolter 1991). What we mean by these statements is that we cannot process any more stimuli and will no longer attend.

There are other people with a severe inability to focus on anything. They appear as though they are scanning the world with no interest. With very careful stimulation, possibly using touch, movement, or music, they can be trained to attend to simple and appealing tasks. This may be for very short periods at first but the length of attention can expand in time. As the ability to attend is expanded through training, riding or therapy, the attention span is lengthened. This refers to the time a particular activity is pursued. It is helpful to understand what help a specific person to attend better. Must all other stimulation be removed? Can attention be gained with the movement of the horse? Does it help to add appealing music? Does talking to this person aid or distract from gaining attention? To understand how the person in question functions best, one must carefully observe the individuals behavioral reactions. The development of attention is followed by the persistence of attention which involves the continued pursuit of an activity in the face of obstacles such as stimulants.

It is important to remember that a lack of attention does not indicate a lack of intelligence or a lack of interest. This is demonstrated by very bright individuals with autism, head injuries or those with learning disabilities who may seem to be "in a world of their own." Treating a person with poor attention as though he or she has limited intelligence, giving him or her overly-simplistic tasks, is degrading and unproductive. It may actually turn the client "off" because of boredom. Remember too, what interests you may not interest your client even if YOU think it should. In Temple Grandin's new book "Thinking in Pictures" she described her ability to think like playing a VCR. She can not process thoughts as most people can and has little access to emotional expressions. BUT she has skills and abilities that most of us do not have. It is best to reserve one's impression and judgements, always focusing and building the client's abilities. We work in an area which is atypical, and with some people who are also atypical. We must be aware that if we are a "low keyed" person we may have difficulty arousing a low keyed child. If we are hyperactive we may overwhelm a hyperactive child.

THE ROLE OF ADAPTATION:
Phylogenetic development, called organic learning by Feldenkrais (1981), begins at conception in the womb and continues until all systems have matured. The infant will make changes or adapt his or her responses to his or her environment. During ontogenetic development this learning process continues. Gilfoyle (1981) points out that the environment continuously provides new experiences to which the individual makes adaptive responses, using previously acquired knowledge for further growth. This maturation process requires a continuous spiraling of change and learning. During this spiraling process of development, primitive movements develop into purposeful behaviors. "Purposeful behaviors are the foundation for the development of complex strategies which are adapted to perform purposeful activities and develop skill." Ayres (1979) defines adaptive response as *"an appropriate action in which the individual responds successfully to some*

environmental demand." Piaget states (Pulaski, 1980), "adaptation is the essence of intellectual functioning, just as it is the essence of biological functioning." According to Piaget, *adaptation* consists of two processes:
- *Assimilation--the taking-in* of nourishment, sensation, or experience.
- *Accommodation--the out-going* or reaction to the stimulation of the environment.

These two processes function simultaneously at all levels of development and learning. We say that in the therapeutic riding environment, the client *assimilates* the movement of the horse through his or her central nervous system and *accommodates* with adaptive postural responses. His or her central nervous system is learning to *balance*. The brain learns to understand what balance is and why is is needed. The individual then internalizes that feeling. The client *assimilates* the therapist's or instructor's words and *accommodates* by sitting back as instructed. This is a social form of adaptation. Initial changes in the organism occur as a result of pleasurable sensation, or to maintain a balance between assimilation and accommodation, as Piaget would say, to "the on-going self-regulating process which he called equilibrium" (Pulaski, 1980). The human organism, as all living things, is never still; there must always be reaction to change, called adaptation, either in the organism itself or to the environment. Feldenkrais (1981) states that when this process is not allowed to develop naturally by being "PUSHED BY PARENTS OR ANYONE TO REPEAT ANY INITIAL SUCCESS, THE LEARNER MAY REGRESS, AND FURTHER PROGRESS CAN BE DELAYED BY DAYS, EVEN WEEKS, OR NOT OCCUR AT ALL". This is an important point to remember. We can allow our clients to develop balance by allowing adaptive responses to occur when they are sliding off-balance on the horse. Let them regain their own balance with no help or minimal assistance. If the side-walker pushes the rider back to the center of the horse, **the rider can be deprived of learning the concept of balance.** This would also apply to other tasks such as mounting, which requires many postural adjustments and adaptation to movement from ramp to horse. *The organic learning process occurs on a neurological basis and must be allowed to progress in its natural patterns. It cannot be subjected to scholastic methods of learning* (Pulaski, Feldenkrais, Ayres, Bobath).

SENSORY INTEGRATION AND ADAPTION
The theory of sensory integration assumes that the active participation in a self-directed activity promotes adaption and in turn causes sensory integration. Adaption is promoted by the person's engagement and active participation in an activity which is self-directed. Adaption is the process of change in the acquisition of skills as one responds to one's environmental demands. It is believed that the adaptive process is driven by the engagement in activity. Sensory integration is the finalizing process of fine tuning the nervous system. One aspect of sensory integration theory assumes that adaptive behavior promotes sensory integration. The therapist encourages and assists a person to perform purposeful activities that in turn cause an adaptive response. This indicates that the person has increased a performance skill to a higher level integrating the individual's sensory, motor, cognitive and psychio-social systems. Occupational therapy also basis it theory on the development of performance skills - from one level of adaption to the next level as integration occurs. For example the child has gained sitting balance on the horse and learns to hold the reins with a gross grasp. As control is gained here, she begins to adapt her fingers so the reins are held correctly between the fingers. From here she begins to fine tune her arm movements so that she can hold the reins still and communicate with the horse with fine
movements of the fingers. She has adapted a gross grasp to fine finger control through integration of the sensory, motor, cognitive and psychosocial systems through a purposeful and goal-directed activity.

THE ROLE OF PERCEPTION
De Quiros (1978) defines perception as the recognition of sensory information which is produced by stimuli from the environment. Affolter (1990) feels that perception is a prerequisite for interaction with the

environment. The search for information is observed in horses and other animals as well as in humans. We perceive through feeling, hearing, seeing, smelling, and tasting. This allows us to: organize information, memorize, acquire knowledge, make judgements and interpretations, make conscious reactions and interact at progressively higher levels.

Form perception (the ability to assess shapes or objects) is developing long before an infant can explore his or her environment with his or her hands and feet. Many children with severe physical dysfunction rely on form perception for much of their knowledge of objects and their environment. Form perception is innate but also develops with stimulation and maturity. Without physical contact with objects, some dimensions are lost. If we look at a mountain covered with trees, we would not understand the formation/shape of the mountain. If we were to go to the mountain and explore the hills, the trees and rocks, we would have a totally different picture in our mind, the next time we see a mountain. The term "perceptual-motor" refers to the perception of the stimuli and the motor response. For example: we hear a voice calling our name, we identify the direction of the sound, we understand what the sound is, and we make a physical response to what we hear. We made a judgement in responding to what we heard.

THE ROLE OF MEMORY

Memory is a major factor in learning and performance. The child explores his or her environment to confront new experience. Memory helps the child to build a reservoir of information upon which to build new knowledge. Memory can be short-term, long-term and/or sensory in nature (Duchek, 1991). Sensory memory is momentary, allowing for interpretation and possible pattern recognition. It is then transferred to short term memory. Short term or primary memory has a limited capacity but can be expanded when information is grouped or clustered (Marsh, 1983). The information in short term can last 30 seconds (Duchek, 1991) before it is stored into long-term memory. Deficits in short term memory may actually be a deficit in attention, organization or metamemory [awareness of one's own cognitive processes.] (Marsh, 1983)

Long-term memory is where permanent information is encoded and stored. Encoding refers to those strategies used to levy a type of organization on the facts to be stored so that they will be easier to retrieve. The ability to sequence plays a role in the retrieval of information. If there is no order to the stored information, it makes it difficult to retrieve or find. Retrieving information from long term memory appears dependent upon the system of encoding and installing used and the depth of processing which has occurred. Memory processes are those cognitive mechanisms that are under our control when dealing with information. When the rider can attend, clearly hear, and is given enough time to **attend, absorb,** think about, and practice information taken in, he or she is more likely to use "deep processing". With this process, he or she will be able to recall the information more readily. Use of visual imagery, verbal associations, key words, or cues can aid in recall from permanent memory.

THE ROLE OF CONCEPTION:

Webster (1966) defines concept as "a generalized idea of a class of objects, a thought, a generalized notion." Experiences are developed into concepts which involve abstract thinking. Children use their experiences in perceiving their object world. They begin to see similarities and differences and will categorize or group things together; they begin to develop concepts. The understanding of concepts begins to develop at about age six years and continues to develop into adulthood. A concept is dependent on thought (Pulaski, 1980). A child can see a dog or horse and can name it as an object. This is considered a concrete object. The dog or horse as a "pet" is a concept of animals as companions, protectors or helpers. The child can see the relationship between a dog as a pet and the horse as a pet so he or she can classify these together. You can only describe this. You can not "draw" it or "see" it. As the children's concepts increase they gain additional experiences and knowledge. As they grow mentally, their concepts become more complex and abstract. Later they deal primarily with relationships. Concepts enable children to develop the ability to anticipate and to predict future events.

When instructing a child, especially one who has learning difficulties or is mentally retarded, it is important to understand his or her level of concept development. If this has not developed well, instructions must be such that they can be visualized in simple terms. For example, how would one present the concept of balance to a small child, or to an adolescent mentally retarded girl? Sally Swift (1985) has developed many images which may be useful in getting the point across. A rag doll might be used to show what happens when the doll is not balanced; it falls off.

THE ROLE OF STRESS AND ANXIETY

Anxiety is a state of being uneasy. Feldenkrais (1981) states "anxiety can be a positive, useful phenomenon. It assures our safety from risking what we feel would endanger our very existence. Anxiety appears when deep in ourselves we know that we have no other choice, no alternative way of acting." An example might be: You are warming up a horse, walking slowly around the area when the horse is startled and runs. This startles you, and you become anxious, but you realize you must pull yourself together in order to control your horse. Your anxiety alerts you to this conclusion.

Stress is the result of being under pressure, strained, tense, or fearful. It is the disturbance of the equilibrium in our life. Selye (1976) divides stress into three stages. The first stage is one of alarm, the second is the resistance stage and the third stage is the exhaustion stage. Stress, at a tolerable level, is present in everyone's life and can help a person to become more alert, to heighten awareness, to function and to perform (Heiniger, 1981). It will challenge an adaptive response at a higher level of function.

Stress affects the whole body, the CNS (central nervous system), the endocrine and immune systems, the cardiovascular, and the respiratory systems. The fight-or-flight reaction which is so well known in horses, is also present in humans. Heiniger (1981) points out the three phases of this reaction in humans. The first phase is increased arousal or alarm reaction resulting in physical or verbal attack. The second phase is the physical fight reaction. The third phase is the flight reaction. This can involve physical withdrawal, or more damaging, emotional withdrawal. It is important to be aware of signs of stress which indicate that clients are overwhelmed by a situation. Too much stress would indicate that clients are inappropriately placed in a situation, or that too much is being asked of them. When working with non-verbal persons, their visible signs of stress are so very important.

Each person demonstrates his or her stress signs and at his or her own rate. Some people can handle a great deal of stress while others respond to seeming non-stress situations with stress reactions. It is not up to the therapist, instructor or the volunteer to make a judgement on the appropriateness of stress since stress is a biological reaction. One can make a judgment on the amount of stress that a person can tolerate without losing the ability to function and learn. Observe the rider and determine which signs of stress he or she may show and under what circumstance this stress appears. Try to stop the activity that produces undesirable stress before it interferes with the activity in progress.

STRESS SIGNS!!!!!!!!!!!!!!!!!!!!!!!!

Muscle stiffness		
Unusual hyperactivity	Vomiting	White face and lips
Loss of color in the face	Damp skin	A startled blank look
Lack of eye expression	Inability to move	Dizziness
Withdrawal of expression	Inability to process	Upset stomach
Drooling	Sudden Coughing	Unusual decrease in breathing
Fear expression	Anger	Fatigue for no reason
Defensiveness	Perspiration increase	Fast breathing

THE ROLE OF PROBLEM-SOLVING

Problem-solving is involved in all performance tasks that are not immediately accessible. If therapeutic riding instructors and therapists intend to help their clients to become more independent through the acquisition of functional horsemanship skills, they need to assist these clients to develop good problem-solving abilities. Learning the process of problem-solving carries over to all aspects of life's skills and therefore reaches far beyond the equestrian arena. Instructors and therapists will recognize that one cannot assist the client in achieving these goals without possessing good problem-solving skills themselves. Problem-solving occurs when one is trying to accomplish a specific goal. Internal organization comes from quality sensory-integrative function which leads to concrete, sequential classification skills. Furthermore, good development at this level leads to abstract, sequential organizational skills. These abilities are the basics to the progression of developing good problem-solving skills (Knickerbocker, 1980). In addition to these basic elements, all the cognitive-related abilities which have been discussed are involved in problem-solving.

A person approaches a situation which requires him or her to make some decisions. He or she must problem-solve in order to move forward. The steps involved (Umphred, 1985) are:

- ◘ The problem must be identified
- ◘ There must be an evaluation of the situation
- ◘ The components of the problem must be analyzed
- ◘ The goal must be selected
- ◘ One must choose the best way to achieve each component
- ◘ One must select the psychological and physical means to achieve each component

PERFORMANCE

Cognitive and problem-solving skills are necessary in order for performance to occur. Additional areas which are involved include decision-making, the initiation of, carry though with, and completion of the task. For example the task of mounting might include:

Jose is sitting on the bench at the stable. He is **aroused** by a sound, he **attends** and identifies a voice. He **adapts** his behavior to locate the voice and hears the instructor ask him to mount the horse from the mounting block. He **interprets** the instructions, maintains **focus**, is **motivated** to follow the directions. He **shifts his focus, initiates** action and **perceives** the location of the horse and mounting block, then walks to the mounting block. Jose must **remember** how to climb the block and **problem-solve** the mounting procedure. He then must initiate the action and **perform** the task of mounting the horse.

Conclusion

Clients who come to a therapeutic riding program , to participate in therapy or graduate to functional skills in horsemanship have a great deal to learn. Any equestrian knows that the only way to be around horses is the safe way. Safety around horses requires a lot of knowledge. There is so much to learn and the staff of a therapeutic riding program has a wonderful opportunity to teach. Some people have a natural gift of passing on knowledge to others but most people need to understand and develop these skills. Teaching a population who may have difficulty learning requires an in depth knowledge of the total process. By understanding the learning process, the instructor and his or her staff have a better understanding of how to communicate with their clients and teach them all they can about horsemanship and related skills.

References

Affolter, F. (1990). *The Use of Guiding as a Perceptual Cognitive Approach.* Course notes.

Ayres, A.J. (1979). *Sensory Integration and the Child.* Los Angeles: Western Psychological Services.

Bobath, K. (1980). *A Neurophysiological Basis for the Treatment of Cerebral Palsy.* Philadelphia: J.B. Lippincott Co.

Cruickshank, W.M. (1967). *The Brain-injured Child in Home, School, and Community.* Syracuse: Syracuse University Press.

De Quiros, J.B.; Schrager, O.L. (1978). *Neuropsychological Fundamentals in Learning Disabilities.* San Rafael: Academic Therapy Publications, Inc

Duchek, J. (1991). Cognitive Dimensions of Performance in Christiansen, C., Baum, C. *Occupational Therapy Overcoming Human Performance Deficits.* Thorofare: Charles B. Slack Inc.

Feldenkrais, M. (1981). *The Elusive Obvious.* Cupertino: Meta Publications. pp 29-37

Gilfoyle, E.M., Grady, A.P., Moore, J.C. (1981). *Children Adapt.* Thorofare: Charles B.Slack, Inc. pp 47-55, 173-193.

Grandin, T., Scariano, M.M. (1986). *Emergence: Labed Autistic.* Novato, CA: Arena Press.

Grandin, T. (1995). *Thinking in Pictures.* Vintage Books, NY

Heiniger, M.C., Randolph, S.L. (1981). *Neurophysiological Concepts in Human Development.* St. Louis: The C.V. Mosby Co. 6,126, pp 177-208.

Knickerbocker, B. (1980). *A Holistic Approach to the Treatment of Learning Disabilities.* Thorofare: Charles B. Slack, Inc.

Lawther, J.D. (1968). *The Learning of Physical Skills.* Englewood Cliffs: Prentice-Hall,Inc. p 47.

Lewin, K. (1935). *A Dynamic Theory of Personality.* New York: McGraw-Hill Book Co.,Inc.

Marsh, G.E., Price, B.J., Smith, T.E.C. (1983). *Teaching Mildly Handicapped Children.* St. Louis: C.V. Mosby Co.

Pulaski, M.A.S. (1980). *Understanding Piaget.* New York: Harper & Row Publishers. pp 109-110

Ross, A.O. (1977). *Learning Disability.* New York: McGraw-Hill Book Co.

Scott, D.H. (1978). *The Hard-to-teach Child.* Baltimore: University Park Press.

Selye, H. (1976). *The Stress of Life, revised ed.* New York: McGraw-Hill Book Co.

Skinner, B.F. (1938). *The Behavior of Organisms.* New York: Appleton-Century Crofts.

Swift, S. (1985). *Centered Riding.* North Pomfret: David & Charles Inc.

Thomas, A, Chess, S., Birch, H.G. (1968). *Temperament and Behavior Disorders in Children.* New York: New York University Press.

Tjossem, T.D. (1976). *Intervention Strategies for High Risk Infants and Children.* Baltimore: University Park Press. pp 152-53

Umphred, D.A. (1985). *Neurological Rehabilitation.* St. Louis: The C.V. Mosby Co.

Webster's New World Dictionary, College Edition. (1966). Cleveland: The World Publishing Co. pp 302,758,833.

CHAPTER 18

TREATMENTS OF CLIENTS WITH SPECIFIC DIAGNOSIS

THE TREATMENT OF HYPOTONIA

Colleen Zanin, M.Ed, OTR

For years now we have seen the evidence of the results of the horse's three dimensional movement and its effect on relaxing spastic or hypertonic muscles. Typically, we can observe a rider with very limited movements in the pelvis or legs, barely, nevertheless able to mount the horse or to separate the legs to straddle the horse. Almost magically the rider sits upright and astride after 15-20 minutes of sensory input supplied through the horse's back muscles. Along with the improvement noted in the rider's balance, the relaxation of muscle tone, particularly in the lower extremities, has helped to put the horse in the same arena as the "Swiss Ball" or "Bolster" as an aid in the treatment of clients with movement disorders resulting from central nervous system damage or dysfunction.

This paper discusses another movement disorder - the flip side of hypertonus - "hypotonia" or low muscle tone. Because the characteristics of hypotonia are often less obvious than hypertonus, they are frequently overlooked. Yet, the improper management of the hypotonic client can be just as harmful, if not more so, as when working with the rider with increased muscle tone.

DEFINITION OF HYPOTONUS
While researching the subject of hypotonia, it was found that the term is frequently misused or used interchangeably with such words as flaccidity, flaccid paralysis, paresis, or weakness. In this paper the term is based on the definition given in *Physiotherapy in Disorders of the Brain* (Carr and Shepherd, 1980). This book describes hypotonus as <u>decreased postural or muscle tone caused by a lesion or lesions in a part</u> of the <u>brain which results in difficulty or inability to move, to sustain a posture against gravity, or to support functional movement.</u> It is not a result of injury to the spinal cord resulting in paraplegia or quadriplegia. The <u>quality</u> of the muscle is associated with postural limpness or a feeling of heaviness when the limb is moved passively by the clinician. There is a definite head lag when the head is lifted against gravity. Hypotonia is frequently seen in diagnoses such as: cerebral palsy, athetoid or ataxia, Down Syndrome, head injury, and various Developmental Disorders.

CHARACTERISTICS OF THE HYPOTONIC PATIENT
The hypotonic patient may have difficulty interacting with the environment due to a limited ability to maintain a secure posture. The limbs and body appear to sink into gravity. There is a lack of joint stability, particularly in the proximal musculature and throughout the midline, which limits dynamic postural stability or graded movement.

Hypotonic clients may appear passive or unmotivated to move. The lack of movement is likely due to the amount of energy that they must expend to move their heavy, limp, limbs. The client has difficulty shifting weight, and has an inability to bear weight through the limbs in normal alignment. Due to decreased sensory awareness, the hypotonic child or adult usually has a high threshold for pain. Therefore, the therapist or instructor must be very aware of pressure sores or over-stretching the ligaments.

TREATMENT OF THE HYPOTONIC RIDER

The treatment of the hypotonic rider is based on the principles of neurodevelopment treatment, an approach developed by the late Karl and Berta Bobath. Several techniques are used to gain joint stability and to improve the quality of the movement patterns.

1. Weight bearing or joint compression is used to increase joint co-contraction and to improve proximal stability.
2. The facilitation of weight shift and balance reactions is stressed during treatment to improve movement transitions.
3. Proper biomechanical alignment of the joints is monitored and facilitated.
4. Training the client to place and hold a limb against gravity is encouraged to promote strength and joint stability.
5. Application of external sensory input, such as tapping or vibration may be used to help activate the muscles.

In addition to these handling or positioning techniques, the therapist's or instructor's use of speech is important. Frequently the correct phrase to trigger a motor response may be found. A rider many not respond to a request when it is phrased one way, but may respond when it is phrased differently. For example, "push" may not get a response, but "reach toward the sky" may get the desired reaction. The rider may want to use his or her own speech while doing a movement. This is often an effective way to reinforce movement because it helps the rider to concentrate and to regulate the movement through auditory feedback.

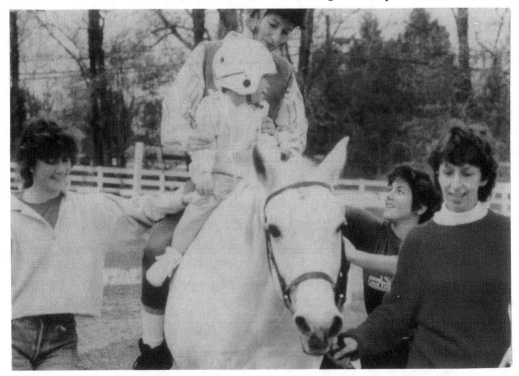

A HYPOTONIC CHILD BEING TREATED BY THE NDT APPROACH

Visual stimulation is also an effective teaching tool. The client can be encouraged to look at the part of the body he or she is trying to move. A mirror can be used to identify a limb. This helps the rider to concentrate his or her attention on movements of the limbs and reinforces laterality and spatial awareness.

PRECAUTIONS OF THE HYPOTONIC RIDER

The hypotonic rider may have more subtle movement problems than the spastic or stiff rider, but he or she is just as much at risk for improper handling and injury while on the horse. Unlike the spastic or stiff child who has a limited range of motion due to tight muscles, the hypotonic child or adult is "hypermobile" and has an excessive range of limb excursions. There is a lack of ligament, muscle, and tissue resistance toward extreme movement ranges. For example, the consistent use of the hip abduction, extension and internal rotation [the usual sleeping and riding position] can create a lack of joint range into hip adduction, extension and internal rotation.

Hip dislocation may also occur when this position is used excessively, or when hip ligaments are excessively weak. Scoliosis may result due to body asymmetries and the effects of gravity on the low tone trunk. A good clinical eye for normal movement and proper alignment on and off the horse is important. To provide a safe and effective therapeutic ride, immediate alterations of improper alignment are vital when abnormalities are observed. If one has any uncertainties, it is best to check with a physical or occupational therapist who has more experience with the hypotonic clients, and/or the client's physician.

References:
Boehme, R. 1987. The Hypotonic Child: treatment of Postural Control, Endurance, Strength and Sensory Organization. Boehme Workshop. 8642 North 66th St. Milwaukee, WI 53223.
Carr, J., Shepherd, RB. 1980. *Physiotherapy in Disorders of the Brain.* William Heinemann Books, London, ASPEN Systems Corp, 1600 Research Blvd., Rockville MD.20850 (2nd Printing)
Cruickshank, WR., Editor. 1976. *Cerebral Palsy: A Developmental Disability*, 3rd ed Revised. Syracuse Univ Press.
Tscharnuter, I., Scherzer, A. 1983. *Early Diagnosis and Therapy in Cerebral Palsy.* Marcel Dekkeer Inc., NY 10016

DUCHENNE MUSCULAR DYSTROPHY

Carol A. Heugel, BHS, PT

WHAT IS IT?

Muscular Dystrophy is not one disease; the term designates a group of muscles destroying disorders, which vary in a hereditary pattern, age of an onset, initial muscles affected, and rate of progression. Duchenne Muscular Dystrophy (DMD) is confined to boys. Its incidence is approximately one in 3500 male births. DMD is inherited as an X-linked recessive trait in half the cases. Otherwise, it is caused by a new genetic mutation. In the X linked type, females carry the defective gene that causes the disorder, but show no symptoms. When a mother carries the gene, her female children each have a 50% chance of carrying the gene also, and each male child has a 50% chance of having the disease. Diagnosis is confirmed through a battery of tests including electromyography (EMS) and muscle biopsies. Changes in the muscle include degeneration of muscle fibers with replacement by fat and connective tissue. In recent years, scientists have identified the gene containing the defects that cause DMD, and a milder form of the disorder, Becker Muscular Dystrophy. Becker M.D. is characterized by later onset and slower progression. This information has helped greatly with definitive diagnoses of affected boys and being able to tell female relatives whether or not they are carriers.

SYMPTOMS

DMD is present from conception, but symptoms are not usually evident until the child is 3-6 years of age. The visible symptoms are a result of progressive muscular weakness that first appear in the proximal muscles (hips, shoulders and trunk). For example, a boy will have difficulty in running to keep up with his peers. He will have difficulty going up stairs, and will take one step at a time, instead of step over step. Eventually, he will have to pull himself up by using the handrail. He will have difficulty coming to stand and will need to use his hands to help himself up, a finding called the Gower's sign. Additional early symptoms include:

1. Walking on tiptoes. This is caused by weakness in the anterior tibial and peroneal muscles.
2. Development of an exaggerated curvature of the lower spine (lardosis) with protrusion of the abdomen.
3. Protrusion of the shoulder blades (winging scapulae) indicate progressive weakness in the shoulder region. This is typically observed 3-5 years after the initial symptoms.
4. Stance will become progressively wider based with hip abduction and external rotation, causing toes to point outward.
5. When ambulating, development of a waddling type of gait.
6. Increasing frequency of falls.
7. When attempting to sit on the ground, a "controlled fall" will be performed.

A tailor sit position is typically used when sitting on the ground, as it provides maximal stability and requires the least amount of trunk control to maintain. Muscles will look healthy, and may be enlarged. This is called "pseudo-hypertrophy," or false muscle enlargement. It is caused by an accumulation of fat. It is often obvious in the calf musculature. Intellectual impairment is common. The mean IQ of boys with DMD is approximately 15-20% lower than that of their peers. Personality patterns are characterized by dependency, withdrawal, passivity, and lack of ambition, attentiveness, and spontaneity.

Inevitably the weakness progresses until the child can no longer walk. He will require the use of a wheelchair for long distances at first, and then for all mobility. The age when a child first requires a wheelchair varies; many children are between eight and ten years old, and most use a wheelchair by age twelve. Initially, a manual wheelchair will be used. Progressive loss of strength in the shoulders and upper arms will occur, until it becomes impossible to lift objects of any weight. Eventually lifting his hands to his mouth unaided will be impossible for the child. Strength in the fingers and hands is retained, but fine motor control diminishes. A motorized wheelchair, which allows independent mobility, is eventually necessary.

As the amount of time a child with DMD uses a wheelchair increases, the weakness of one group of muscles, but not of their antagonists (opposing muscles), results in permanent shortening of the stronger muscles. This leads to the eventual development of contractures (joint tightness), especially in the hips, knees and ankles. He also develops more curvature of the spine, side-to-side, called a "scoliosis." His weight tends to increase as the level of activity decreases, and the caloric intake remains the same, or more commonly, increases.

TREATMENT
Once a definitive diagnosis is made, boys with DMD are usually seen by a variety of medical and health professionals, including an orthopedist, a neurologist, and physical and occupational therapists. Medical treatment and therapy are aimed at slowing the progression of the disease. Affected children will still develop marked disability even if all known therapeutic measures are followed, but they will experience less physical and emotional discomfort, remain mobile longer, and their lives may be prolonged for several years. Treatment, including therapeutic use of the horse, can make a difference. The idea of a "normal" activity will be enthusiastically received by the child as well as his family, who have been suddenly thrust into a medical abyss.

USE OF EQUINE-ASSISTED THERAPY
When a child with DMD is referred to your program, having open communication initially with the primary physician and therapist will be important. Communication should continue as the disease progresses, with increasing muscle weakness and decreasing function. While the child is still walking independently, allow him to participate in as many activities as your program allows. Your goal will be to keep him at his present level of function for as long as possible. Caution must be used to prevent fatigue. This could hasten the breakdown of muscle fibers, which lack normal regeneration capabilities. Ultimately, this could actually accelerate the muscle weakening process and should be avoided.

TACK OPTIONS
One may choose to use a bareback pad or saddle. Both have benefits. A bareback pad allows for a multitude of positions and transitions, including side and backward sitting, as well as vaulting positions. When use of a saddle is desired, dressage or all purpose types may be most beneficial, as their seat design will help to keep the pelvis in a neutral alignment. Use of synthetic saddles has been found to be beneficial. The saddle's fabric provides friction with the rider's clothing and thus reduces slipping. As decreased range of motion of the calf musculature (plantar-flexors) becomes more of a concern, use of stirrups, positioned under the ball of each foot, can help. Sidewalkers can provide traction at the heels to provide a prolonged stretch.

CHOICE OF HORSE AND TEAM
A good team is imperative to really safe and effective equine-assisted therapy. An appropriate horse is an extremely important member of the team and thus must be assessed carefully. The ability to stand still during

the transfer is essential. A strong back is necessary to prevent strain as the rider's size increases. Wide-backed horses are desirable to provide a good base of support for the rider. Adjustability of the horse's stride length is desirable.

MOUNTING AND DISMOUNTING

Initially, when mounting, allow as much independence as possible. A stair step type of mounting block should be sufficient, with assistance provided only as necessary. As weakness in the hip extensors (gluteus maximus) progresses, more assistance (at the hips) will need to be provided. The child will exhibit a progressively wider-based stance (with hip abduction and external rotation) to maintain standing and walking balance. The steps can still be used as long as the child is ambulatory, but must be wide enough to accommodate the increasingly wide stance.

The dismount can be performed by having the rider lean forward, then helping his right leg back and over the cantle of the saddle and the rump of the horse. Then, have the rider lie prone over the saddle/barrel of the horse and slowly lower him down to the ground, feet first. Use the front of your body and the side of the horse to "sandwich" the rider for greater control. When the rider initially begins to use a wheelchair, this dismount can continue to be used by having the wheelchair brought next to the horse before dismounting and having the child pivot to sit in the chair.

There are a variety of ways to mount once the child is dependent on a wheelchair. Available equipment and staff as well as personal preference may all have a role in the decision making. A well-equipped facility may have access to an overhead lift system. If the child is to be physically lifted up onto or off the horse, care must be taken due to shoulder girdle weakness. This is shown by Meryon's sign when lifting under the armpits, the child will slide through the lifter's hands. Therefore, if lifting from behind the child, have the child cross his arms across his chest. The lifter can place his or her arms around the child and across them in front of the rider's chest, then grasp the rider's wrists, keeping the rider's arms close to his body, to provide stability and prevent sliding

If a wheelchair mounting ramp is available, a standing pivot transfer, performed by a knowledgeable person using good body mechanics, can be made from the wheelchair at the top of the ramp. An assistant will stand on the off (right) side of the horse, elevated to provide adequate height (is on a step-type mounting block). The horse leader stands in front of the horse to ensure the horse stands perfectly still during the mounting process. When preparing for the mount, ensure the wheelchair brakes are locked. Assist the child to scoot to the edge of the seat. Place your knees to the outside of his to prevent excessive abduction of his hips. Lift him from his hips into extension to stand, then pivot around to have him side-sit upon the saddle. As soon as possible, complete a "crest type mount." Lift the rider's right leg over the neck of the horse to achieve a straddle seat position. Initially, he may be anxious. Transferring from the low, stable, supportive wheelchair onto the much higher, less supportive, dynamic back of the horse is an intimidating experience for any wheelchair dependant rider. As soon as possible, take just a few steps away from the mounting ramp. Be cautious of the rider's foot and leg on the side of the mounting ramp that it does not become caught or left behind. In just a few moments, the rider should adapt to the horse's movements and feel comfortable and confident and ready to "walk on".

Dismounting may require some "creativity". One method is like a reverse of the mounting process, but away from the mounting ramp. Have two persons at the near (left) side of the horse and one on the off side, while the horse leader ensures the horse stands still. Place the rider's wheelchair, facing forward, directly at the horse's near side. The primary instructor/therapist should stand behind the chair, facing forward, and an assistant should stand in, front of the chair, facing the rider. A third person on the far side of the horse should assist the rider to lift his right leg over the neck of the horse. The rider should then cross his arms in front of his chest so the primary instructor or therapist can reach around the rider's sides from behind, cross his or her arms in front of the rider's chest, and grasp the rider's wrists. The assistant standing in front of the wheelchair can hold each of the rider's legs behind the knees. Together, the two persons on the near side of the horse can slowly lower the rider directly into his chair.

MOUNTED ACTIVITIES

The movement of the horse at the walk provides passive movement of the pelvis and facilitates active reactions through the trunk. Since the muscle weakness occurs proximally in the hips, trunk and shoulders first, these are the areas that initially will benefit the most from equine-assisted therapy. Activation of the trunk is a primary goal, and can be achieved in a variety of ways. A rider should be discouraged from using his hands for support in order to encourage maximal trunk activity. He may use his hands to hold reins. Playing games, such as tossing and catching a ball or ring toss keeps hands occupied as well as further enhancing use of trunk musculature while reaching out in all directions. Overhead hand activities are especially encouraged early on as this achieves active shoulder mobility, lengthening through the rib cage and allowing for maximal pulmonary (lung) expansion as well. The rider's arms may tire easily, though, in this position and he may rest his hands on his head. Be careful, as he could end up with the weight of his arms pushing down on his head and collapsing through his trunk. Verbal or physical prompts can be used to maintain upright position. Stop this (or any) activity when he tires.

To accentuate postural control in the sagittal plane (front to back), transitional work and riding on gentle inclines are useful. Halting from the walk, decreasing the stride length or slowing the pace are examples of downward transition which facilitates an anterior (forward) position of the pelvis and activation of the back extensor muscles. Walking down a hill also encourages this. Walking on from a halt, increasing stride length or pace (upward transition) or walking up a hill causes the pelvis to tip back into a posterior tilt and activates abdominal muscles as the rider adapts to the positional change. Be cautious not to over challenge the rider. He will use his hands to support himself and maintain his balance, rather than his trunk musculature. Together, these activities encourage a neutral position of the rider's pelvis, which is necessary for proper trunk alignment.

Lateral control, in the frontal plane, can be facilitated by having the horse walk in circles or serpentine patterns. This challenges trunk control through enhanced weight shifting to the side toward the outside of the circle. Care should be taken to make the circles as round and symmetrical as possible. The smaller the diameter of the circle, the greater the challenge. The ½ circles of the serpentine, alternating directions, should be equally sized. If the rider can tolerate it, sitting sideways on the horse also provides an enhanced lateral weight shift, primarily on the caudal (tail end) side.

As the disease progresses, alterations must be made to accommodate the rider. Sidewalkers now play a vital role and must be attentive. They can provide traction at the riders heels (while stirrups are used and properly positioned at the balls of the feet) to assist with lengthening of the calf musculature. Grasping the heel of the shoe is easy and can be pulled down, when the rider's heel pulls up. The removal of shoes while mounted is one way to deal with this while providing better visual feedback for the instructor/therapist. Sidewalkers can also provide assistance at the rider's knees, helping to keep the rider's hips in adduction and internal rotation provide assistance at the rider's knees, helping to keep the rider's hips in adduction and internal rotation (out of his typical "frog-legged position"). The goal is to keep the rider's inner thighs in contact with the saddle. Having the rider actively squeeze with his legs activates weakening hip musculature (adductors and internal rotators) while providing the horse with a cue for an upward transition.

Use of hands by the rider for support at the pommel will eventually be needed at the start of the session. The horse's strides should be slow and even. After a few minutes the rider will accommodate the movement and more challenge can then be provided as tolerated. This can be accomplished by having the rider place his hands on his thighs or hold the reins (attached to the horse's halter, preferably not a bit), and by lengthening the horse's stride. Exercises (ideally in a game playing atmosphere) for active or active-assisted mobility of all extremities can be performed. Encourage reaching in all directions to facilitate use of both arms and providing more challenge to the trunk. Be especially careful not to over challenge, as the child cannot maintain trunk control as easily as before. Use of the trunk through the dynamic movement of the horse provides the assistance needed in maintenance of postural control, thus slowing the progression of scoliosis (spinal curvature) development as well as allowing for maximal pulmonary function. This is difficult to achieve in any other therapeutic setting. Besides, on the back of a horse the exercises are fun and it is great for self-esteem.

UNMOUNTED ACTIVITIES

Once a child is wheelchair dependent he will need to learn the safest positions for himself and his wheelchair around the horse that will allow him the easiest access to the horse. This requires problem solving, which can then carry over to other settings. Grooming the horse from the wheelchair encourages active use of the young man's arms. There are few activities that necessitate having his arms over his head. This will assist him in prolonged maintenance of dressing/undressing and other self care skills. The higher the horse's body part, the higher he must reach. Brushing is more difficult than using a curry comb, because he has to lift the brush off with each stroke, requiring more active shoulder control. Remember that the horse has two sides. Take advantage of both of them during grooming, encouraging the use of both arms.

The horse's legs offer the different challenge of having to lean over to reach. This activity can provide a carry over into maintenance of the ability to retrieve dropped objects (Author's note: Many boys with DMD acquire service dogs, like Canine Companions, as their disease progresses, to assist with jobs like retrieval of dropped objects). When cleaning the brush with the curry comb, one may see a tendency for the boy to stabilize his elbows on his thighs or arm rests. By doing this he is using only his wrists and fingers, the distal areas (farthest from the trunk) that maintain strength and function the longest.

DETERMINATION TO CONTINUE EQUINE-ASSISTED TREATMENT

Continuance of therapeutic use of the horse for the person with DMD is determined by his medical condition and the capabilities of the individual riding facility. As some scoliosis progresses, a surgical fusion with steel rods is often performed to prevent further curvature. This may be a contraindication for riding, but time spent with horses need not end. He can still do grooming from his wheelchair if physical assistance is provided to help him maintain shoulder elevation. Use of the hands remains and activities such as tack cleaning offer a pleasant task. Driving a wheelchair accessible cart (with good shock absorption) may also be a possibility.

DISEASE PROGRESSION

With additional weakness of the chest muscles, the young man will have difficulty breathing deeply or coughing effectively. Even minor colds and chest infections have a high chance of leading to pneumonia. Severe respiratory problems mark the disease's final stages, usually claiming the lives of those affected during their twenties. The heart muscle is often affected, and some may die of cardiac failure.

Over the past few years, encouraging research advances have been made. There is hope that in the near future, treating the disease will be possible. For more information about DMD or any other Muscular Dystrophy, contact: Muscular Dystrophy Association, 3300 East Sunrise Drive, Tucson, AZ 85718-3208; 1-800-572-1717

HIPPOTHERAPY AND AUTISM

Hana May Brown, PT

Autism is a broad spectrum disorder that usually involves one or more of the sensory systems. The presenting signs are often contradictory and vary from individual to individual. The person may be hyper-reactive or hypo-reactive, and may often exhibit components of both sensory states. For example, a person with hyper acuity (increased sense of hearing) may actually experience pain from a sound considered to be within the "normal" range of tolerable sound. The person may not present any form of interaction and/or eye contact. Conversely, the person might exhibit attention-seeking behaviors and use eye contact as a form of communication. Diminished tactile sensation may make the autistic person relatively pain-free and unaware of serious injuries. However, this same person may be extremely sensitive to light touch and certain textures. Dr. Temple Grandin who is autistic, learned as a child that deep pressure has a calming effect. As an animal behaviorist and one who designs equipment for handling livestock, she has developed a "squeeze machine," patterned after a cattle chute, as a treatment modality.

All senses may be affected. Some autistic people state that looking at a particular color is painful. Some people have taste and tactile problems in their mouths and will eat only foods with certain flavors and consistencies. Most clinicians discover that they cannot wear perfumed products around these clients. Sight, hearing, taste, smell, and touch are special senses that are stimulated by the environment. The information that comes from within the body - muscles, tendons, and joints - tells where the body is in space and is called proprioception. How the body reacts to gravity and movement is determined by the vestibular system input. How all the sensory systems react in response to external and internal stimuli depends on the person's ability to process the information. It appears that much of the autistic person's communication problem comes from difficulties in processing

The Diagnostic and Statistical Manual of Mental Disorders (DSM-IV), gives a general definition of autism with a variety of criteria and guidelines necessary to give the diagnosis of autism. My experiences over the past seven years of working with young autistic children have clearly demonstrated that each child is uniquely different in type, degree, combination and number of diagnostic criteria. While it is often difficult for the label of "autism" to be accepted, it should be strongly stressed that the most important reason for giving the diagnosis is to enable the client to receive all therapy services necessary for effective treatment. This program should include physical therapy, occupational therapy, speech therapy, and appropriate schooling because autism is such a broad spectrum disorder that extensive services are necessary. The most important thing to remember in treatment is that each situation is different and requires a treatment program specific to that individual. There are now some basic techniques and therapies that will benefit all autistic individuals. These approaches usually involve the use of structured environments and visual cues for teaching and communication. However, none of these methods will effectively work unless the client is initially engaged through awareness, compliance, acceptance of interaction, and some form of communication (signing, "talker", picture board, or some vocalization). Fortunately attitudes and approaches toward the treatment of autism have changed drastically. Clinicians are realizing that many negatives and self-limiting behaviors can be altered to allow the client to become more socially adapted, and consequently, more socially accepted. One of the most significant and widely accepted ideas is that an early childhood program is the key to greater success in the treatment and development of the autistic child.

Dr. Temple Grandin states that she owes much of her success to a firm but loving nanny who "grabbed her by the chin and yanked her into reality." This intrusive approach is the basis for the form of therapy I have used with autistic children for the past seven years. Most autistic children seem to have a problem with change and transition. Therefore, when the client arrives at the facility for the first time, one might see some sort of oppositional behavior. Some clients will have tantrums, withdraw, and/or drop to the ground in an avoidance posture. This type of behavior will almost always become even more severe when one tries to put on the riding hat or hip belt. One must persist. It may take several adults to accomplish this task, but it must be done. In the majority of our clients this behavior stops when they are on the horse and move out. (Obviously it is of the utmost importance that one has a truly reliable, trusting, and trustworthy horse.) The first session should involve only walking the horse while one provides some calm, simple narrative about what is occurring. This should last at least fifteen minutes even if the client has not calmed down. If the agitation persists, try to find the most positive behavior, i.e., quiet for a minute, then give lots of praise and remove him from the horse, all the while praising and narrating what he has done. When possible, prepare the client for the end, e.g., *"One* more time around and you are finished." Use signs if indicated. End the session with praise and a positive attitude.

Throughout the past seven years, 99% of our clients have dramatically improved by the second week. Hats and belts go on and smiles appear. Now we begin gradually to introduce "intrusion." Intrusion seems to work in many ways. It can bring a client "back" from withdrawal and it can also expand his world.

The client's posture is a strong indication of the level of engagement possible. If one sees "sloppy" posture and "empty eyes," one will know that initiating any type of communication or interaction will be difficult. Therefore, something must first be done before you can continue the session. We have found that we can consistently engage the client after we have used some sort of intrusion into "their world." This intrusion can be accomplished by introducing a simple change in their environment. Having the client ride backwards or sideways is usually enough change to cause a reaction that may vary from a state of wariness to a state of extreme agitation. You now have a new starting point for engagement. You have intruded into their world and made them aware that you are there with them. Because this intrusion is done while the client is in a positive environment - on the horse - the change is ultimately accepted. While this procedure may seem very painful to the client at first, it has consistently been demonstrated that this experience is a building block for new experiences to follow. Each session progresses past the previous negative reaction because the horse has been accepted as a positive reinforcer by the second session. What seems to occur thereafter is that the client is able to accept more and more intrusion when he is on the horse.

Another form of intrusion is the basis for "teaching" interaction. This is done by having two clients ride together, on a bareback pad, face to face. Initially there might be strong gaze avoidance and attempts to minimize physical contact. Strong, alert side-walkers are definitely required. Eye contact can be developed through games, such as asking for the color and number of eyes of "your friend."

Physical contact can also be achieved through games that involve touching the other person's hat, nose, and ears. Making the horse move out at a faster pace introduces a challenging situation that causes both riders to hold onto each other. Again narrate the situation positively."You are riding with your friend." Often verbal prompts are necessary to get them to hold on when the clients are still not aware of where their bodies are in space. Holding hands, with a physical prompt when necessary, while singing a song such a variation of "Ring around the rosy" works well with young children. Eventually the "face to face" segment becomes an enjoyable game for most clients. Carryover of this social interaction has been observed in the classroom following these sessions.

Through my experience as a classroom teacher, physical therapist, and therapeutic riding instructor, I have seen that an experiential-based approach has been the most successful form of therapy for the autistic client. By exposing the client to more and more new demands of the world, social adaptations can be developed, especially in the younger child. Without socially appropriate behavior, the autistic person cannot realize the full potential of his strengths. The family, school and community can more readily include an autistic person when the behaviors are not difficult, outlandish, self-destructive, or dangerous. While therapeutic riding or hippotherapy does not cure autism, it does bring about some important behavioral changes. Furthermore, it enriches the client's life through the joy of being with horses and special people who care.

THERAPEUTIC RIDING AND HANSEN'S DISEASE

Beatriz Berro Marins, MS, OT, ST

Hansen's disease (leprosy) still exists in various countries and, therefore, it is necessary for all professionals dealing with this malady to understand it more broadly in order to develop an all-inclusive body of work which comprises prevention, guidance, treatment, and socialization. Leprosy is a chronic, infectious disease which specifically attacks the trunk of nerves and the skin. It is caused by the <u>Mycobacterium Leprae</u> microorganism, also known as Hansen's bacillus. Until 1874, the disease was thought to have various origins, including being of a hereditary nature.

Some cases have sequelas (deformities or functional disabilities) and cause serious emotional disturbances. A person's social life can be jeopardized due to the slowing down of productivity. The diagnosis of leprosy is achieved by a clinical examination that includes:

- Dermatological tests.
- Oeurological tests (by verifying lesions to nerve trunks).
- Ophthalmological.
- Complementary exam (histomine, pilocarpine, or acetycholine tests).
- Lab tests (bacterioscopic, bistopathologic).

Following these procedures, each case is classified in order to establish the therapeutic course of action. The classified types include:

<u>Virchowian</u>
Numerous maculas, ill-defined, asymmetrical and reddish. Presence of nodules, reddish lesions, spissated nerve trunks, and positive bacterioscopy

<u>Tuberculoid</u>
Few maculae, asymmetrical, raised and dry, alterations in their color, red or pallid.

<u>Indeterminate</u>
Lasting from 3 to 6 months. Only maculas of undefined borders and smooth surface, appreciable loss of sensitivity, and negative bacterioscopy

<u>Dimorpha</u>
Numerous maculas of irregular shape or well-defined symmetry, some cases with unaffected nerves, and bacterioscopic test either positive or negative.

The inclusion of a patient in a therapeutic riding program will depend primarily on the stage of illness since <u>it is contraindicated in acute cases</u> and in <u>the presence of ulcerations</u> (open lesions).

During therapeutic evaluation, an examination of the anesthetized areas, attrition sites and pressure points, abnormalities, equilibrium and vision, must be made. Occupational therapy contributes enormously towards the facilitation of physical activity by using a variety of techniques, and towards the acquisition of socialization skills including daily living activities, leisure, recreational, and work habits. Therapeutic riding is a managed activity, allowing the patient to become aware of his or her limitations, thus favoring self-esteem. The physical alterations caused by the disease can be intense and painful, impairing social and work-related performance, and causing a relational distancing from the environment in which the patient lives.

The therapeutic merits, and reaction to them, will depend entirely on the approach maintained by the therapist to the patient.

Alterations that can occur include: reduced sensibility, pain, articular restraints, deformities, open lesions, articular debility, dry skin, paresis or paralysis, and edema. Precautions that need to be taken include observation of skin, hands, feet and eyes.

Numerous disabilities observed in Hansen's disease are the consequences of nerve lesions involving the 5th cranial nerve pair - the eyes, 7th pair of cranial nerves - the facial nerve, the medial nerve, the ulnar nerve, the peroneal nerve, the tibial nerve, and the radial nerve. The brain and the spinal marrow are not affected.

It is important to understand the evolutionary process of the disease and its sudden worsening and take appropriate actions during therapeutic riding.

The deformities resulting from nerve lesions progress in the following ways:
The eyes may demonstrate insufficient blinking, irritation and infection, and loss of vision.

The hands may develop clawed fingers, loss of sensitivity, and sweating. The skin of the hands may develop sores and fissures clawed fingers, rigidity in thumb flexion. The bone may show resorption (disappearance of bone) and excessive scaling and loss of soft tissues.

The feet may develop clawed toes, foot drop (plantar flexion), or loss of sensitivity and sweating. The skin of the feet may develop sores and fissures, foot drop, and inverted and can develop bone resorption and scaling and loss of soft tissue.

Hansen's Disease must be recognized in terms of its lesions (both symptoms and signals) in order to provide the data to the therapist so that he or she can preventing further relapses. In therapeutic riding, extra precautions must be taken in the face of exposed lesions. Appropriate materials must be utilized in order to prevent skin attrition because of sensitivity problems. Proper clothing must be worn as well as to avoid ulcerations. Clothing includes slacks, leggings, shoes with flexible toes and foot position, soft glove to allow for thumb flexion, and a helmet which is always requires. Sunglasses help to protect the eyes. Special tack and materials may include sheepskin pads, horsecloth and thick foam pad, reins that are covered with suitable material, and special stirrups.

The objective of therapeutic riding is to keep the patient active in order to preserve or improve articular mobility in places where paresis or muscular paralysis exist in the upper limbs - the hand, and lower limbs - the feet, and to improving blood flow and lymphatic drainage. The therapist must be aware of signs of lesions, hot spots, spissated skin nodules, pressure points, sensation of pain to the touch, edema, stiff, and scaling skin or fissures. Certain adjustments must be made through occupational therapy in order to prevent deformities or the development of new lesions. For the hands with large contractures, the use of reins specially equipped with leather loops and covered with flexible material to avoid attrition. (figure 1.) For hands that are clawed yet have mobility, wrap the reins with expandable material such as foam or neoprene. This helps tp promote increase of articular amplitude of the fingers (metacarpophalangeal, proximal and distal interphalangeal (figure 2.)

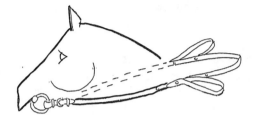

FIGURE 1. REINS WITH LOOPS

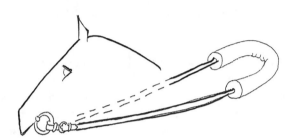

FIGURE 2. PADDED REINS

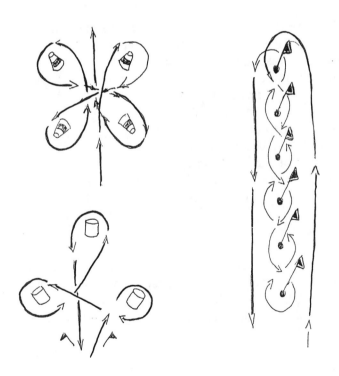

FIGURE 3.
THE OBSTACLE (BARREL, CONES, POST, ETC.) CAN HAVE DIFFERENT STIMULI, SUCH AS COLOR, NUMBER, SHAPE, ETC. -EXERCISES CONDUCIVE TO SELF-ESTEEM.

The increase in muscle strength of the hands can be stimulated using directional commands for the horse to turn left, right, and stop, which also promote manual prehension and sensitivity. The path that the horse takes must include various circular figures with changes in direction and halts For this activity gloves would not be used as protective cover.

For foot drop use stirrups to avoid plantar flexion. Work the foot and ankle muscles, exercising and stretching the calf muscles. For foot drop flexible shoes are not used.

As changes occur due to closing or blinking eyes, care must be taken to avoid drying or irritation to the eyes which can lead to serious lesions that can even cause loss of vision. Sunglasses should be used for protection.

The treatment program is based on case-by-case examination, with reference primarily to development in the following sequence:
- Insensitivity of the palms/fingers
- Insensitivity of the plantar surface and toes
- Clawed hands, moveable or slightly rigid
- Insensitivity of eyeballs and weak palpebra muscles
- Intense pain in nerve trunks and/or eyes
- Foot drop.

The main objectives of therapeutic riding through purposeful movement include:
- Increase and or the maintain of articular amplitude.
- Develop or increase equilibrium reactions.
- Mobilization of the joints - the feet (toes, tarsus, and ankle), hands, (ulnar, medial and radial movements), fist and forearm.
- Increase and or maintain muscular strength.
- Elongate contracted muscles as in the calf.
- Avoid the development of new deformities.
- Develop self-confidence and self-esteem.
- Increase vision muscles strength.
- Increase attention span and sensitivity.
- Exercise stumps
- Care for hands, feet and eyes.

The usage of therapeutic riding by patients with Hansen's Disease is delicate because of the consequences of the illness. The working to develop equilibrium, posture, changes of direction and speed from stop/go commands, and different paths, offers excellent muscular and emotional results. These activities gives the patient self-confidence and awareness of his or her body which is often 'forgotten' due to the loss of sensitivity and/or the privation of limbs (stump).

Providing animal hygiene such as bathing, brushing, and other grooming activities makes the patient take care of him or herself. This is generally ignored because these people may not have a neat appearance owing to their socio-cultural background and their limited means. The transfer of benefits obtained through therapeutic riding can be applied to activities of everyday life. Contraindications must be carefully followed in order not to aggravate the patient's clinical situation.

CONCLUSION

Therapeutic riding has a fundamentally important role to play in leprosy due to its interactional function between two living beings. This eases the emotional adjustment of the patient who is so adversely affected by visible and painful body lesions and is alienation from work and society. In addition the patient is subjected to the threat of clinical relapses. All these factors also affect family members.

Refferences:

The Leprosy Mission. Preventing Disability in Leprosy Patient - The causes and degrees of disability in Hansen's Disease. London.

The Manual for the Control of Hansen's Disease. (1983). Washington, DC.

Summary of the technical manual for technical assistants in Hansen's Disease. (1989), Tavares de Macedo, State Hospital, Brazil

Woullacott, M. (1989). Postural control mechanisms in the young and old, in P.W. D., Duncan.

Beatriz Berro Marins
Rio de Janeiro, Brazil

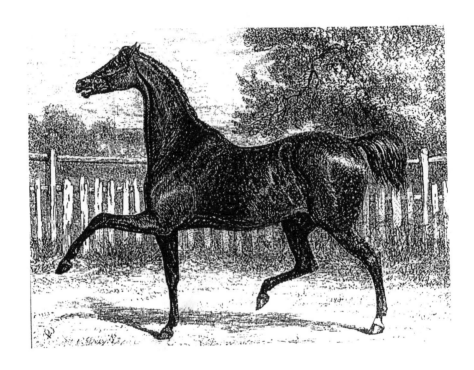

CHAPTER 19

PHYSICAL THERAPY

A COMPARISON OF CHANGE IN FLEXIBLE KYPHOSIS PRE- AND POST- HIPPOTHERAPY--A RESEARCH APPROACH

Elizabeth A. Baker, PT

Hippotherapy has achieved tremendous popularity which continues to grow in many countries. As clinicians we see the benefits and improvements achieved through the use of hippotherapy. As clinicians it is our responsibility to know what changes hippotherapy can facilitate in what client populations. Only then can we say with confidence that it is the treatment of choice. But this means research, which means time, effort, and usually money. Our challenge then is not only to do the research that validates hippotherapy as a treatment technique, but to find ways to make doing that research possible. Research at the level of the individual clinician can be made significantly easier by the use of single system research.

Single system research design looks at small groups or a single subject. The intervention, as well as the outcome, is studied and may be modified as one would do during treatment. The emphasis is on knowledge for immediate practical use; the costs are small, and the procedures can be easily included as part of the clinical routine. This method of research relies on variations within an individual or small group to make inferences about the performance of an individual or small group. It appears ideally suited to therapeutic riding, as it is to physical therapy, because it allows one to study small client groups or individuals such as are seen in treatment every day. But it also allows one to legitimately document findings, so that this information becomes retrievable from the professional literature.

In hippotherapy, the three dimensional movement pattern imparted to the rider by the walking horse is thought to improve the proximal motor control of clients with disorders of movement, such as cerebral palsy. Many such clients demonstrate low muscle tone in the trunk accompanied by increased muscle tone in the extremities. They often show a sitting posture on and off the horse that includes an exaggerated but flexible kyphosis or rounding of the entire trunk, with forward head, rounded shoulders and a posteriorly tilted pelvis. The stabilizing extensor muscles of the posterior trunk will be weakened and difficult to activate when allowed to remain in the lengthened state that exists in the kyphotic, flexed trunk; they must be placed in a shortened range and activated there to be strengthened. The movement of the horse coupled with other facilitation techniques is thought to be effective in correcting this posture and allowing this strengthening to occur. The constant, precise and rhythmic movement of the horse is also thought to provide the additional sensory input needed to maintain the well-aligned posture, allowing the client to experience and practice normal balance and movement skills. The therapist should see an improvement in the client's alignment off the horse, but more importantly, the improved posture should result in functional and noticeable gains in everyday life, such as better balance and extremity use.

From 1985 to 1990, the author was the physical therapist for a therapeutic riding program at a residential facility for adults with developmental disabilities. Since many of the clients with motor deficits showed the flexible kyphosis previously described, hippotherapy was used as a part of the physical therapy program to activate their trunk musculature and improve alignment and trunk control, so that normal trunk equilibrium reactions and extremity use could follow. It was difficult to assess the change in trunk posture in the sagittal plane by observation alone, as the changes were often subtle. A review of the available literature in English indicated that measurement of posture immediately pre- and post- hippotherapy sessions was relatively unexplored. However clinicians support the belief that hippotherapy improves posture based on treatment observations. The author decided to investigate changes in trunk posture as viewed from the sagittal plane. Specifically the research problem addressed was to determine whether hippotherapy would change the flexible rounded or kyphotic posture while on the horse; how static sitting affected the same postural problem; and how this would be measured.

Methodology

The hypothesis was that a decrease in flexible kyphosis as measured while still on the horse, in those with this postural problem associated with neuromotor dysfunction, would result from hippotherapy. Four clients were selected to participate. Three were already involved in a physical therapy program on and off the horse to improve some aspect of ambulation: one was in a hippotherapy program to develop preliminary skills on the horse prior to progressing to therapeutic riding. Each participant was an adult with developmental delay; they had varying degrees of retardation; their motor deficits also varied. All demonstrated poor alignment in the trunk from the sagittal view, specifically an increased rounding or kyphosis that was flexible.

The research design used was alternating treatment, with the subjects serving as their own controls. The treatment sessions consisted of the subject mounting the horse followed by immediate use of a measurement tool to record the initial degree of kyphosis. The subject was then treated in an individualized hippotherapy session. When the therapist felt that the optimum benefit from the session had been achieved which was typically after fifteen to twenty minutes, the treatment was stopped and the measurement tool was used again prior to the dismount. In the controlled, or non-treatment sessions, the client sat on a bolster in an approximation of the mounted position for fifteen minutes. The measurement tool was used at the beginning and at the end of the fifteen minutes while the client was seated on the bolster.

The measurement system consisted of a tool worn by the client. The tool was a somewhat flexible plastic strip with three-inch screws projecting from it. The tool was worn on the back and secured by straps which were elasticized for comfort and to accommodate movement. It was applied from the seventh cervical vertebrae down and aligned with the posterior midline of the trunk. The plastic strip itself was broken in one place with an elastic insert to accommodate the elongating and shortening of the spine associated with movement. During all sessions it was closely monitored for position and adjusted if needed. Immediately before and after hippotherapy, but while the client was still on the horse, a slide photograph was taken of the client wearing the tool. The slide was later developed and projected onto white paper using a straightedge, the screws at the approximate upper and lower thoracic spine were traced onto the paper and extended until an angle was formed. Angles were then measured and compared. It had been previously established that when a normal subject was sitting more erect, the angle would be more acute, such as 45 degrees, and when the spine was rounded the angle was larger, such as 70 degrees. Reliability was partially addressed by having one person, the expert, consistently apply the tool and complete all measurement procedures. To be recorded as a positive or negative change, the difference in angle measurements had to be greater than five degrees.

Results
Consistent with single system research, the angle measurements before and after treatment were compared. Each subject was treated as an individual; the clients' results were not treated as group results. One client, JS, achieved a more upright posture in 8 out of 10 treatment sessions: during the other two sessions there was no change. The second client, ST, achieved a more upright posture in 6 out of ten sessions. The third client, JS, achieved a more upright posture in 6 out of ten sessions. The fourth client, RW, achieved a more upright posture in two out of ten sessions. In the non-treatment sessions, there was no improvement in posture seen; rather there was a tendency for the posture to worsen and become more rounded.

Conclusions:
Three of the four clients showed the desired result from the treatment sessions, and thus supported the hypothesis; all were either the same or worse in the non-treatment sessions, as expected. The client who showed the least improvement while on the horse did demonstrate pelvic rotation and has progressed to assisted ambulation, a new skill for him. It may thus be said that in three of the clients studied, hippotherapy did produce the desired changes in posture. It is suggested that the client who showed less improvement in posture did so because his kyphosis was less flexible than the other clients, and was accompanied by a structural scoliosis. This project sparked great interest for this author and others working in the research, because the single system design was simple and appropriate for very small numbers of clients, and was relevant to the individual client. It is acknowledged that changes in posture occurring while on the horse are difficult to assess objectively. Further research in this area is needed to enable clinicians to predict that hippotherapy is the treatment of choice.

Presented at the VII International Congress on Therapeutic Riding, August 1991, Denmark

HIPPOTHERAPY WITH THE CONSIDERATION
OF REMEDIAL EDUCATION

Gundula Hauser, PT, Special Educator

In the past, modern physics has demonstrated that the universe is a dynamic whole which cannot be divided and in which all parts interrelate and react to one another. This idea of systemic interrelatedness of all living organisms has become part of today's scientific thought. The same holistic approach can also be found in the field of social education where a human being is perceived as a mind-body (or bio-psychological) entity.

At the beginning of the **Modern Age**, philosophy introduced the separation of body and spirit in medicine which led to a body of research solely tied to body chemistry and function. This is not plausible. For a long time, remedial education has been connected too closely with scientific medicine. Under the new holistic approach it may be more aptly called "educational therapy" which includes the total mind/body concept.

Hippotherapy--physiotherapy on horseback--tends to use a neurophysiological treatment approach modeled after Bobath or other similar methods. This opens avenues of learning and experimenting which, due to movement restrictions, are usually closed or not part of a spontaneous experience. A physiotherapeutic approach that includes visual-spatial experiences may raise certain aspects to a conscious level when it is combined with active movement. Movements and their patterns occur in the form of actions and reactions. Lorenz (1973) called this "pattern matching." The execution and the end result of a movement depends on the connection with and the differentiation of a "mental image" and an "outward reality." This involves the whole personality.

With physically disabled children, the main focus of this paper, the physiotherapeutic treatment has the above task and function. Every therapeutic approach which does not deal with the whole person is a failure. It simply cannot work when the focus remains on the physical disability or isolated physical functions. Especially in hippotherapy, where the therapeutic helpmate is a horse, therapy does not have to be limited to the physical defects. Therefore, a background in social education may provide helpful insights for use in this treatment method.

Many approaches, based on different training methods, provide insight into the mind-body relationship. As a physiotherapist, this author primarily relies on a medical and kinesiological approach. As a special educator, this same author plans which cognitive goal she wants to introduce and how she wants to direct the child toward it. Central to her work is the sensory approach. Each of the senses must be addressed and brought into consciousness. This begins with seeing, hearing, smelling and touching, and it includes the vestibular and proprioceptive senses. Much too often, these last two sensory systems are not taken into consideration.

When a child approaches a horse or is led to it, the author attaches great importance to the fact that the child looks at the horse, establishes contact, and talks to it. The child perceives the reaction of the animal to his or her attentions whether it is manifested in a look or a turning of the head or ears in his or her direction. Furthermore, the author likes to let the children put their ears against the horse's side to listen to the sounds in its stomach and to try to perceive the heartbeat. This approach to the horse is carefully measured but intensive and even includes perceiving the horse's smell. In addition, the child touches the horse using gentle strokes from the shoulder to the neck and nostrils.

When the child finally gets on the horse's back, he or she literally loses the ground under his or her feet. For a child with vestibular dysfunction, this can be a rather unpleasant experience. But the fun of sitting on the horse's back helps him or her accept and overcome this initial difficulty. On horseback, the child may listen to the horse's steps, the rhythm of the walk or trot. With each step the child's joints and muscles must adapt to his or her moving support: the horse's back. The child may be asked to carry out some of the exercises with his or her eyes closed to eliminate one of the senses. This, in turn, stimulates the tactile and proprioceptive senses and produces an increased awareness of his or her own body and the ongoing movement. In the area of social interaction, hippotherapy entails a meeting of two living beings, as manifested by the child/horse relationship. As mentioned above, the child is encouraged from the beginning to make contact with the horse. His or her ability to relate to others is important for the development of his or her self-image. Unlike the people around him, the horse is not concerned with physical defects. This may be very important to many children with disabilities as they often meet people with frightened or worried expressions or encounter other negative reactions to their physical defects.

The therapeutic exercise of lying prone or supine on the horse creates an intense contact which further enhances the child/horse relationship. Many children express this by saying, "You are so warm and soft," or "Your mane tickles my nose," and other expressions. As often as possible, the child decides when to walk or trot. A well-trained horse that reacts appropriately to the child's commands, allows the child to experience cooperative behavior. The therapist is involved in the child's socio-emotional development by helping him or her improve his or her relationship with the horse. As a result he or she becomes part of the confidence-based relationship, child-horse-therapist.

Client-centered conversation may be used as part of an introduction. This is an approved technique used in psychotherapy. If possible, the child should be prepared for the experience on his or her way to the horse. This may include a discussion of what the child will tell the horse or what exercises he or she wants to do this time. He or she should also have the opportunity to decide beforehand, if he or she wants to try a new exercise or if he or she wants to continue with the familiar ones. In any case, the child must be given the opportunity to free him or herself from all emotional and mental preoccupation with his or her daily life to be free for new experiences on horseback. In therapy the feelings and experiences are made conscious through the dialogue. Soon the child will enjoy expressing him or herself with phrases such as, "The horse pushes me, hop, hop, hop," or "The horse rocks me, back and forth, back and forth," verbally reproducing the rhythm of the horse's steps. The child thereby connects his or her experiences with words which also improves his or her later recall. In the discussion following the therapy, therapists do not only reflect the content of the session, they go beyond that and try to make the child recall what he or she felt, smelled, and heard through the use of visualization and imagery.

Exercises to increase relaxation similar to the ones used in psychotherapy can be used on the horse. The author, for instance, likes to have the child lie down backwards on the horse. This means, the child's head is on the croup, and his arms point to the horse's tail. The author then proceeds to let the child experience the first steps of a modified autogenic training: the experience of heaviness and warmth. This gives the child the ease to let his head, body, arms and legs sink heavily into the soft coat of the horse. Additionally, the experience of warmth is made more readily accessible by the warmth of the horse's body.

The child's positive behavioral responses can be reinforced by therapists. Through dialogue and visual-motor experiences, the child is able to learn, especially in the area of social interactions. The therapist demonstrates different movements and stimulates the child with the help of mimicry and gestures to copy his or her movements in mirror symmetry. In addition, any arising anxiety on the part of the child at any time during the therapy must be accepted and dealt with by the therapist. It should be mentioned that by training the proprioceptive and vestibular senses alone, the child will get an improved body scheme. This leads to greater self awareness and ultimately to an improved self image.

A well-developed self image will result in greater self-confidence, and with that the child will become less fearful. When these initial problems and fears have been overcome, the therapist can create new demands and new goals thereby leading the child, step by step, toward a fuller, more satisfying life.

Through hippotherapy, children with disabilities can discover the often unknown pleasure of being physically active. When steady problem solving, together with positive reinforcement through successful experiences lead to an increase in motivation and in the pleasure of learning, the child is ready to learn new skills and to reach toward the next higher level of function. It is, of course, not possible or even necessary to use the whole range of therapeutic approaches in any one session, but a background knowledge or some training in special education and psycho-therapeutic techniques are desirable for physiotherapists, especially for those working with children.

In Austria and many other countries, more emphasis is placed on separating hippotherapy and the psycho-educational aspects of therapeutic riding than on finding ways of connecting these two methods. This report is designed to do away with all fragmentation and to give prominence to the connecting element - the child as a mind/body entity, in short: the total child.

Reference
Lorenz, K. (1973). Die Ruckseite des Spiegels, Munchen, Germany.

Gundula Hauser
Wein, Switzerland

NDT AND HIPPOTHERAPY: A LESSON REVIEW

Joann Benjamin, PT

Physical and occupational therapists have many treatment techniques they may use to treat a client effectively. They will generally choose techniques with which they are most familiar and which they judge will be the most beneficial to the client.

Neurodevelopmental treatment (NDT) is one technique which has been used extensively in the therapy clinic. The therapists who use this approach will have had training beyond that received in school, for working with children and adults. NDT is commonly utilized with clients who have neurological disorders. Let us review a single lesson in which the equine-assisted therapy will take an NDT approach.

Audrey is an eleven year old girl who had a traumatic brain injury (TBI) two years ago when she was struck by a car. She was a typical nine year old prior to the accident. She is still very active, bright, personable and loves animals. Audrey's mother is interested in having her daughter ride in a therapy program. She has obtained a referral from Audrey's pediatrician and from her therapists.

The physical therapist (PT) in the program evaluated Audrey and reports the following: Audrey has functional use of her left side. The muscles on her right side are tight and resist stretching (hypertonus). Audrey carries her right arm close to her chest with elbow bent and hand fisted (flexor pattern). She stands 'crooked,' leaning to the right, and has difficulty rotating to the left (right trunk hypertonus). Audrey can walk for short distances (10-15 feet) with her mother's help or with a cane. Her steps are unequal and her balance is poor. She exaggerates stepping with her right leg and tends to turn her ankle under. This walking pattern gets worse the further she walks.

The therapist explains that this client demonstrates abnormal postural tone. Normal tone is "muscle tonus high enough to maintain posture against gravity, but low enough to move through it" (Sherrington, in Bobath, 1982). In other words, muscles need to have enough tension to support the body upright without being so tense that movement cannot occur. Audrey is unable to move easily against her tense muscles. his prevents her from effectively adapting to changes in position (balance) or from initiating voluntary smooth movements. When she has an increase in her effort to move, as when she walks, she repeats the abnormal movement patterns which increases the amount of muscle activity. Her nervous system is unable to control the excessive muscle activity and therefore her muscle tightness increases; this further restricts normal movement. This is now a vicious cycle.

Audrey also lacks symmetry in her posture and in her movements. The therapist explains that this is, in part, a result of Audrey's asymmetrical muscle tension; it is greater on the right than on the left. She has shown this posture for two years. Her sensory feedback system (proprioception) has adapted to this posture and accepts it as "normal." When Audrey is placed in proper alignment, she feels off balance. The same holds true for her movement patterns. She has moved in abnormal patterns for so long that the sensation of this movement has repeatedly entered her nervous system. Audrey no longer recognizes normal movement patterns as correct.

According to NDT theory, "normal movements need a background of normal tonus" in order to exist (Bobath 1982). Therefore, the "aim of NDT treatment should be to change the abnormal patterns of movement (Bobath 1982)" or to break the abnormal cycle of movement and sensory feedback. The control of abnormal activity results in the ability to develop normal postural responses, to initiate functional movement and to experience the sensation of normal movement. Through the experience of normal movement, one hopes that Audrey will develop more appropriate muscle activity: both automatic (unconscious) postural responses and voluntary movement.

Specific NDT handling techniques are applied by the trained therapist to decrease abnormal muscle tone and to encourage (facilitate) normal movement. The therapist works with a team of assistants (sidewalkers, a horse handler) who are critical to the success of the session. Awareness of NDT principles and objectives makes every team member a contributor to the therapy experience.

In Audrey's case, as soon as she arrives at the arena the therapeutic riding team should begin to involve her in activities appropriate for her. Because Audrey will show signs of increased tone when walking a long distance, she is encouraged to use her wheelchair instead. With activities such as grooming, she will perform tasks which are a challenge, but not so difficult that they induce stress (increased tone). Throughout, Audrey should be positioned so that she can participate in activities while maintaining midline, not turning or leaning to her favored side.

When she is ready to mount her horse from the ramp, she will require assistance - enough help so that she is not struggling, yet, allowing her to do as much of the mount as she is able. The therapist positions Audrey on the horse in a symmetrical posture which will help to prevent abnormal patterns. Additionally, the therapist will avoid positions that cause Audrey discomfort, as pain will increase her muscle tone.

When Audrey is comfortable astride the horse, her right leg is flexed more than her left. Even so, the therapist is certain to check that her weight is distributed evenly on her seat bones so that she can have a solid, midline base of support. Her trunk is supported by the therapist who facilitates symmetrical posture. Audrey has her hands on a weight bearing platform (a firm foam roll) at the horse's withers. This helps to encourage an upright trunk (shoulders over pelvis) while providing sensory input through the arms. Weight bearing will help to normalize tone in the limbs as well as in the trunk.

The therapist has the horse handler work the horse at a rhythmic walk along the rail as horse, rider, and therapist accommodate each other. They begin to the right, with gentle turns at the corners, because Audrey is stronger in this direction. The movement of the horse, the weight bearing of the arms and trunk, along with reflex inhibiting techniques by the therapist all help to decrease Audrey's muscle tension. As Audrey's muscle tone decreases towards normal, her position on the horse improves; her pelvis, with the therapist's facilitation, begins to move into a neutral posture from a slumped position (posterior pelvic tilt). Her right leg positions more easily downward without squeezing the horse (adduction), her right arm shows less fisting of the hand and supports more weight. Audrey is more symmetrical from left to right; she now sits easily in midline. Her body is more supple and she now moves in rhythm with the horse. As she feels a decrease of muscle tension (hypertonus), the therapist chooses to facilitate greater postural response from Audrey. The therapist asks for changes of direction, turns across the arena. Turns by the horse require Audrey to lengthen her trunk, primarily on the long side of the turn. The therapist can help facilitate this truck elongation in conjunction with the horse's movement. Elongation and shortening of the trunk are essential for activities such as reaching and walking.

The therapist now has Audrey work on skills to enhance upper-trunk-on-lower-trunk movement such as twisting, bending forward toward the horse's neck, and side bending. The horse generates lower-trunk-on-upper-trunk movement as the therapist manually facilitates postural control and stability of the upper trunk in good alignment. The therapist concentrates on the child's trunk control because the trunk is the basis for all other movement. Audrey has been moved through a symmetrical, midline position. The movement of the trunk is over a stable base of support (pelvis) in good alignment (neutral pelvic tilt). Audrey begins to demonstrate improved trunk mobility as a result of her increased trunk stability. Both mobility and stability are directly dependent on normal muscle tone.

As Audrey develops better control in her trunk, the therapist is able to concentrate more on her arms and legs. Her right arm and leg may well have relaxed simply due to the decrease in hypertonus achieved in her trunk. Further decrease in muscle tension is achieved through handling methods (reflex inhibiting positions). As the decrease in tone occurs, the therapist will be facilitating muscle activity in the limbs. She asks Audrey to perform skills, and assists as necessary. The therapist is looking for Audrey to achieve successful movement without inducing abnormal patterns. The child, with her therapist's help reaches out and touches parts of the horse, plays with a ball and handles large rings. At the end of the lesson, Audrey is integrating several of the skills the therapist helped facilitate. For instance, as Audrey places a ring in a mailbox she demonstrates:

- A stable base (pelvis) in neutral alignment
- Weight shifting toward the mailbox which requires elongation of the reaching (weight bearing) side, and shortening of the opposite side of the trunk
- Movement of the upper trunk on the lower trunk
- Voluntary, controlled movement of the arm
- Resumption of midline posture upon completion of the task

At the end of the session, Audrey dismounts to the ramp. The therapist chooses to have Audrey dismount by bringing her right leg over the horse's neck and turning to sit on the horse sideways before standing on the ramp platform. The sidewalkers are careful to help support Audrey's trunk, and the leader is careful to monitor the horse from the front. It seems Audrey requires much less assistance than when mounting . She is able to initiate lifting her leg over the horse's neck, her trunk muscles show greater control in this off-balance posture. The therapist then has Audrey walk to her wheelchair. She continues to monitor the effort that Audrey must put forth to walk and facilitates when needed. This gives the therapist a chance to see what functional gains Audrey has made as a result of her riding session.

The riding session has been successful in achieving certain neurodevelopmental objectives appropriate for this child. Audrey's muscle tone is decreased to the point where more normal movement can take place. Audrey has an improved sense of midline orientation, she is comfortable when positioned in midline and her postural muscles help to maintain a symmetrical alignment. The increased stability of her trunk allows her to gain more active function of her trunk and extremities.

During the session the horse provides the child with a tremendous amount of sensory input through movement. By inhibiting her abnormal tone to allow freer movement, the therapist helps Audrey to integrate the movement stimuli received from the horse. Her normal balance reactions are encouraged as the horse moves. The horse is the three dimensional movement stimulus, the therapist is the facilitator. Audrey benefits from the influence of both.

The therapist will take a similar approach on subsequent sessions, increasing the challenge as Audrey progresses. The therapist schedules Audrey twice per week, for 30 minute sessions. Re-evaluation is ongoing though she will formally re-evaluate Audrey at the end of eight weeks to determine continuation of the program. She will also contact Audrey's primary therapists to monitor progress in other areas, and to integrate functional goals for Audrey with theirs.

As Audrey continues her therapy, one can expect to see improvements throughout her trunk and limbs. She will demonstrate improved stability and midline orientation, as well as increased control of the trunk and extremities. Improved function, both on and off the horse is the ultimate goal. All along, the horse and the therapist will work closely to provide Audrey with sensory input, and a means through decreasing her abnormal movement to integrate those sensations to reproduce the normal movement Audrey once knew.

References:
Bobath, B. (1982) *Adult Hemiplegia: Evaluation and Treatment.* 2nd ed. London: Heinemann.
Bryn Mawr Rehabilitation Hospital. Physical Therapy Department, 414 Paoli Pike, Malvern, PA. 19355 USA. 215-251-5560.

ASSESSMENT AND ADAPTATIONS IN RIDING THERAPY FOR THE CLIENT FOLLOWING A CEREBRAL VASCULAR ACCIDENT

Victoria Haehl, MS, PT
Diagrams by Victoria Vallee

A cerebral vascular accident (CVA) or stroke occurs when circulation of blood to a part of the brain is disrupted. This condition has a high incidence among both young and old but is more common in adults. Changes in a person's physical, emotional, mental, speaking and writing abilities may occur. Blood supply to the brain can be altered by:

1. An arteriosclerotic thrombosis--an artery becomes slowly clogged with a clot.
2. An embolism--a blood clot travels from another part of the body and becomes lodged in an artery in the brain.
3. Intercranial hemorrhage--due to hypertension (high blood pressure), an aneurysm, or atrioventricular malformation (Biery et al, 1989).

In humans one side of the brain controls function on the opposite side of the body. A person whose CVA occurred in the right side of the brain will demonstrate a weakness on the left side. This is called a left hemiparesis or hemiplegia. Though most persons who have a CVA will have either a right or left hemiparesis, each one will be different depending on the type and location of the insult, the size of the area involved, the length of time from onset, and the age and physical condition before the onset.

In addition to difficulties with weakness, a CVA can cause problems with regulating the muscle tone or tension that provides a normal muscle with a state of readiness. The tone may be abnormally high, low or fluctuating. An individual may demonstrate different tonal quality in different parts of the body, and it may vary depending on the person's body position. Spasticity refers to a muscle's response to quick stretch, and this may be observed or felt as resistance. The terms "tone" and "spasticity" are frequently used to describe motor control difficulties that arise following a CVA. Although each rider with a CVA is different, there are some alterations which occur that can be generalized. These are listed below.

Left brain injury:
1. Decreased control and sensation on the right side of the body
2. Speech and language impairment
3. Decreased memory related to language
4. A slow and cautious style of interaction with the environment

Right brain injury:
1. Decreased control and sensation of the left side of the body
2. Decreased ability to judge space and size
3. Left side neglect or inattention to the side
4. Decreased memory or decreased attention span
5. A quick and impulsive style of interaction with the environment

ASSESSMENT

Persons entering a therapeutic riding program should be carefully evaluated. It is important to look at how the head, arms, trunk and legs work as a whole, not as separate parts. The same need for the holistic view is especially true for the person who has suffered a cerebral vascular accident. Although it is tempting to focus attention solely to the side of the body with less control, therapists' and instructors' observations should be all-inclusive. Reference should also be made to the report of the physical and occupational therapists, as well as the speech pathologist, who have been working with the rider to glean any pertinent information. If a therapist is available at the therapeutic riding facility to perform evaluations, a full evaluation can be undertaken. Figure 1 shows an example of an initial therapeutic riding physical therapy evaluation.

PHYSICAL THERAPY (EQUINE-ASSISTED THERAPY) EVALUATION
(evaluation for physical therapy treatments)

DATE OF EVALUATION _____

NAME _____   BIRTH DATE _____

DIAGNOSIS _____

MEDICAL HISTORY (medical history: seizures, surgeries, accidents)_____
_____

HIP X-RAY, MEDICATION, ASSISTIVE DEVICES USED_____

W/C _____   BRACES _____   SPLINTS _____

A. MOTOR BEHAVIOR
  (purposeful vs random responses to handling, reflex activity [ATNR, STNR], grasp-voluntary vs involuntary, coordination, respiratory, gross oral motor function).
_____

B. MOTOR FUNCTION ABILITY

HEAD CONTROL
sitting _____ supported _____ unsupported _____
standing _____ supported _____ unsupported _____

BED MOBILITY_____
ROLLING _____
SUPINE TO SIT _____
SIT TO SUPINE _____

GAIT _____
TRANSFER
  car _____
  sit to stand _____
  stand to sit _____
  posture _____
  sitting _____
  stand _____

Figure 1.

296

C. BALANCE   (equilibrium reactions, righting reactions, sitting, standing, static, dynamic, quadruped)

_____

_____

| D. TONE | E. RANGE OF MOTION |

neck _____

trunk _____

right U E _____

left U E _____

right L E _____

left L E _____

F. COGNITIVE/PERCEPTUAL

expressive speech/language   _____

language comprehension   _____

hearing _____

following commands   1 step_____, 2 step_____, 3 step_____, complex_____

attention span   poor [0-1 min]_____, fair [1-5 min]_____, good [5+ min]_____

frustration tolerance   poor_____, fair_____, good_____.

problem solving   poor_____, fair_____, good_____.

cooperation   poor_____, fair_____, good_____.

G. SPECIAL CONSIDERATIONS

_____

_____

H. CHANGES OBSERVED WITH INITIAL TREATMENT

_____

_____

RECOMMENDED PROGRAM

frequency and duration   _____

hippotherapy   developmental vaulting   remedial vaulting   other _____

helmet   sidewalker   1 or 2, backrider _____

mounting: ramp   block   leg up   vault on _____

assistance needed _____

longeing: therapeutic longeing   ground driving   longeing/circle _____

dismounting: ramp   block   slide off   assistance needed _____

Long term goals (6 months)

_____

Communication should be ongoing between the therapeutic riding team members and any active rehabilitation team members to make the experience most beneficial to the rider. The physician who makes the referral and signs the authorization should certainly receive periodic updates on the client's progress. It is often useful to invite members of the rehabilitation team to a hippotherapy session to observe. Prior to the initial session, invite the rider to tour the facility and possibly observe hippotherapy in action. This may be a suitable time to screen the rider and describe the purpose of hippotherapy/therapeutic riding.

Some additional concerns that should be noted if present on the initial assessment include hypertension, heart problems, osteoarthritis and back problems such as degenerative disc disease and stenosis. The rider's physician should be consulted if any questions arise. Also, your facility should have a list of conditions that contraindicate participation in riding therapy. Further be aware that individuals with CVA disabilities may become more stiff and sore following riding sessions, thus requiring additional warm-up/cool-down time and shorter riding sessions.

THE IMPORTANCE OF OBSERVATION

Learning to be a good observer is key to the assessment of riders on and off the horse. "How are they sitting in the car when they arrive?" "How do they get out of the car?" "Is assistance required?" "Are they ambulatory or in a wheelchair?" "Do they use a cane?" "Does walking on uneven ground look like a new experience for them?" and "Do they seem fearful in the unfamiliar surroundings?" Observing their first visit to the barn can provide very useful information in determining riding strategies and goals. It can indicate how best to assist the rider and what horse and equipment may be the most appropriate for him. After meeting the rider, his family and friends, and concluding parts of the initial evaluation, have the rider indicate what he hopes to accomplish during the hippotherapy/therapeutic riding sessions. Your goals should be made with this in mind. As in any therapeutic setting, goals can be altered as progress is made or interests change.

The individual who has had a cerebral vascular accident resulting in a hemiparesis may demonstrate limitations in the joints, pain, changes in sensation and an impaired ability to feel where a body part is (proprioception). The physical therapist's evaluation should be able to provide specific information regarding the rider's physical status, but an observation of the rider on the horse provides other critical information.

TRUNK AND HEAD

An important observation to make on or off the horse is, "What is the trunk (top of the shoulders to bottom of pelvis) doing?" An optimal view of the rider's trunk and upper extremities can be made by seating the rider on a pad or sheepskin and surcingle. Weather and provision for modesty permitting, have the client disrobe as much as possible (provide T-shirts) so that you can see his posture before the horse moves. This is important because the horse's movement may have the most impact on the rider's trunk. As stated by Detlev Riede, MD, in his book, *Physiotherapy on the Horse*, "according to Baumann (1978), Kunzle (1979), and Kluwer (1983), the three dimensional movement of the horse's back simulates the human gait." During normal gait the trunk moves in anterior/posterior, lateral, rotational, and superior/inferior directions (Figure 2).

The movement of the horse provides the rider's trunk with the components of normal human gait and positions him in a more normal upright posture which is difficult to duplicate in the therapeutic setting. Although the rider is sitting, the lower extremities are allowed to partially extend, unlike sitting in a chair. The lower extremities are brought closer to the plumb line of the pull of gravity on the horse than in sitting, making the posture resemble standing. In addition, the freedom of the lower extremities allows them to react to the movement of the horse and rider's trunk, resembling the demands of movement during gait (Figure 3).

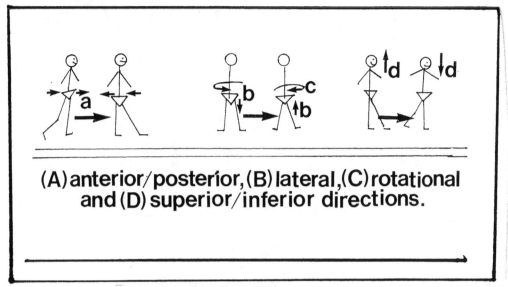

(A) anterior/posterior, (B) lateral, (C) rotational and (D) superior/inferior directions.

FIGURE 2.

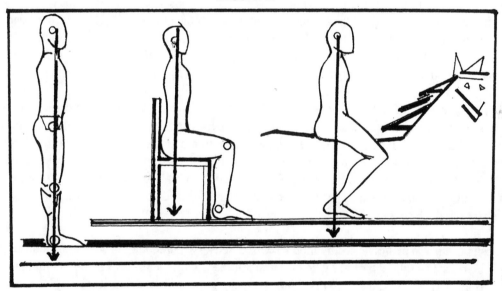

FIGURE 3.

A variety of trunk postures can be observed. If a video camera is available, it may be useful to film the rider from all angles to capture what your eye might miss. The rider may also find this interesting. But do not be surprised if he is somewhat shocked. Most people have no idea what they look like in action. Figure 4 illustrates some common poor postures observed. Standing directly behind the horse enables the therapist to see the asymmetries that frequently accompany a CVA. While these result from one side of the trunk function better than the other, remember that the whole trunk is reacting to the effects of the CVA, not only the hemiparetic side. Make sure both sides are carefully assessed.

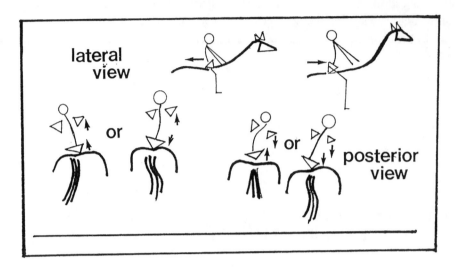

FIGURE 4.

In addition to the anterior/posterior (front to back) and lateral (side to side) postures and movements, it is also important to get an idea of what the rider would look like if you observed him from above. This would give important information regarding trunk rotation. Alternately it is beneficial to "feel" what the rider looks like. Place your hands on the pelvis. You can "see" by feeling if one side is in front of the other (lower trunk rotation). Hands on the back of the ribs below the scapula demonstrate that the upper trunk is rotated. Now have the horse walk on and observe the impact of the horse's three dimensional movement on the client's trunk.

Although this description of assessment provides clues for observing the rider for specific body parts, it is important to step back frequently to observe the whole. Many persons with hemiparesis will have problems with disassociation. Disassociation can be described as the ability to move one body part separately from another. Examples of disassociation are the ability to move the scapula on the thorax or move the lower extremity on the pelvis without moving the entire trunk. Problems with disassociation can best be seen by looking at the person as a whole. The therapist may see that the movement of the horse assists in disassociating body parts while the client passively sits on the horse.

The head position can also be influenced by motor control, sensory, perceptual or visual difficulties. Take note of whether the rider has full or partial range of motion in the neck. Due to any one or a combination of these factors, the rider may not hold his head in midline (center). A head-forward posture may be a result of poor postural habits acquired from prolonged sitting following the CVA.

UPPER EXTREMITIES
The postures that the upper extremity assumes are numerous. An important observation to be made is at the shoulder. Due to abnormal positioning of the scapula and humerus, impaired motor control and soft tissue changes, the glenohumeral (shoulder) joint may become subluxed. This is a mal-alignment in which the head of the humerus can move interiorly, anteriorly or superiorly relative to the scapula. If the rider is unaware of this condition or is unable to inform the instructor or therapist, the limitation can be detected by feeling the top

of the shoulder joint on both shoulders and observing the position of the scapula on the thorax. It is advisable to discuss this situation with the physical or occupational therapist treating the rider. Looking below the shoulder, be aware of the position of the arm in relation to the body. Is it held behind, out to the side, or in front of the trunk? How does it change when the rider and horse begin to move? Pay particular attention to the hand; the wrist and fingers may be good indicators of how the client is reacting to the riding challenge. Clawing of the fingers and flexing of the wrist generally accompany the rider's sense of compromised balance or mal-alignment of the shoulder or trunk. (Similar changes can be seen in the toes and ankle).

Observe carefully the effect of the movement of the horse on the posture of the upper extremity. If it appears to become increasingly tight, it may be necessary to reassess the present activity, if improving posture is a goal of that session. It may also indicate that it is time for a break, a change in activity, or that the rider is fatigued. Continue to evaluate, observe and modify as the session progresses. Be aware that movement of the horse and movement of any part of the body can affect other parts of the body. This can especially be seen in the upper extremity. Pain should be closely monitored and avoided. If it persists or increases, riding may need to be discontinued until the therapist can further evaluate and treat the problem.

LOWER EXTREMITIES

Evaluating the lower extremity is sometimes difficult due to clothing: pants, boots, braces and equipment (i.e., stirrups, leathers). When making your initial observations and for periodic follow-up, it may be beneficial to use a sheepskin or pad secured by a surcingle. Remove braces and roll up pant legs. Knowing how the lower extremity reacts to the horses's movements, changes in direction, and halts gives a better understanding of how the legs will posture in the stirrup or brace. If the rider can wear shoes (no boots or brace), the ankle can be assessed more clearly. Make observations, as for the trunk and upper extremities, from all angles. Follow this by observing the whole body, horse, and lower extremity relationship. A common posture for the involved foot is one of supination, in which the ankle turns in, the bottom of the foot points down and in. The toes may also claw. This posture may affect the type of stirrup chosen. A broader surface of support in addition to a variety of aids that can be placed on the ankle or foot may be beneficial to improve the posture. (Some suggestions are discussed in the treatment section.) The physical therapist working with the client may have some suggestions.

Balance should be assessed off the horse in a variety of positions: sitting, standing, and quadruped (hands and knees). On the horse, take note of the rider's trunk posture as well as any need for the support of his hands and/or from the sidewalker to maintain himself. Also record what the horse's walk is like, including its speed, amplitude and what direction of movement seems most prominent. How the rider tolerates this movement reflects his balancing capabilities.

During the observation/evaluation process the horse has already initiated the treatment session. The instructor or therapist need only facilitate this. In the beginning of each session, a warm-up period is advantageous. The horse should have received some conditioning or warm-up time prior to the rider mounting. Generally, it is best to start with riding long straight lines along the outside rail of the arena in both directions to make the rider feel more secure, balanced and prepared. This will also give the instructor time to quickly reassess posture and balance. The horse can proceed at a slow, medium or fast walk, depending on the rider's balance. Vary the horse's stride from short to extended. The rider may be more comfortable starting the session holding onto the surcingle handle with one or both hands. This makes the rider less tense and more able to feel the movement of the horse.

TREATMENT STRATEGIES TO FACILITATE RIDING

This description of various treatment ideas will address a rider who is on a horse with a surcingle, pad or sheepskin, the horse driven from behind with long reins (or being led) and two sidewalkers. Certainly, a saddle would not interfere with many of the activities proposed and may improve the rider's balance enabling him to perform more challenging activities. If stirrups are used for lower extremity weight bearing and the posture of the foot continues to change significantly, i.e., toes pointing down with heel up (plantar flexion of the ankle) or the bottom of the foot turning inward (supination), alternative positioning or equipment should be considered. A variety of ankle-foot-orthoses (AFO) are prescribed following a CVA. Some allow for motion at the ankle joint. The articulated AFO has hinges at the ankle to allow dorsiflexion (Figure 5). Other AFO's, depending on their rigidity, may also provide some support but allow for the movement necessary. Be careful to observe where the orthotic device ends under the foot. This may interfere with weight bearing on the stirrup in the proper portion of the foot. If the foot does not plantarflex excessively, but instead the sole turns inward (straining the lateral structures of the ankle and placing the ankle at risk for injury) an ankle airsplint may be of assistance (Figure 6). This support straps on with Velcro, does not limit dorsiflexion or plantar-flexion and limits medial/lateral movement at the ankle. There are also elastic wrap supports, which may be all that is required.

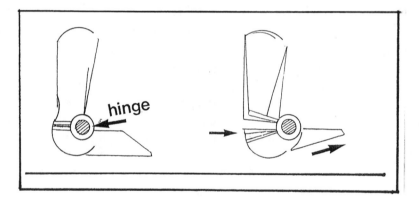

FIGURE 5.

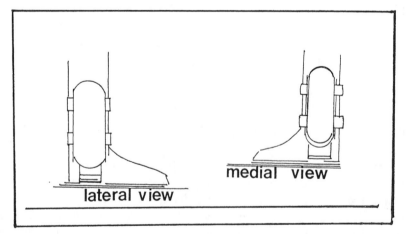

FIGURE 6.

Stirrups may be modified to fit the needs of the rider. The Devonshire Boot is a covering that encloses the front portion of the stirrup to prevent the foot from sliding through. Stirrup modifications such as rubber wedges should not be used without consulting a physical therapist. Remember that as the rider becomes more accomplished on the horse, these additional supports may need modification or may no longer be necessary.

When the lower extremity is not supported by a stirrup it is free to swing with the movement of the horse. This may assist in pelvic-lower extremity disassociation resulting in freer movement at the hip and ultimately better gait for the rider. The abducted slightly externally rotated position of the hip on the horse may improve the hips' range of motion. At a walk the pelvis is also being passively moved on the femur which passively mobilizes the hip joint. Relaxation of tight muscles of the hip, knee and ankle may be observed as the client continues during a session or series of sessions. By observing the rider from behind, an appreciation of leg length (reflecting tightness in muscles or pelvic obliquity) may be obtained. Changes in riding direction, doing circles, serpentine, figure eights, and lateral work may influence the lower extremity therapeutically.

The physical therapist may have some specific techniques that can be performed during the riding session for handling the hemiparetic lower extremity. For example, if the lower extremity tends to pull up, forward and inward; the therapist can give a gentle, slowly sustaining slight down and out pull above the knee, and a downward pull behind the heel momentarily at the halt; this may assist in relaxing the tightened muscles. The therapist should be consulted prior to actively manipulating the rider's extremities.

Following a CVA, as noted in the assessment section, the upper-extremity may assume a variety of postures that are related to the position of the trunk, the available range of motion in the joints, muscle tightness, motor control, sensation and, usually, the anxiety level of the rider. After the initial warm-up walking on the long sides of the arena, if the rider has been instructed in any self range of motion that can be performed sitting, this

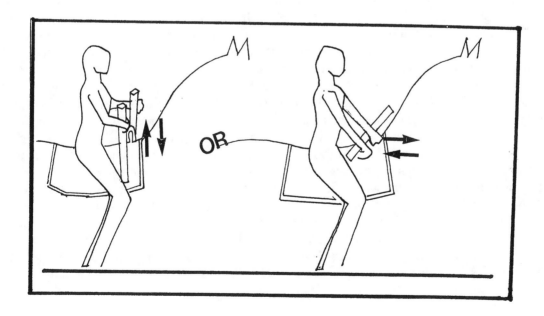

FIGURE 7.

303

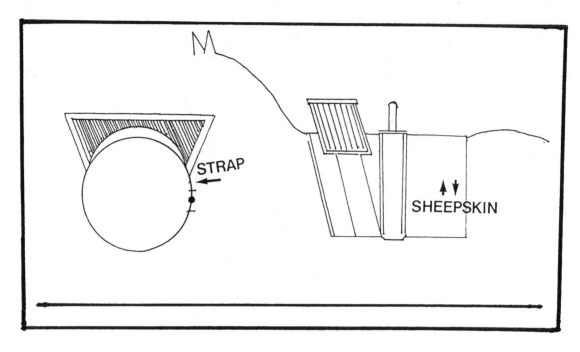

FIGURE 8.

may be carried out by the rider with the horse halted or at the walk, if feasible. It may also be helpful for the rider to perform some weight-bearing activities on the upper extremity as the horse walks on or at the halt. Positions can vary depending on the upper extremity. Some suggestions include placing the hands on the thighs, on the horse's neck, on the surcingle handle, or on the shoulders or arms of the sidewalkers. Dowels may also be positioned to allow weight bearing (Figure 7). If the rider is able to tolerate riding backward weight bearing with hands on the horse's haunches can be a great position. There is a lot of movement, proprioception and scapula/thoracic disassociation provided to the upper extremity and upper trunk in this posture. Frequently the upper extremity cannot fully extend at the elbow, wrist or fingers or does not have the control to maintain an extended position. It may be useful to use assistive positioning such as the upper extremity weight-bearing platform developed by Susan Christie, physical therapist, and rehabilitation engineer at Bryn Mawr Rehabilitation Hospital in Malvern, Pennsylvania (Figure 8). It enables the rider to weight bear on a solid surface without fully extending the joints in the upper extremity. There are also a variety of plastic balls that can be placed between the rider's thigh and the body of the horse, at the surcingle handle or on the platform that may assist the positioning of the wrist and fingers. If the rider is more involved in controlling the movement of the horse, adaptive reins such as the ladder reins or Humes reins and adaptive gloves may be of assistance. These must be carefully monitored so there is not the danger of an inability to release if the rider needs to dismount in an emergency. Various non-weight-bearing activities that include the rider supporting his own upper extremity, and reaching in all available pain-free directions, may assist in function. Allowing the arm to swing freely at the side may also be beneficial. This is what arms normally do during gait. It may be the only opportunity that the rider has to experience this normal movement response, since usually a cane is in the hand of the stronger arm.

POSITIONING ADJUSTMENTS

A major impact of the horse's movement can be seen in the rider's trunk. Frequently following the initial few minutes of warm-up, the rider may be feeling a need to adjust his seat. Or it may be suggested to improve the symmetry, which will alter his experience of the horse's movement. Many times in therapy, improving symmetry of the trunk is a goal. The postural control of the trunk, head, and neck is key in the rehabilitation of the rest of the body. As the horse walks and the rider's pelvis is moved, the remainder of the trunk (spine, ribs, scapula and clavicle) reacts to these movements. These movements should be encouraged (not necessarily exaggerated) to insure the rider is not "fixing" or holding the pelvis. By observing the trunk, the instructor or therapist can decide what horse movement may be most beneficial to the rider. Transitions within the walk from slow to fast to slow, as well as to halt and back to walk, can assist in facilitating control anteriorly and posteriorly by activating the abdominals and the back extensors. The abdominals are often weaker on the affected side, which may cause the trunk to rotate back or ribs to flair as the rib cage loses it abdominal anchor (Ryerson, et al 1988). Abdominal control is very important to trunk control. Various figures can be used to move the pelvis laterally or rotate one side forward in relation to the other. By sitting on the horse yourself, you can feel which side of your pelvis or which scapula is tending to lower or raise, and which side of your trunk is working harder to stay symmetrical or balanced on the horse. Use your imagination; try various moves to help with trunk control--side pass, shoulder in, and obstacles for the horse to step over. Using poles to create labyrinths for the horse to walk through combines transitions, changes in directions and amplitudes of movement. Changing the rider's position will also place new demands on his trunk, i.e., backward, sitting sideways, or forward, with both legs toward one side as if riding side saddle. The horse's movement will move the pelvis in relation to the upper trunk. Also encourage the upper trunk to move on the pelvis in a controlled way rotating in both directions, while the horse proceeds through a variety of changes and directions. Have the rider reach forward to either of the horse's shoulders or up the horse's neck on either side. By experiencing all of these movements yourself on the horse you will be familiar with the specific demands placed on the rider. The qualities of rhythm, timing and speed of movement may also be affected by a CVA. These may be improved by the work on the horse. Make sure that the rider is breathing normally and is relaxed at all times. This work to affect the trunk is of key importance, and cannot be duplicated in any other therapeutic setting.

The rider's head posture should also be addressed. There may be other factors beside the hemiparesis which contribute to the abnormal posturing of the head. With certain visual disturbances the rider may have limitations in the range of vision which may affect head positioning. The rider may also have a limited awareness or attention to the hemiparetic side, termed "neglect." Frequent changes in direction, circles and other figures, while instructing the rider to look in that direction with eyes and head forward may help this problem. Having dressage letters or other visual cues in the arena, or playing catch, may also be beneficial in promoting good head movement.

As the rider has been proceeding to move in response to the movement of the horse and in response to verbal cues from the instructor or therapist, staying on the horse has always been a goal. Fear of falling, especially for older individuals who have frequently experienced falls, may be strong. Side walkers, a well-trained horse, driver or instructor, and therapist can all help to ease this fear. This will allow the rider to not tense his muscles, to get better balance and react to the changing demands placed upon his vestibular, oculomotor and neuromuscular systems. As the rider sees himself better balanced on the horse, he may also see an improvement in his balance off the horse, sitting, standing, and walking. Biery and Kauffman (1989) cited studies conducted by Hall, Hulac, and Myers (1983) and Fox, Lawlar, and Luttges (1984) showing improvement in balance from riding. Biery and Kauffman went on to examine the effects of therapeutic riding on the balance of eight individuals with mental retardation. By measuring their balance in a variety of postures off the horse in standing and quadruped position prior to and after a six month therapeutic riding program, the authors were able to document improvements. Each instructor is encouraged to monitor each rider's physical and functional status so that similar data can be gathered to support the use of the horse in the rehabilitation process.

MOUNTING AND DISMOUNTING

Since many disabled persons cannot mount and dismount in the usual ways, various aids and adaptations may be needed to make those activities possible. A ramp and mounting platform are desirable when dealing with adult riders. Children are more easily assisted by lifting them onto the horse from the ground. Additional factors such as pain, joint instability, and limitations in the available range of motion may impair mounting from the ground. If a saddle is being used, slightly lowering the stirrup and assistance from the side walkers may be all that is necessary. When using a mounting platform, a variety of techniques may be used. The physical or occupational therapist working with the rider may be of more assistance in recommending a suitable transfer technique, especially if the rider is to be transferred from a wheelchair. If the rider is in a wheelchair, either that individual or a family member should be able to tell which direction of movement--left or right--is easiest. When assisting the rider in a wheelchair it may be safest and more practical to remove the footrest and the arm rest closest to the horse. Make sure that good body mechanics are used. The therapist's back should not be compromised.

If the rider has limited ambulatory skills, it may be best to have him first sit sideways on the horse prior to swinging one leg over the neck of the horse. Be prepared to support the trunk and assist the lower extremity swinging over the neck. The rider will typically lose his balance backward and may not have sufficient hip range of motion to complete this mounting technique. If the rider is able to balance a short time on one leg with some support, an alternative method is to have the rider face the head of the horse, hold on to the handle of the surcingle or to the therapist and swing a leg over and sit. It may be easiest for a rider to stand on the stronger leg while swinging the involved lower extremity over the horse. Dismounting can be performed either way. It is helpful to have a chair on the platform so that the rider can sit after the ride.

CONCLUSION

This discussion has considered the physical assessment, observation, treatment and benefits for the client with CVA and his response to the horse in equine-assisted therapy. Look at the rider as a whole, consult rehabilitation team members and set obtainable goals with the rider. During and after treatment observe the rider's response to the horse, monitor for ill effects as well as the positive responses seen, and adapt the activities appropriately. But do not forget to help your riders have some fun and then watch their self-esteem rise.

References
Baumann, (1979). *Therapeutic Exercise on Horseback for Children with Neurogenic Disorders of Movement.* 3rd International Congress. England.
Biery, M.J., Kauffman, N. (1989). **The Effects of Therapeutic Horseback Riding on Balance**. *Adapted Physical Activity Quarterly.* 221-229.
Bobath, B., (1978), *Adult Hemiplegia, Evaluation and Treatment.* Second Edition, London: William Heinemann Medical Books Limited.
Carr, S., Gordon, G. H. (1987). *Movement Science for Physical Therapy and Rehabilitation.* Maryland, Aspen Publishers.

Conti, D. (1984). *Post-Stroke Adapted Exercise Program.* (Informational Pamphlet): American Heart Association.

Davies, P. (1985). *Steps to Follow: A Guide to the Treatment of Adult Hemiplegia.* Germany: Sprirges-Verlag.

Fox, V. M., Lawlar and Luttges, M. W. (1984). "Pilot Study of Novel Test Instrumentation to Evaluate Therapeutic Horseback Riding" *Adapted Physical Activity Quarterly.* 1, 30-36.

Hall, S. J., Hulac, G. M., and Myers, J. E. (1983). *Improvement Among Participants in a Therapeutic Riding Program.* Unpublished manuscript, Washington State University, April.

Kluwer, C. (1982). On the Psychology of Riding/Vaulting. *Proceedings of the 4th International Congress.*

Kunzle, U. (1982). The Effect of the Horse's Movement on the Patient. *Proceedings of the 4th International Congress.*

Riede, D. (1988). *Physiotherapy on the Horse.* Wisconsin: Omnipress.

Ryerson, S., Levit, K.(1988). *Physical Therapy of the Shoulder.* New York: Churchill, Livingstone, Chapter: The Shoulder in Hemiplegia, 105-131.

Ryerson, S., Levit, K. (1988). *Physical Therapy of the Foot and Ankle.* New York: Churchill, Livingstone, Chapter: The Foot in Hemiplegia. 109-141.

Documents in these Proceedings. *Sixth International Riding Therapeutic Congress.* (1989). Toronto: Canada.

Haehl, Victoria, PT, BS. NDT certified (adult). consulting--All Seasons Riding Academy and other Bay Area therapeutic riding centers; member--NAHRA, Bay Area Equines for Sports & Therapy.

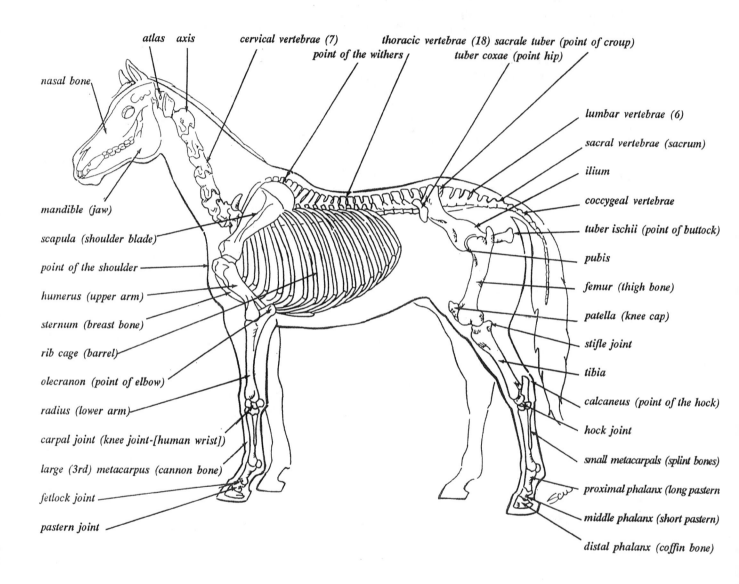

atlas   axis

cervical vertebrae (7)

thoracic vertebrae (18) sacrale tuber (point of croup)

point of the withers

tuber coxae (point hip)

nasal bone

lumbar vertebrae (6)

sacral vertebrae (sacrum)

ilium

coccygeal vertebrae

mandible (jaw)

tuber ischii (point of buttock)

scapula (shoulder blade)

pubis

point of the shoulder

femur (thigh bone)

humerus (upper arm)

patella (knee cap)

sternum (breast bone)

stifle joint

rib cage (barrel)

tibia

olecranon (point of elbow)

calcaneus (point of the hock)

radius (lower arm)

hock joint

carpal joint (knee joint-[human wrist])

small metacarpals (splint bones)

large (3rd) metacarpus (cannon bone)

proximal phalanx (long pastern)

fetlock joint

middle phalanx (short pastern)

pastern joint

distal phalanx (coffin bone)

308

A HIPPOTHERAPY TREATMENT PROGRESSION

Barbara Heine, PT

Marcus, aged 6 1/2, has a diagnosis of cerebral palsy of the spastic quadriplegic type. He presents the typical forward flexed kyphotic posture and an excessive posterior pelvic tilt. His hip flexors are moderately tight and he has increased tone in hip adductors and internal rotators. He ambulates with a reverse walker using his upper extremity strength to "pull" himself along. Trunk strength and trunk/pelvic dissociation are poor. He can bench sit independently but is unable to do so with an erect trunk and neutral pelvic (see Photo 1). His treatment plan includes short term goals of independent transitions on the horse at the walk, and maintenance of an upright midline trunk with a neutral pelvis for 20 minutes, including changes in direction and tempo. Long term goals include bench sitting with an erect trunk and neutral pelvis, sit to stand without assistance using lower extremities only, and walking with bilateral canes for 50 feet. Marcus receives physical therapy and occupational therapy twice a week through the State school system and one weekly 30 minute hippotherapy session.

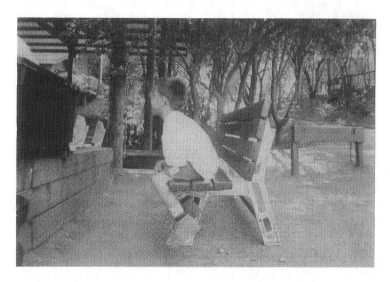

PHOTO 1.

Marcus commenced hippotherapy in 1994. For the first 24 sessions he required backriding to provide sufficient support at the pelvis and trunk for the facilitation of an upright midline position. He progressed to sitting astride with maximal assistance from the therapist on the ground and has improved to the point where he currently requires minimal assistance or contact guard only.

Each hippotherapy session begins when the therapist assists Marcus in walking from the bench outside the arena to the mounting block. The horse chosen for Marcus is an 8 year old thoroughbred/quarter horse mare. Her narrow base is well suited to Marcus's adductor and internal rotator tone. In addition, the mare has a ground covering walk that can be precisely graded to produce the exact amount of perturbation required to address the client's needs at any given time during the treatment. The equipment of choice is bareback pads: specifically, a 1" thick felt shock-absorbing pad to protect the horse's back, 1 thick foam pad for client comfort, and 1 large white cotton over pad, all held in place by a plain surcingle with sheepskin covering the D-rings and hard leather edges. The horse is controlled for the session with long lines and wears a snaffle bridle with a flash noseband and side-reins (see Photos 3, 9 & 11).

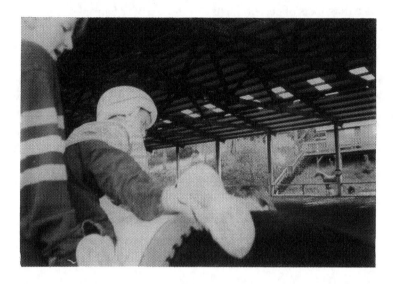

PHOTO 2.

To mount the horse, Marcus is lifted from the mounting block and placed in a prone position over the horse's barrel. With moderate assistance he transitions from prone to sitting astride facing forwards. The transition focuses on motor planning, trunk/pelvic dissociation and appropriate weight shifting (see. Photo 2). Facing forwards does not facilitate a neutral pelvis and in (Photo 3) it is clear that although Marcus's sitting posture has improved slightly, he still exhibits a kyphotic trunk and a posterior pelvic tilt. Facing forwards is, however, the initial position of choice secondary to increased tone in hip adductors and internal rotators. It is necessary to have Marcus in this position for approximately 10 minutes during which time the rhythmic movement of the horse and the stretch provided by the position will produce sufficient reduction in tone to enable Marcus to transition to facing backwards. In these first 10 minutes, the therapist provides verbal and tactile cues to encourage trunk extension and independent sitting with hands on thighs. It is critical at this stage to keep the horse's tempo slow so as not to compromise Marcus's ability to maintain midline head, neck and trunk alignment. The position is maintained until Marcus exhibits trunk/pelvic dissociation and hip abduction, external rotation and extension has increased.

In Photo 4, Marcus transitions to facing backwards. This position facilitates an anterior pelvic tilt by "tipping" the client forward and facilitating the trunk extensors. It is the combination of the upward slope of the horse's withers and the close proximity of the surcingle to the base of the sacrum, that causes a displacement of the center of gravity, anterior to the base of support. This activates an extensor response and a subsequent anterior pelvic tilt. In Photo 5, Marcus's initial reaction to this displacement is to "prop" with his fingers, but it does not take him long to accommodate posturally and assume an excellent upright position with his bands on his thighs (Photo 6).

Note that sitting backwards requires a greater degree of hip abduction and external rotation. Clients with excessive lower extremity tone and/or limited range of motion, must be carefully assessed before utilizing this position. Sufficient range of hip motion must exist to "straddle" the horse comfortably. Forcing the position will cause discomfort and/or pain and may result in exacerbation of tone and increased likelihood of hip subluxation.

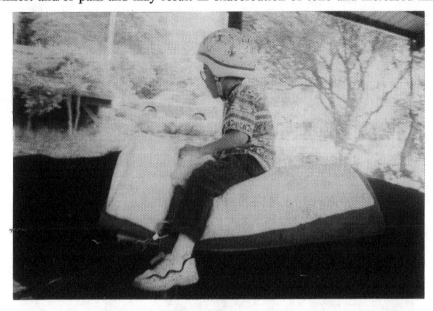

PHOTO 3.

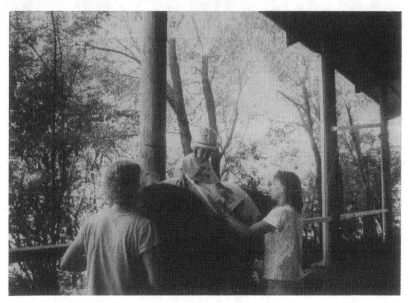

PHOTO 4.

The next 10 minutes are spent in the backward sit position. The treatment foci include trunk rotation and bilateral upper extremity reaching activities, with the overall goal of distal mobility and proximal trunk stability. Compare Photos 7 and 8 that were taken a few minutes apart. Photo 7 shows the first reaching activity; Marcus has difficulty with trunk rotation and selective muscle control. The effort of reaching (clearly seen on Marcus' face) has resulted in loss of balance, slumped posture and exacerbation of upper extremity flexor tone. His reaching arm is flexed at the wrist and elbow, while the left arm is in a moderate guard position and trunk/pelvic dissociation is poor. Photo 8 of a subsequent reaching activity, just minutes later, shows considerable improvements in posture, trunk rotation, balance and upper extremity function. During the last five minutes of the backward sit position, Marcus is engaged in upper extremity activities. Photos 9 and 10 show Marcus reaching for and catching a ball with an upright trunk, no loss of balance and excellent functional use of upper extremities.

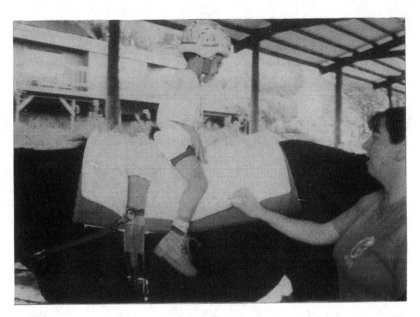

PHOTO 5.

In the last 2 minutes of the session, Marcus transitions to quadruped with minimal assistance while the horse continues to walk. Quadruped increases proprioceptive input and is an ideal position to facilitate co-contraction at hips and shoulder girdle . In addition, Marcus enjoys the challenge of successfully achieving this higher level balance skill. From quadruped, Marcus returns to sitting astride facing backwards and dismounts from that position. In Photo 12, Marcus dismounts with contact guard by leaning forward, swinging one leg behind him and sliding to the mounting block. Note the excellent upper extremity function

For the duration of the 30 minute session, the horse remains primarily on straight lines as, at this stage in the treatment plan, changes in direction compromise Marcus's ability to remain in an upright midline position. The horse's tempo however, is increased gradually as the session progresses to provide a graded increase in postural challenge. During transitions, the tempo is slowed to allow for the successful and safe execution of the activity.

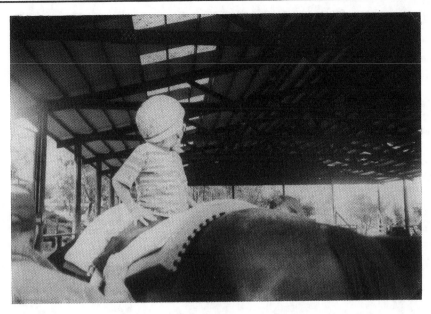

PHOTO 6.

Photo 13 shows Marcus bench sitting immediately following the treatment, holding a carrot for Java, his therapy horse. Note the enormous improvements in postural control, trunk and head alignment and upper extremity function as compared to Photo 1.

Marcus loves to "ride" and is thus highly motivated in this setting. His parents report that this enthusiasm is not always seen in other clinical environments. Hippotherapy is ideal for a child like Marcus who has been, and will be, in therapy for many years. As Marcus progresses, the hippotherapy treatment plan will be modified to provide a continuing challenge in this highly motivating setting.

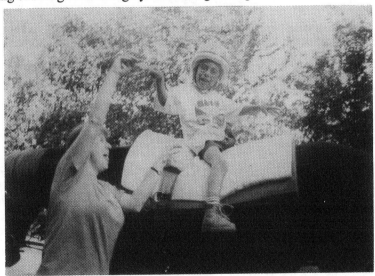

PHOTO 7.

Summary of a Thirty Minute Treatment Session	
Walk into arena and mount	2 minutes
Facing forward	10 minutes
Transition	1 minute
Facing backward	10 minutes
Transition to quadruped	I minute
Quadruped	4 minutes
Dismount and walk out of arena	2 minutes

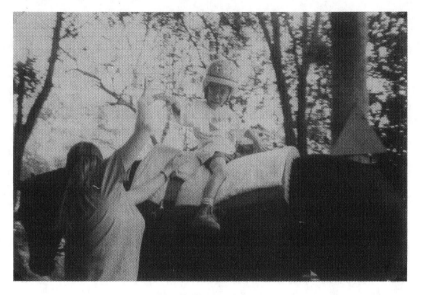

PHOTO 8.

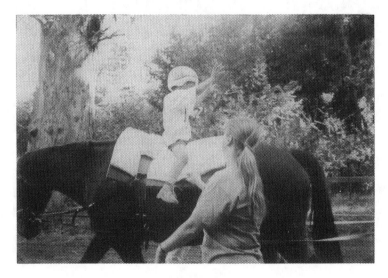

PHOTO 9.

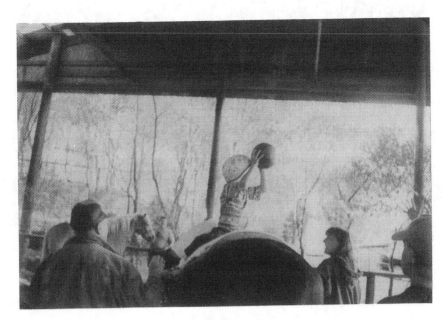

PHOTO 10.

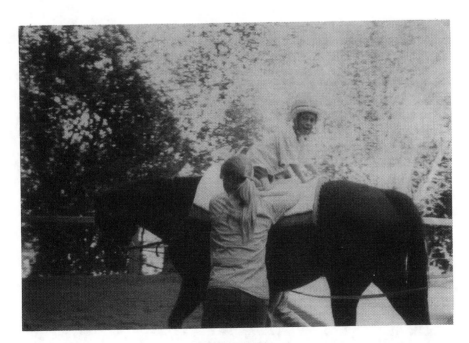

PHOTO 11.

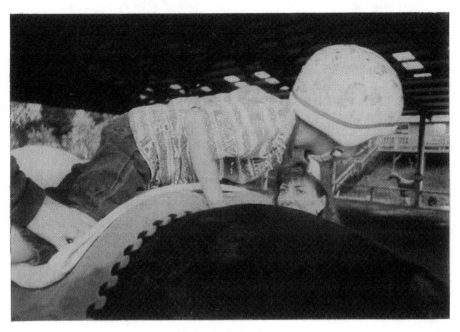

PHOTO 12.

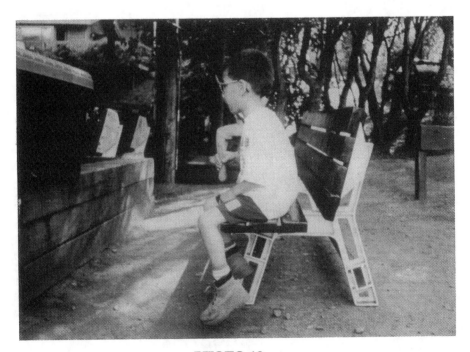

PHOTO 13.

THE REHAB RANCH: A RESIDENTIAL RIDING THERAPY CAMP

Kate Zimmerman, MBA, PT

THE DREAM

In the summer of 1980, the author was sitting on a deck overlooking San Francisco Bay with a fellow therapist and future partner, tossing around ideas on how to combine the therapy they had been performing at Children's Hospital Medical Center (CHMC), in Oakland, California, with their favorite outdoor activities. They decided to investigate the possibility of running a summer camp for children with physical disabilities, which set in motion a series of events leading to the creation of a non-profit corporation called REHAB CAMPS, INC.

The author had been introduced to the concept of therapeutic riding through a course at All Seasons Riding Academy (ASRA)* where she spent three months cleaning stables, riding, and learning how to work with disabled children astride the horse. As a physical therapist, she found it very exciting to use the horse as a treatment modality as well as an adapted recreational activity, and gained the knowledge of the value of the horse in therapy. At the time the notion of the camp had developed, horses became the main focus that would be initiated during the camp experience.

THE BEGINNING

The next year, professional friends were signed up to be on the board of directors of REHAB CAMPS, INC. Funds were raised from a variety of sources, grants were written, and pleas were made for donations from local corporations. In the fall of 1981, the earnest planning of the camp had began. Staff was recruited from local therapy programs, and a site and clients were all that was needed now. The camp began in June, 1982, and continued for four years. Some clients came back each year. It was an immensely gratifying learning experience at best, a tiring and frustrating one at its worst.

THE SITE

Initially, the group explored the possibility of renting established camps with riding facilities. These were all too expensive for REHAB CAMP's fledgling budget. Through the contacts of ASRA, the group found a riding enthusiast who held the lease on a riding concession at the Grant Ranch, in Hall's Valley east of San Jose. The use of the site was a donation for the first year's operation. There was open land for tents, primitive showers, stables, and a riding arena. After a survey of Grants's Ranch for wheelchair accessibility by a team of physical therapists, it was decided that this site was suitable. The team readily agreed to the free use of the land.

A ramp was constructed for wheelchair users. Barbecue pits were built. A portable shed and an above ground pool were purchased. To augment the one public restroom on the grounds, Porta-potties were rented. A member of the Board of Directors obtained the use of a recreational vehicle for the executive staff, and tents for campers were obtained from the U.S. Army. Refrigeration was another problem, but the team managed the first year with one refrigerator and a couple of big ice chests. The group simply made the operation work.

* All Seasons Riding Academy, Fremont, California.

The second and third years that the camp was in operation were much easier as the host of the camp added facilities. A barn was built which was used for the director's living quarters and office. A netting and tarp covered area was built for eating and daytime activities that made campers and ranch staff more comfortable. The fourth year was the most comfortable of all. Because of an increase in funding, the group was able to rent a real camp with a pool, cabins, and indoor toilets. There were some steep hills at this locations but with paved paths. Wheelchair users needed to have someone to help push them up the hills. A real benefit of renting an established camp was that the proprietors provided meals and a program director to augment the group's staff.

THE CAMPERS

The first year, from connections at CHMC, a group of 16 clients was selected for the first two-week session of the camp. In selecting the client/campers, finding a homogeneous group that could participate in activities together was of primary concern. The actual physical diagnosis was not as important since the director felt that establishing common ground for developing relationships in the weeks to come was more important.

The author had been a camp director at a large camp which accepted clients with a mixture of cognitive and physical disabilities. Through this experience she had learned the difficulties of program planning for groups too diverse to engage in similar activities or even to engage each other in relationships. As both the author's and her co-director's specialty was physical therapy, their focus became primarily clinical for boys and girls with physical disabilities. Another criteria for client selection was age. The clients needed to be old enough to spend two weeks away from home. The age ranged selected was from seven to sixteen years.

A review of the camp records indicates that the acceptance policy was liberal. During the four years there were clients who were blind and those who were severely disabled, needing one-on-one attention. Other clients had only mild disabilities and could assist in the care of the dependent campers. Clients' diagnoses included spinal muscle atrophy, cerebral palsy, spina bifida, equinus varus (club foot), closed head trauma, polio, and muscular dystrophy.

THE STAFF

Recruitment and selection of counselors evolved around identifying people with an interest in working with young physically challenged campers. The staff found the local colleges fertile ground, especially those with therapy, special education, and recreational therapy programs. Word was spread among professional co-workers and friends. A warm response ensured, and offers were received for volunteers. The staff included high school students with riding background, therapists with years of pediatric experience, and the mothers of the executive staff. A pediatrician joined the staff at the camp the first year and remained with the group as a consultant in the years to follow. Including the executive staff, the group always had at least one-on-one staff-to-camper ratios. Counselor-to-camper ratio was from one-on-one to one-on-three depending on campers' needs and abilities.

Due to the needs of the campers, the group recruited at least two nurses per session to help with potential problems that could and did arise. In the first year of REHAB CAMP, the staff found the camp needed the two nurses almost all the time in dealing with constipation, seizures, pressure sores and sunburn. The University of California San Francisco Hospital was the main source for nurses. The first year REHAB CAMP was fortunate to find an experienced rider who was also a nurse, and she later became a co-director of the program. It was surprising to find such a wealth of experienced and willing people, once the needs for staff was made known to the community.

CAMP PROGRAM AND TRAINING

REHAB CAMP program planning differed from that of the usual summer camp for disabled children in that it tried to focus on physical therapy in combination with recreation. Arts and crafts programs were taught by occupational therapists and occupational therapy students with an emphasis on cognitive learning. A purely recreational program was also offered with activities like dances, campfire sings, and story telling. The physical therapy staff provided pool and riding programs with an emphasis on physical therapy.

Training for the staff consisted of one to two day on-site sessions prior to the camp openings. The staff was trained in areas of:

- basic health care
- CPR (cardiopulmonary resuscitation)
- the nature of disabilities to be seen
- the general schedule of camp days
- the activities offered
- brainstorming on programming ideas
- campfire songs and stories
- campers profiles specific to the counselors assigned to them

The directors had produced manuals for reference for all the counselors. In addition, the directors sent out information about each camper to the staff prior to the first meeting. The directors made every attempt to cover all possible areas of concern to the staff, including job descriptions and schedules of a normal camp day. Each counselor reviewed the charts of the campers assigned her. The first year, young camp volunteers and executive staff did it all: camper care and attention, food buying and cooking, horse care and preparation, tent set up and maintenance, and a major part of program planning and implementation. The second and third years, we had additional assistance. This left more time for the executive staff to plan and implement the programs and made an enormous difference in the quality of the camp.

A DAY AT CAMP

A typical day's schedule at camp:

6:30 am	out of bed for staff and counselors.
6:30-7:30 am	readying campers for breakfast.
7:30 am	breakfast, announcements, and a brief staff meeting.
8:50-9:00 am	preparing for morning activities
9:00-10:30 am	activities began with choices of:

- riding
- arts and crafts
- individual therapy/group exercise
- swimming

10:50- Noon	rotating groups, same activities offered
Noon-1:30 pm	lunch and clean up
1:30-2:00 pm	rest and organization for afternoon activities.

2:00-3:00 pm	rotating groups in the same activity
3:00-4:00 pm	same as above, plus fishing
4:00-5:00 pm	rest and prepare for dinner
5:00-6:30 pm	dinner
6:30-7:00 pm	free time
7:00-8:30 pm	campfire activities/special dances

The stated schedule proved to be demanding for both campers and counselors and in later years it was amended to give more time between activities and for meals. The staff learned to make allowances for the most disabled persons in the group. This included cutting back on the number of activities offered to give everyone, especially staff, more time to breathe and relax.

This was the planned schedule. The staff had to make allowances for the weather. Because there was a lake in Hall's Valley, lake activities were incorporated into the daily schedule. Some campers caught fish which were cooked for dinner. The fourth year's site of REHAB CAMP had to adapt its activities to the schedule of an established camp of which it was a part. Nevertheless, most of the therapy activities were accommodated along with the many other activities the management had to offer.

THE RIDING PROGRAM
The first year the riding program consisted of simply getting everyone used to a horse and also to the use of a horse as a therapeutic modality. The approach was very basic--teaching care of the horse, grooming, bridling and saddling. The riding program focused on learning the basic commands of walk, halt, trot, turns, and simple patterns.

In the years to follow, a surcingle was used for a vaulting program, and backriding was used to facilitate reactions in therapy. Both recreational and therapy sessions were incorporated, with different goals for different campers. For therapy sessions, a longe line and a surcingle were used, with two side-walkers, an occasional backrider, and a therapist in the ring at all times. Altering the gaits of the horse was used to facilitate equilibrium reactions and for trunk strength; prone work across the horse, and sitting to kneeling exercises were performed for strength and balance. The use of a longe line gave more control over the horse and provided more security in trying the different gaits. The covered arena at the Grant Ranch provided a controlled environment for the horses and riders.

For the recreational program, one-fourth of the campers could ride alone while the rest of the campers needed at least a leader. Many needed sidewalkers. In years two and three, there were more horses to choose from and the staff screened and trained the mounts to suit the individual needs of the campers. The author had received additional training in New York with Barbara Glasow (Winslow, NY Clinic 1982). This contributed greatly to the approaches used in years two and three.

The fourth year, REHAB CAMP used the horses provided by the YMCA camp. While this may sound ideal for a riding camp, it was not the optimal arrangement for a therapeutic program. It was necessary to screen each horse and train the ones that were suitable for disabled riders. The riding director and her YMCA staff adapted to this new approach well and were trained to help.

SUMMARY

The four years that the Rehab Camps were in operation were exciting times. The directors created as they went along, evaluating, criticizing, changing, and improving from year to year. They accomplished what they set out to do, which was to prove that recreation and therapy can be combined in an outdoor setting where clients stay for an extended period of time. Changes noticed in the campers included:

- ☻ increased self confidence
- ☻ increased physical abilities
- ☻ improved attitudes toward the therapists and therapy
- ☻ increased ability to take care of themselves
- ☻ increased ability to ask for help when it was needed

During the camp's concentrated weeks noticeable changes can be seen in both the campers and the staff. The directors watched themselves grow, as they dealt with the challenges of creating something from nothing. They dealt well with problems and avoided serious problems or accidents. What was learned during these years was:

- ☻ the complexity of the daily lives of the clients, their challenges, and how immense their needs were.
- ☻ the value of dedicated professional directors who have time to lend to such a worthwhile project.
- ☻ the value of the volunteers who contributed their time to make the project become reality.
- ☻ the value of dreams and of individual visions of potential reality.
- ☻ the value of the blind faith that sometimes, somehow things will work.
- ☻ to prepare for the worst, yet hope for the best.
- ☻ to know that everything that can go wrong will.

Camps like Rehab Camp need to happen. Pediatric therapy must be taken out of the white-walled clinics and made a part of our client's live. Having the responsibility for clients for two weeks is an enormous undertaking which requires a lot of work and planning, but it is one of the most gratifying experiences this author has had in her therapy career.

SMALL ARENA

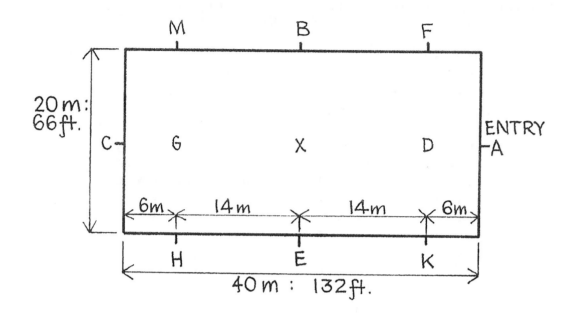

LARGE ARENA

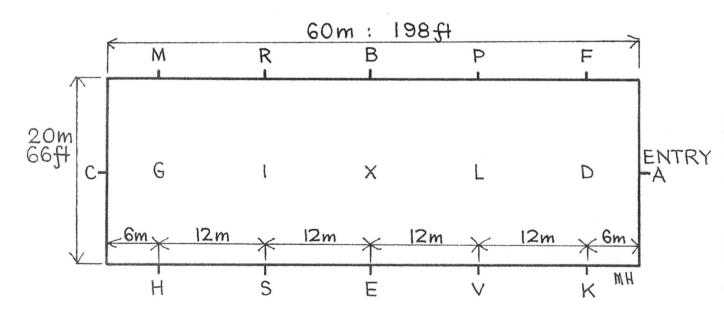

EXERCISES FOR EQUESTRIAN

Mary Beth Walsh, PT, BHSAI

Equestrians are a unique group of athletes who require a specific regimen of exercises to meet the challenge of all riding including dressage, hunt seat and vaulting. For physically challenged riders, it is especially important that the riders prepare their bodies for riding by performing the appropriate stretches prior to getting into the saddle. Special consideration for each individual's postural reflexes and tonal patterns should be adapted to the stretches performed. Consultation with the riders' physical therapists is encouraged to maximize the quality of stretching. In all forms of riding, flexibility and strength are essential prior to putting their feet in the stirrups.

The following pages describe a comprehensive fitness program for all riders. Special emphasis is placed on the lower abdominal strength and pelvic mobility for dressage riders, and on back extensor muscle strength in order to maintain a solid hunt seat position. Vaulting requires both flexibility and great strength of all muscle groups in order to execute set maneuvers. Daily performance of these exercises is necessary to achieve the best results for flexibility, strength and motor learning. Flexibility exercises should be done prior to riding. Cross training in sports that improve pelvic and low back mobility and improve strength in the legs and abdomen are also beneficial for riders. Some of these sports are swimming, cycling, dancing, gymnastic, cross country skiing and climbing the stairmaster. For dressage riders, practicing the hula hoop (even when sitting on a stool) is highly recommended for improving muscle tone and coordination.

Prior to starting an exercise program within your program, it is important that one understands how to stretch properly. There are a few important points that should be remembered. Remember to relax, to breathe throughout the exercise, to focus on the muscles being stretched, to make the stretch smooth-steady stretch and to avoid pain. Program instructors should request assistance from their physical therapy (or occupational therapy) consultant, to help adapt exercises to special riders with unique needs but remember that everyone, including the staff, profits from proper stretching. Remember, too, that all these exercises are not suitable for every rider.

Please note that although these exercises are designed for the rider, some may not be appropriate for **all riders.** Always contact the rider's physician, physical therapist, or the program's consulting physical or occupational therapist prior to initiating this exercise program.

WHY STRETCH**
Stretching, because it relaxes your mind and tunes up your body, should be part of your daily life. You will find that regular stretching will do the following things:
- Reduce muscle tension and make the body feel more relaxed.
- Help coordination by allowing for freer and easier movement.
- Increase range of motion.
- Prevent injuries such as muscle strains. (A strong, pre-stretched muscle resists stress better than a strong unstretched muscle.)

- Make strenuous activities like running, skiing, tennis, swimming, cycling, and horseback riding easier because it prepares you for activities; it is a way of signaling the muscles that they are about to be used.
- Develop body awareness. As you stretch various parts of the body, you focus and get in touch with them.
- Help loosen the mind's control of the body so that the body moves for "its own sake rather than for competition or ego.
- Promote circulation.
- It feels good.

Reference
Sections and exercises noted with asterisk ** are excerpted from Bob Anderson's book *Stretching* (1980)--reprinted by permission. Anderson, B., Anderson, J. (1980). *Stretching*. Shelter Publications, Inc., P.O.Box 279, Bolinas, CA 94924.

LOWER EXTREMITY FLEXIBILITY

Quadriceps Stretch

The quadriceps are the muscles in the front of the thigh. Flexibility is necessary for pelvic mobility and to allow legs to be held in proper, aligned position while riding.

Perform standing or kneeling, grab the ankle and relax hip forward. Hold position for 30 seconds. Repeat 5 times. You will feel a stretch in the front part of the thigh and hip.

**

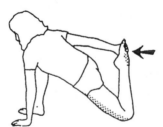

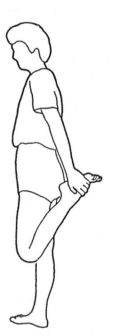

Calf Stretch

The muscles in the back of the calf need to be flexible in order to keep your heels down and your feet in the stirrup. Simply lunge forward and keep your back heel in contact with the floor as in this picture. Hold 30 seconds. Repeat 5 times.

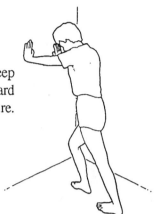

Combination of inner thigh, quadriceps, calf stretch, low back. Hold position for 30 seconds. Repeat 5 times. Nice quick "pre-riding" stretch.

**

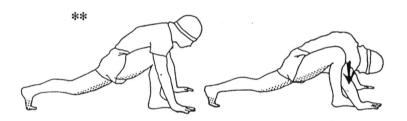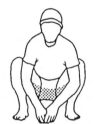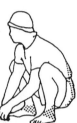

Hamstring Stretch

The hamstrings are muscles in the back of the thigh. These muscles will restrict pelvic movement if not flexible.

Start by stretching one leg out in front of you as the picture demonstrates. The calf muscle can be incorporated by using a towel to pull up on the foot. Hold for 30 seconds. Repeat 5 times.

**

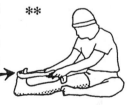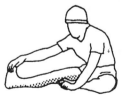

Progress to both legs in front.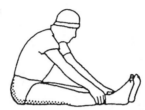

Next, sit down with your legs straight and feet upright, heels no more than six inches apart. Bend from the hips to get an easy stretch. Hold for 20 seconds. You will probably feel this just behind the knees, and in the back of the upper legs. You may also feel a stretch in the lower back if your back is tight.

Remember to bend forward from the hip as if it were a hinge.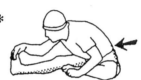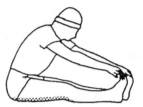

Think of bending from your hips without rounding your lower back.

If your hamstrings are particularly tight and the above positions put too much strain on the low back, perform the stretch by leaning against a wall. Hold for up to 1 minute. Repeat 2 to 3 times.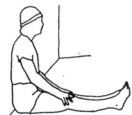

Inner Thigh Stretch

The inner thigh muscles perform a "gripping" or "squeezing" legs together while contracting. This contraction is necessary to stabilize the lower leg and pelvis while in 2-Point, but must be supple and flexible in Dressage to allow the pelvis to be relaxed in the saddle. If these muscles are not properly stretched prior to riding, the pelvis will not be allowed proper flexibility and a bumpy ride is in store for the rider.

** Remember—no bouncing when you stretch. Find a place that is fairly comfortable that allows you to stretch and relax at the same time.

**

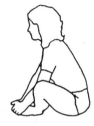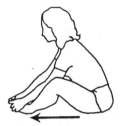

Begin the stretch by sitting with the soles of the feet together. Pull the feet together. Pull the feet close to your body.

** If you have any trouble bending forward, perhaps your heels are too close to your groin area.

If so, keep your feet farther out in front of you. This will allow you to get movement forward.

** Variations:

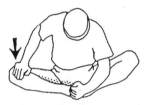

Then gently press down on the knees. Start by stretching one knee. Hold for 30 seconds. Repeat 2 to 3 times.

** Hold on to your feet with one hand, with your elbow on the inside of the lower leg to hold down and stabilize the leg. Now, with your other hand on the inside of your leg (*not on knee*), gently push your leg downward to isolate and stretch this side of the groin. This is a very good isolation stretch for people who want to limber up a tight groin so that the knees can fall more naturally downward.

To Stretch the Groin Area

**

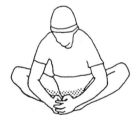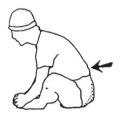

Then progress to stretching both knees down. This can be done by pressing your elbows into your knees. Hold for 30 seconds. Repeat 2 to 3 times.

HIP AND LOWER BACK STRETCHES

Double Knee to Chest

This exercise helps to stretch out the long broad muscles that surround your spine. Relax and pull your knees up to your chest, and hold for 10 seconds. Repeat 10 times.

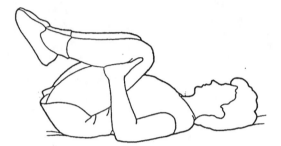

Then progress to a **piriformis stretch.** This muscle is deep in your buttocks. Simply pull one leg diagonally across your body, keeping your hips on the mat. Hold up to 30 econds. Repeat 5 times.

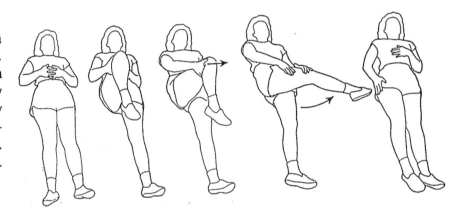

Hip Flexor Stretch

The hip flexors are in front of the hip at the top of the thigh. In order to maintain a long leg on the horse and good pelvic mobility, these muscles need to be stretched. Hold position 30 seconds. Repeat 5 times.

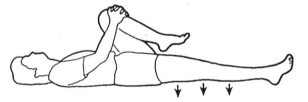

Start by pulling one knee to chest, pushing down on opposite leg.

Again, hold the stretch up to 30 seconds, repeat up to 5 times.

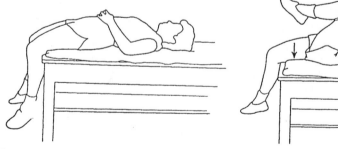

Progress to letting one leg hang over mat.

PELVIC TILT

The pelvic tilt is performed to increase the mobility of the low back. The exercise utilizes the lower abdominal muscles to pull the seat underneath you. The muscles relax, allowing the low back to gently arch again. Performing the pelvic tilt is similar to the movement necessary to "go with the movement" of the horse, especially in the sitting trot.

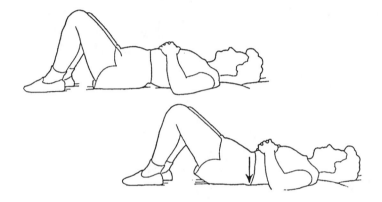

Perform by pulling up with the lower abdominals, pressing the low back into the mat. Perform 10 times.

Pelvic Tilt with Wall Squat

Lean against a wall, squat down to about 45° to 90° and hold. While holding, perform a series of 10 pelvic tilts as shown above. Repeat at different levels of squatting, increasing the time held in the squat position up to one minute.

* This exercise is particularly good to improve strength and mobility for the Two-Point position.

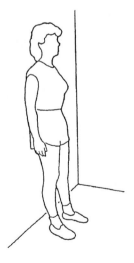
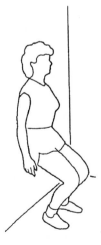

LOW BACK FLEXIBILITY

To improve the mobility of the low back and pelvic tilt, sit and have a friend assist you in rocking your pelvis back and forth while you maintain an upright posture. The movement is the same as a pelvic tilt, perform by tightening and relaxing your lower abdominal muscles. Repeat 10 times.

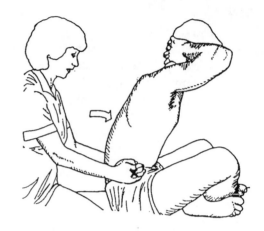

Cat and Camel Exercise

Perform a series of pelvic tilts, rounding your back **as an angry cat** and then **arching your back as a camel.** Repeat in succession up to 20 repetitions.

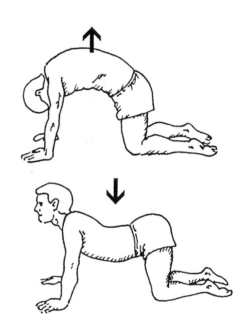

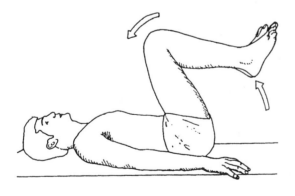

Lower Abdominal Lift

To perform the lower abdominal lift, first perform a pelvic tilt, flattening the low back into the mat. Hold legs up at 90° to the body, then by contracting the lower abdominal muscles, lift and lower the pelvis off the mat. Repeat in 2 to 3 sets of 10 repetitions.

Abdominal Strengthening

The best way to strengthen the abdominal muscles is to perform "curls" described below. The muscles are necessary to assist in supporting the back and promoting good posture.

Perform abdominal exercises daily in sets of 10 repetitions. Increase the number of sets performed as the exercise becomes easier and you can maintain good form.

EXERCISES FOR THE ABDOMINAL MUSCLES:

The abdominal muscles are the strength center of the body. They are essential for endurance. They help keep your back free from pain, assist in proper movement, easy elimination of waste, in rhythmical breathing, and in standing erect. But few of us have ever felt the energy that goes with strong abdominals.

"Sit-ups" are generally considered the best exercise for strengthening abdominal muscles. Yet sit-ups offer little in the way of rhythm and can cause severe strain. Because of this, many people understandably detest sit-ups.

The straight legged sit-up is potentially dangerous for the lower back for this reason: your abdominal muscles can raise your body off the floor to about a 30° angle. To raise any further activates the primary hip flexor muscles, which are attached to the lower back. This puts severe stress on the lower back.

Bending your knees will relieve much of the strain in your lower back. The bent knee sit-up is good, as long as you do each sit-up fluidly and mentally concentrate on the abdominal muscles. Be careful of this exercise because people generally do too many repetitions, and when tired, jerk up quickly, which stresses the lower back.

The developmental exercise I do recommend for strengthening abdominals without straining the lower back is the *ab curl*. Here the upper body is curled forward no more than 30° and the lower back remains flat.

** Here are three exercises and one variation that will work the upper, lower and sides of your abdominals. If your abdominals get tight doing these, just relax and straighten out your legs, put your hands over your head and reach in the opposite direction with a controlled stretch. Hold for 5-8 seconds. This should stretch the abdominals and relieve any tightness that might occur.

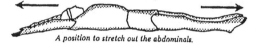

A position to stretch out the abdominals.

The Abdominal Curl (Ab Curl)

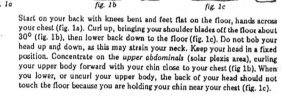

fig. 1a   fig. 1b   fig. 1c

Start on your back with knees bent and feet flat on the floor, hands across your chest (fig. 1a). Curl up, bringing your shoulder blades off the floor about 30° (fig. 1b), then lower back down to the floor (fig. 1c). Do not bob your head up and down, as this may strain your neck. Keep your head in a fixed position. Concentrate on the *upper abdominals* (solar plexis area), curling your upper body forward with your chin close to your chest (fig 1b). When you lower, or uncurl your upper body, the back of your head should not touch the floor because you are holding your chin near your chest (fig. 1c).

The Elbow-Knee Ab Curl

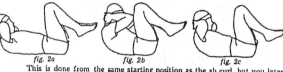

fig. 2a   fig. 2b   fig. 2c

This is done from the same starting position as the ab curl, but you interlace your fingers behind your head about ear level and raise your feet off the floor. Using your abdominal muscles, hold your upper body at about a 30° angle off the floor (fig. 2a). Now, bring your elbows forward, touching about 1-2 inches above the knees (fig. 2b). Uncurl as in fig. 2c, then raise your elbows and knees again as in fig. 2b. Your lower back should be flat at all times during these abdominal exercises.

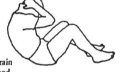

UPPER BACK MUSCLE STRETCHING

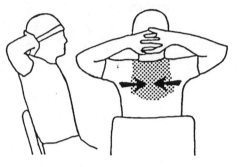

Pectoral Stretch

The pectoral muscles are located in front of the chest. When these muscles are tight, they prevent you from keeping your shoulders back. Stretch these muscles with hands behind head as in Figure 1 or with arms at side as in Figure 2. Pull back as far as you can. Hold 10 seconds. Repeat 5 times.

** **Figure 1**

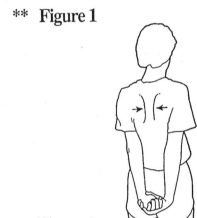

Figure 2

To strengthen upper back muscles to promote good posture, start by lying on mat with arms over edge. Raise and lower arms, pulling shoulder blades together with every arm raise. Increase resistance by adding small weights to hands. Repeat 10 times.

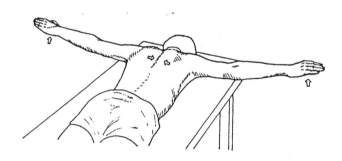

Progress to raising arms and trunk as in this picture. Perform slowly and hold for 5 seconds in the raised position. Repeat in 4 sets of 5 repetitions.

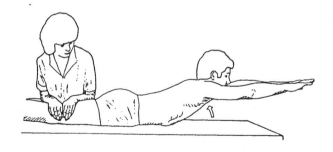

SHOULDER AND BACK FLEXIBILITY

Low Back and Shoulder Stretch

Sit on your heels, bend forward, stretch your arms overhead, hold for 30 seconds. Repeat 2 to 3 times. You'll feel this in the shoulders and low back.

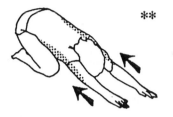

Side Stretch

Stretch as in Figures 1 and 2. Hold for 10 to 30 seconds. Repeat up to 5 times.

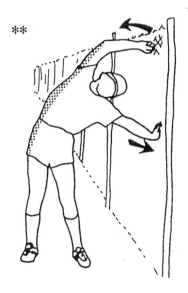
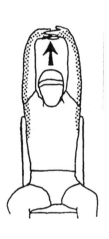

Figure 1   Figure 2

Tricep Stretch

Position arm as in the picture and pull elbow as shown. Hold for 10 to 30 seconds. Repeat up to 5 times.

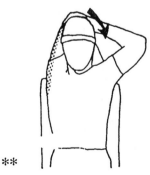

LOW BACK EXTENSION EXERCISES

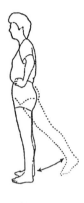

Leg Extensions

To begin to strengthen the back muscles, perform these leg lifts. Increase the difficulty by adding ankle weights. Repeat 3 sets of 10 repetitions.

Back Bends

Hold hands on hips, gently arch back, hold for 1 to 2 seconds. Repeat 5 times.

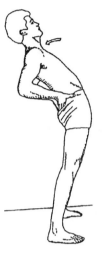

Or

Leg Extension

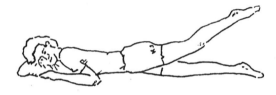

Progress to performing lifts while on your stomach. Again, add ankle weights (up to 5 pounds). Perform in multiple sets of 10 (i.e., 2 sets of 10, progress up to 5 sets of 10 repetitions).

Perform lying on stomach as in a **press-up**. This is a nice warm-up to improve low back flexibility. Make sure you keep your hips on the mat. Hold 10 seconds. Repeat 10 times.

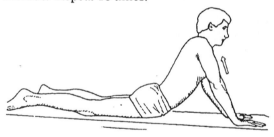

*Total Back Extension (The Swan)

Figure 1

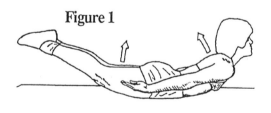

Begin with arms at your side

* These exercises are especially good to prepare for Two-Point and jumping.

Figure 2

When you are really strong, progress to raising all four limbs and your trunk off the floor. Hold position 5 seconds and relax. Progress to arms over head. Repeat 10 times.

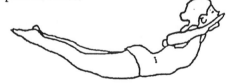

334

CHAPTER 20

OCCUPATIONAL THERAPY

SENSORY INTEGRATION DEVELOPMENT

Jill Standquist, OTR/L, NDT

The infant uses reflexes and information from his senses of:	To develop these sensory motor abilities:	He uses sensory motor abilities to learn more concrete concepts and to develop:	He uses perceptual motor skills to accomplish an automatic level of function in:
TOUCH	BODY SCHEME	EYE HAND COODINATION	ACADEMIC LEARNING
			READING
MOVEMENT	REFLEX MATURATION	OCULO MOTOR CONTROL	WRITING
			NUMBERS
GRAVITY	CAPACITY TO SCREEN	POSTURAL ADJUSTMENTS	SPELLING
	SENSORY INPUT		
HEARING		AUDITORY - LANGUAGE	ACTIVITES OF
	POSTURAL SECURITY	SKILLS	DAILY LIVING
TASTE			
	AWARENESS OF TWO	VISUAL - SPATIAL	ABILITY TO
SMELL	SIDES OF BODY	PERCEPTION	CONCEPTUALIZE
VISION	MOTOR PLANNING	ATTENTION CENTER	INDEPENDENT
		FUNCTIONS	WORK HABITS
		MASTERY OF	BEHAVIOR - ABILITY TO
		ENVIRONMENT	FORM MEANINGFUL
			RELATIONSHIPS

SENSORY MOTOR PHASE
0 - 12 months

PERCEPTUAL MOTOR
PHASE
1 - 5 years

LEARNING PHASE
(cognitive or intellect)

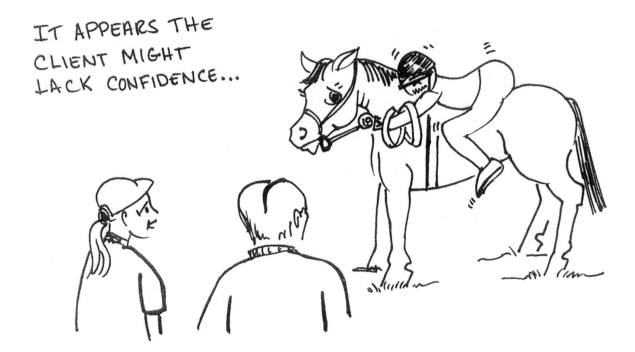

SELF-CONCEPT IN CHILDREN AS IT AFFECTS LEARNING

John H. Brough, OTR

One of the most important and least understood areas of development is the affective area or *"the way I feel about myself"* (Piers). Professionals talk about self image, self concept and their importance but little is really known about how such feelings develop. Self concept is a complicated system composed of many sub-systems. The perception of self-worth is elusive and complex. The following breakdown, showing six factors, is taken from the **Piers-Harris Children's Self Concept Scale**. The six factors give a good view of the important parts of a child's feelings about himself.

The areas measured are:
- Physical appearance and attitudes
- Anxiety
- Intellectual and school status
- Behavior
- Popularity
- Happiness and satisfaction

In the areas of **physical appearance and attitudes** the child is assessed on his or her feelings related to:
- General looks
- Does he or she see him or herself as strong?
- Is he or she important in class?
- How does he or she feel about his:

> Eyes?
> Hair?
> Face?
> Figure?

What does he or she perceive his or her classmates think about him or her in the areas of:
- Ideas?
- Leadership?
- Popularity?

In the critical area of **anxiety**, the child is assessed as to:
- Shyness
- Perseverance
- Nervousness
- Amount of worry
- How well does he or she sleep?
- Test taking (how he or she feels about it)
- Feelings of fear

Testing these concepts gives an idea about the degree of anxiety or stress to the body that can be caused by poor self concept, a perception that can radically change performance. A child with a high degree of anxiety is most likely ruled by the sympathetic division of the autonomic nervous system. This means that his or her brain has "downshifted" and he or she is basically working at the most primitive level. Cortical function is repressed and learning may not be possible.

The area of **intellectual and school status** is evaluated in the following areas:
Does the child feel that he or she is:
- Smart?
- Capable of creating good ideas?
- Liked by the teacher?
- Good at school work?
- Important?
- Popular with peers?

The area of **behavior** is evaluated in many ways. The child's **relationships** are rated in the following environments: school, family, home, with peers, with other people. The tester examines how well the child works and what the trouble areas are in the above situations. The behavior the child describes may or may not be the truth, but it is important to remember that the significance is how he or she **feels** about him or herself and his or her behavior.

Popularity is rated on his relationships in school and peer group--with boys and girls. Popularity can also be looked at in the extended family.

Happiness and satisfaction is rated in all areas. Evaluation is made as to whether or not the individual feels happy, likes the way he or she is, feels lucky and cheerful. Also examined is if the child wishes that he or she were different, or wants to change. The most important fact to remember is that the relationship of how the child feels and what the truth actually is may be either erroneous or very accurate. The child's self-concept comes from how he or she feels, not necessarily from the truth. The self-concept is very important and may greatly influence the course of therapy. A positive and accurate self-image can speed the learning process. A negative self-image, whether accurate or inaccurate, can slow down or completely hinder the self-concept. To build a good concept, it is necessary to give the individual accurate and concrete feedback. One should help him or her develop positive attitudes to replace his or her negative ones and tap any or all of his or her sensory avenues as aids in developing the necessary precepts upon which he or she can build his or her self-concept.

References
Piers, E., Harris, D. *The Piers-Harris Children's Self Concept Scale.* (The Way I Feel About Myself). Nashville: Counselor Recordings and Tests.

GROOMING AND TACKING-UP AS AN ACTIVITY USED FOR TREATMENT IN OCCUPATIONAL THERAPY

Judy Hilburn, OTR

A Therapy Experience

Max, tall for his age, was a handsome four year-old, with big brown eyes and coppery hair. Blessed with high intelligence and advanced verbal skills, he talked excitedly and incessantly about his many super heroes and their grand and varied adventures. But ask Max to climb the `tower' or `leap a small building' in a single bound (playing out his fantasies), and he would fail miserably. Max's big brother was excelling in school. His little brother was running circles around him. Max's parents were baffled. Then the bi-monthly children's clinic came to town. During the clinic it was discovered that this gifted child had a learning disability. Max was hypotonic and afraid of heights. He shuffled rather than ran. When he did try running, he did so with arms pinned at his sides, his shoulders fixed for extra control; even then with this extra control, Max appeared to be on the verge of tumbling forward.

Max was unable to enjoy the playground like the other boys. In the classroom, things were no different. Manipulating a crayon was beyond his capabilities, since his eyes and hands had offered little help in developing visual-motor skills. Being a bright boy, Max was able to cover up most of his shortcomings---but not for long. His gravitational insecurity would soon win out. Max was admitted to a pre-school program where he received occupational therapy with a sensory integrative emphasis, for several months.

When a small hippotherapy program was established in town, Max's parents requested that he be considered for it. Indeed, he was. Combined with clinical occupational therapy, hippotherapy filled in the gaps, and his treatment program was enriched. Max was first involved with grooming the horse to improve his tactile responses and motor planning skills. He also began to use the mounting block to reach the top of the horse. At first he could tolerate only the lower step because of his gravity insecurity. Max then began to assist in leading the horse from the stall. His interest in the horse helped him challenge his fear of movement and soon he had the courage to mount the horse with help. Max continued to progress over the months to come and soon was able to ride alone in the ring. Everyone stood back and watched Max's failures slowly turn into successes. Before a horse can be used in a hippotherapy program or in a therapeutic riding program, it must be regularly groomed and tacked up. Many hours are spent by stable staff providing these needs. Why not use these as treatment activities for selected riders in a therapeutic riding program? Occupational therapists will find that horse grooming and tacking-up are easily adapted for the treatment needs of clients with disabilities.

To begin, equipment required for such activities would be: curry combs, brushes of varying sizes and textures, a hoof-pick, a halter, ropes, a saddle blanket, a saddle or surcingle, a cinch/girth and a bridle. The horse to be groomed must be under the control of a riding assistant at all times, but can be positioned so that riders of all sizes, either ambulatory or in wheelchairs, can participate.

There are factors inherent in the activity of grooming and tacking that address frequent needs in persons whom occupational therapists treat, namely occupational role development and occupational performance. These functions involve activities that require one to involve himself in setting realistic goals and making decisions.

Grooming and tacking-up require these skills. The client will also develop safety awareness, and recognize established routines while working around a horse and caring for him.

Due to the fact that these activities integrate the demand for various senses and skills, there is a continuous overlap in therapeutic effects. For example, the areas of gross motor function, muscle tone and co-contraction of muscles can be influenced by heavy work patterns while a client carries a grooming kit, saddle blanket or saddle. Or, if a platform or mounting block is used during these activities, a client may have the opportunity to "practice" climbing or jumping skills (jumping off the block). If a client is advanced enough in his or her horse skills to begin leading the horse to the grooming area, then ambulatory skills could be influenced. A client may need to walk over uneven terrain or execute stops, starts and turns. A client must match his or her own rate, rhythm and sequence of movement to that of the horse. The author has noted that most of the time, her mare changes her way of walking to accommodate her "challenged" handler's gait.

A client's upper extremity strength and range of motion can be facilitated by brushing a horse, since anti-gravity, resistive movement patterns are inherent in this activity. Tightening cinch/girth straps will also affect strength of the upper extremities. Bilateral upper extremity integration and coordination can be facilitated by using two grooming implements at a time. For example, a client may hold a curry comb in one hand and a body brush in the other, alternating the use of each tool as it is appropriate. While assisting with lacing/adjusting a cinch-strap, reciprocal, hand-over-hand movement patterns are involved.

Similarly, fine-motor development can be affected in many ways. For example, activities of daily living (ADL) skills are improved by the ability gained while manipulating buckles on halter, bridle or girth; or rein and lead-rope snaps; or while brushing mane/tail. Pincer grasp is increased while picking a horse's loose hair out of curry comb or body brush. During combing of a mane, a client may use his or her fingers as the comb. Such an action is effective as an active-resistive exercise for strengthening the hands. Establishment of dominant/non-dominant hand patterns can be affected by these brushing/combing activities since they are rich in spatial sequencing patterns. One can see this as a client may handle the brush with his dominant hand while being encouraged to use the non-dominant hand as a support/assist by resting it on the horse's body. The same situation can also be duplicated while a client is helping to tighten a latigo cinch.

Establishment of hand dominance can be facilitated while the client is leading a horse, carrying the lead rope properly (i.e., one hand holding excess rope coiled, while the other hand holds the rope near the snap end). This activity can be adapted for the right or left-handed client. For such adaptations to occur it is obvious that the therapy horse must be accustomed to being led from either side. Tactile perception for fine-motor control is enhanced because the lead-rope is being held on the diagonal against resistance. Hypotonicity of oral musculature can be improved during highly resistive activity using the hands, such as pulling on the latigo girth during cinching of the saddle, or while using a hoof pick to dig out debris imbedded in the hoof. (Oral musculature and hand function have an associated reaction).

Postural responses are facilitated whenever a client must reach high spots, either during grooming or tacking-up, when needing to get up on tip-toes to brush the horse's back, or to help adjust the saddle or blanket. Equilibrium responses are elicited when a client bends over to brush the horse's belly or legs, or to reach for the cinch. When appropriate, a client may assist with picking out the horse's hooves and in so doing, the vestibular system is again stimulated because of the bending position he must assume. Leading the horse also affects postural control. Such an activity requires the client to use trunk rotation, and separation of head, eyes, and upper extremities.

Grooming and tacking are activities which lend themselves well to a high level of tactile input. Grooming implements are made of varying textures. For example, brushes are stiff or soft, curry combs are made of rubber, plastic, or metal. As far as tack goes, there are ropes of nylon or cotton; ropes are braided, round or flat; reins are of cotton webbing or leather. The horse himself has a myriad of varying textures. The mane and tail are coarse; body hair can be furry or smooth; the muzzle area is velvety; hooves are hard and rough. A groomer comes in touch with all these areas.

Development of cognitive perceptual skills is also easily worked into the grooming/tacking activity. Spatial terms are an integral part of these activities, such as brushing the horse **on top** of his back, or **under** the girth area. The individual can start brushing from **front** (neck area) to **back** (hind quarters). He can learn that saddle blankets go on **under** the saddle. Body scheme concepts are continually used as the person brushes **softly on the horse's face** and **carefully** around his **eyes and ears**. He or she will learn to be sure to brush the **"off"** or **right side** of horse also. Comparison of human body parts to the horse's parts can also be easily done. The horse has a scrape on his **knee**, just like a child sometimes gets on his or her knees. While leading the horse, a client is faced with such "body-map" dilemmas as where to stand (right or left side, or in front of the horse), how close to stand to the horse, how fast to walk, and how to get both the horse and himself safely through a gate, or barn doors.

During grooming, enhancement of tool use and motor planning is seen. The client will realize how the rubber curry comb is to be used in order to remove dried mud, or during tacking-up, how is one going to get the awkwardly shaped saddle or vaulting surcingle onto the horse properly positioned. The activity of grooming and tacking-up easily lends itself to developing direction-following and problem-solving skills. Tacking-up requires that specific sequences be followed; that is, the saddle blanket must be placed under the saddle, or the girth must be tightened before mounting. Such questions as how does the horse pick up its hoof for cleaning, or how does one keep the reins from dragging on the ground, facilitate the use of problem-solving skills. Other cognitive areas such as ideation, sequencing, and programming are enhanced when various questions arise. "In which corral is my horse?" "How will I get him out of the corral?" "Will the horse come willingly?" "What equipment will I need?"

Opportunities to use communication skills are many, both verbal and non-verbal, when dealing with the horse. Simply looking for and greeting the horse encourages communication. Communication is facilitated when various verbal and body cues are used for leading/halting the horse, finding ways to praise the horse either by patting or verbalizing "good girl". Some horses will actually seek out the client with a look or movement which might suggest: "Rub-me-here," or "Who are you, brushing me so nicely?" And each of us has seen every horse non-verbally (or verbally!) say "Where's my carrot?". Such demonstrative body language by the horse is hard to miss and the client usually has no choice but to respond.

Benefits in the area of social-emotional development are many and inherent in the activity. There is the arousal of nurturing instincts of the client toward the horse. Several needs of the horse may be met such as brushing away a bothersome fly, cleaning off dried mud from the girth area to prevent chaffing, or removing twigs from the mane or tail. The client finds he or she must be attentive to the horse's likes and dislikes, such as ticklish spots to be avoided during grooming, or taking care of that itchy spot behind the ear. The client is made aware of his or her own behavior and how it might affect the horse, such as learning that running and jumping around could startle the horse or that jerking on the lead rope or hitting the horse may scare him. The client learns to understand "others'" behavior (the horse's) when he or she has to deal with a horse that momentarily balks, or veers off course while being led. The client learns what pleases the horse (grain, hay or carrots) and how the horse acts to get that treat. Self-esteem is enhanced when he or she is successful in controlling such a large animal as the horse. He or she receives approval when he or she sees the horse properly prepared for riding. Finally, the caregiver of the client sees the positive effect. The treatment setting has usually been the clinic or hospital, with clients surrounded by wheelchairs, crutches, and walkers, but it is now the great outdoors where one is surrounded by fresh air, trees, birds, and horses, viewing people who are busy, working with their horses. The caregiver happily sees his son (or daughter, husband or wife) as a part of this active, bustling environment.

Conclusion

A frame of reference is a body of hypothetical assumptions and principles that give unity and direction to practice and research. It provides the basis for treatment - in this case the treatment used by occupational therapists. The major frames of reference used by occupational therapists include (Christiansen & Baum, 1991):

- Cognition & Activities
- Sensory Integration
- Spatio-temporal Adaptation
- Human Occupation
- Adaptive Responses
- Facilitating Growth & Development
- Role Acquisition
- Occupational Behavior

The approach to treatment involved in all of these frames of reference can be applied within the equine setting. Using the focus of the horse and the manipulation of the environment to meet the specific treatment needs, the occupational therapist has at her disposal many functional and meaningful activities. These therapists carefully select activities to allow clients to adapt behavior as they confront disabilities and to organize sensorimotor systems for function and skills.

Reference
Christiansen, C.. Baum, C. (1991). *Occupational Therapy, Overcoming Human Performance Deficits.* Thorofare: Slack Inc.

COGNITIVE REHABILITATION AND GAMES *
A Therapeutic Horseback Riding Perspective

Kathryn L. Splinter, MOT, OTR/L

According to Hopkins & Smith (1983) cognition is the conscious process of awareness by which knowledge is acquired through perception, memory, and reasoning. It includes the ability to think, know, and understand objects and their relationships to oneself and the environment. Common disabilities in cognition may include difficulties with memory, problem solving, sequencing, and attention span that affect an individual's daily functioning.

Closely linked with cognition and a person's ability to perform a task is behavior (Allen, 1992). Observations of behavior are used to identify an individual's ability to process information. Within the therapeutic riding session, the instructor or therapist can readily pick up indicators as to a person's cognitive functioning. As one participates in a therapeutic riding session, the instructor may encounter a rider's resistance to certain activities. No one likes to do something that they cannot do. Two possible explanations are possible for one's resistance to performing an activity: motivation and ability. The therapist or instructor must distinguish between *will not* and *cannot*. Therapeutic horseback riding is intrinsically motivating, but some of the tasks or activities we ask our riders to do may be difficult. One must separate what may be due to a lack of motivation, or an inability to understand & to perform a task. Keen observation and assessment is necessary for determining the cognitive-behavioral functioning of an individual.

An individual may be referred to a therapeutic riding program because of a cognitive disability, but more commonly seen is a referral for a specific medical diagnosis, usually relating to a physical or psychosocial disability. During the therapeutic riding sessions, cognitive problems are often observed and it may become apparent that the cognitive disability is the limiting factor to activity or task performance. Cognitive disorders or disabilities can greatly affect the performance of individuals in everyday activities. Thus, whether or not a cognitive disability has been identified formally in the referral, it may still be the primary consideration or problem. Of course, within the lesson format, cognitive and behavioral issues can be addressed in conjunction with other problem areas, such as sensory-motor or psychosocial.

Cognitive disorders or disabilities can be defined as difficulties in information processing due to brain impairment. This difficulty in information processing alters a person's experience of and response to environmental or internal stimuli, interfering with the performance of daily living tasks. How well a person functions is largely determined by the quality of thought required to perform functional activities. Cognitive disorders may include problems in awareness, orientation, attention span, concentration, sequencing, memory, problem-solving, decision-making, abstraction, and organization. Disorders in cognition may be global or specific in nature. They may be due to an affective disorder, developmental delay, or organic impairment.

* Editor's note: This article can address clients receiving cognitive therapeutic intervention by occupational therapists or adaptive educational intervention. The approach may differ dependent on the orientation and training of the professional providing the service. The author has tried to address both fields.

Problems are often observed in those with mental retardation, psychosocial dysfunction (ie, schizophrenia or bipolar disorders), head injuries, and cerebrovascular disorders (Reed, 1991). Related cognitive or information processing problems may also be seen in those with cerebral palsy, multiple sclerosis, learning disabilities, and many others.

It is the intent of this paper to focus the reader's awareness on the cognitive problems that become visible as one works with a rider or student. Certain approaches or methods of teaching make a tremendous difference in providing a therapeutically beneficial and enjoyable session for a person with a cognitive impairment. Possible activities or adaptations will be discussed that may assist the therapeutic riding instructor, and as a result, the rider, to be more successful. (The term *rider* is used loosely to mean rider, driver, student, client, or participant in off-horse activities.)

Within the field of cognitive rehabilitation, two different approaches are most widely recognized: remedial and adaptive (Trombly, 1996). The remedial approach attempts to affect specific cognitive functions and assumes that treatment will stimulate recovery of the central nervous system. The adaptive approach utilizes alternative strategies or changes in the environment to bypass the disability in order to facilitate adequate function. The adaptive approach is the most applicable to therapeutic riding as the environment is very adaptable and compensatory techniques can be used. Because the therapeutic riding setting is not clinical, but can focus on real life activities, generalization or transfer of the learned adaptive strategies for performing a task to everyday life activities is often discovered after an individual participates in therapeutic horseback riding.

Almost any activity used for therapeutic riding can be adapted to facilitate cognitive processing. For example, initially a ball may be seen only as a sensory-motor activity as it is tossed to the rider. To address the cognitive problem of memory for example, the instructor may ask the rider to identify the color of the ball, the size of the ball, where the ball is, and then place the ball out of sight. The same questions may be asked of the rider at the end of the lesson, or at the next week's lesson to assess memory. Adaptive cues may be to line up two or three different balls and ask the rider to identify which ball was the one that was talked about earlier.

Often an individual with a disability may have difficulty responding quickly to questions or commands of the instructor (seen with developmental delays, cerebral palsy, etc.). Allowing a greater length of time after giving a command or asking a question, can allow that individual enough time to cognitively process the information and respond verbally or motorically. Simplifying commands to one, two, or three steps can significantly help in the rider's ability to respond correctly. To increase the difficulty of the activity, increase the number of steps; to simplify for success, decrease the number of steps.

The most commonly encountered types of disabilities or problems within the therapeutic riding lessons may include difficulties with memory, sequencing, following directions, problem-solving, or attending to a task. Each of these cognitive problems is relatively easy to work with within the therapeutic riding lesson. Following is a sampling of these cognitive problem areas and examples of activities to enhance the cognitive functioning. In no way is this meant to be a comprehensive list, but only a beginning or a spark to ignite your own creativity and understanding for dealing with cognitive disorders.

Memory:
1. Discussing and pointing out parts of the horse (or saddle, bridle, grooming tools, or gaits) is an excellent activity for encouraging memory. This may be done on or off the horse, with paper and pencil, or with sticky dots or labels on the horse.
2. Remembering and stating names of the other riders and volunteers is another activity that can carry on from one week to the next week's lesson. Adaptations may be to call a person's name as the ball is tossed to that person, or to only ask the rider to remember their horse's name, or a side walker's name.

Following directions:
1. An obstacle course: set up obstacles (poles, barrels, buckets on fences, colored chalk on ground, imaginary obstacles (i.e., a river to cross, a mountain to climb, etc.)) Vary directions to accommodate for slower cognitive processing, i.e., start with one, two step directions and increase to multi-step directions. Adapt with a leader that others in the class can imitate.
2. Any multi-task activity such as "pony express." Mail boxes are set up to which riders have to pick up and deliver a letter. The rider may even be assigned to write a letter to a fellow rider to be delivered at the next week's lesson.
3. Developing riding skills entails a multitude of directions to follow. The instructor gives the commands for a basic walk-trot-whoa lesson. To increase the difficulty, the instructor may add circles and diagonals, progressing to a simplified dressage test.

Problem solving:
1. An obstacle course (as above), but with a focus on the rider determining own paths around or over obstacles. Create a story or situation where all riders must work together to successfully complete an obstacle course.
2. "Around the world" can be used to encourage problem solving. Instead of commanding each step, the instructor asks the rider to tell or show how to turn to various positions on the horse. This also addresses motor planning.

Sequencing:
1. Dressing or tacking up horse. This may be facilitated by step-by-step photos or drawings for riders to sequence on the poster or imitate on the horse. Items of clothing (i.e., hats, large coats, socks, ties, ribbons, etc.) may be placed on horse for an afternoon of fun. Numbering the clothing items or tack can provide cognitive cues to the rider.
2. Riding the barrels: This activity involves numbering or lettering various barrels or points in the arena. The rider must sequentially ride to each point. An activity basket or card may be placed at each point or barrel that the rider must perform (i.e., brush your horse with the brush in the basket, or pat your helmet with your left hand).

Attention span:
1. "Do you see what I see?" This activity entails focusing one's attention on various objects in the environment. It may be led by the instructor or the rider can focus and direct their own attention. Objects may be set out to discover, or things in the natural setting may be pointed out, (i.e., a spotted horse in the next pasture, an airplane overhead, a flower). Using other senses besides vision can be helpful, (i.e., a soft cloth, a stiff brush, a good smelling bean bag).

2. Red light/Green light: This child's game can be varied to facilitate attention using verbal, visual (a sign), or hand signals. Varying the environment or activity by changing direction or adding ground poles for visual structure also helps to keep attention.

Below is a summary of activities for use with cognitive disabilities:

NAME OF ACTIVITY			GOALS ADDRESSED	ADAPTATIONS / PROPS	SAFETY & PRECAUTIONS
1) Activity baskets: ball, beanbags, clothes pins, bubbles, horseshoes			Body movement: crossing midline rotation, gross/fine motor, oral motor. Problem solving Sequencing Motor planning Riding skills	Position of baskets (high or low) Position of horse Use of volunteers, parents Ball, beanbags, bubbles, clothes pins, bucket, horseshoes, baskets, etc.	Horse with baskets & equipment. Explain purposes of activities.
2) Activity cubes			Riding skills. Sequencing. Follow directions	Interactional or individual. Activity dice or a cube.	Space for activity.
3) Around the World			Body movement: motor planning, crossing midline, balance, coordination Sequencing	Western vs English vs. bareback pad.	Support of side walkers
4) Ball Toss			Body movement: rotation, crossing midline, motor planning. Sequencing. Social interaction.	Medium or large ball. Prompt names. Arrange in circle, or line.	Horses must be ok with ball & close proximity to other horses.
5) Barrels			Riding skills. Unilateral reach. Sequencing.	Barrels. Buckets on top with brushes, horseshoes, or potatoes. Numbers or letters on barrels.	Watch spacing for side walkers.
6) Do you see what I see?			Observation skills. Memory. Social interaction. Attention span.	Stationary, or moving. Make sensory (touch/smell instead of visual) Set out objects to find.	If moving, leader may guide horse
7) Dressing your horse			Dressing skills (buttoning, tying, donning, doffing) Memory. Sequencing. Organization skills.	Paper/poster activity. Imitate or sequence photos of tacking horse. Tacking up own horses. Clothing (hats, ties, coats, socks, ribbons)	Horse needs to be calm with items of clothing or equipment. May bridle ahead of time.
8) Follow the leader			Build self esteem, self confidence, independence Problem solving Riding skills: guiding	Lay out possible course. Leader/side walker may coach. Rotate among riders.	Watch for spacing & direction. May need to redirect.
9) Go Fish (for questions on paper, velcro fish, or horseshoes)			Motor planning. Cognitive: horse knowledge, memory, problem solving	Bucket, magnet on fishing pole. Adapt question difficulty Weight, build up fishing pole.	Comfort of horse with fishing pole.

NAME OF ACTIVITY		GOALS ADDRESSED	ADAPTATIONS / PROPS	SAFETY & PRECAUTIONS
10) Horse puzzle		Cognitive skills: memory, body part identification Horse knowledge: body parts, color & markings, breeds	Paper/poster activity.	Good for rainy days.
11) Mother, May I?		Counting steps. Sequencing. Verbal skills.	Adapt to rider's needs.	Spacing of horses.
12) Name: parts of horse grooming tools, colors, sizes, names of people or objects		Memory Demonstrate use of grooming tools	Sticky dots. Paper & pen activity. Brushes, hoof pick, etc.	Horses need to be ok with bits of paper stuck to them.
13) Red Light/Green Light		Riding skills: walk on, whoa, trot Attention span. Follow directions. Competition.	Verbal. Walk on, Whoa sign.	Spacing of horses.
14) Relay races.		Riding skills: guiding skills. Problem solving. Competition.	Adapt creatively (Buckets with objects, poles, tag, vary speed)	Watch speed, spacing, activity.
15) Rings.		Body movement: reaching, stretching. Identifying colors, sizes, shapes.	Rings, handkerchiefs, small balls, flags, etc.	Comfort of horse.
16) Trail ride		Riding skills: guiding. Identify objects in environment. Feel & hear movement/rhythm	Adapt to goals.	Check out area for unknowns.

Conclusion:

Becoming well recognized and documented are the physical and psychosocial benefits of therapeutic horseback riding for those with disabilities. Psychosocial benefits are especially documented in human interest articles where the emotional impact on riders with disabilities and on those observing are greatly touted and photographed. Classic hippotherapy focuses primarily on physical components of posture, balance, mobility, and function for its definition (AHA, 1993). As a person is never a component, but a composite of the whole, one must look to the holistic benefits of relating to a horse: physical, psychosocial, cognitive, emotional, sensory integrative, and recreational. Thus, many goals can be addressed at once, and the task of the observer, instructor, or therapist is to tease out what may really be going on with a rider during participation in an activity. Cognitive and behavioral disabilities or problems may be addressed separately, or along with other areas of concern. Therapeutic horseback riding activities are tremendously adaptable to meet the needs of those with disabilities. They are holistic and functional, facilitating transfer to everyday activities. Therapeutic riding keeps the "fun" in "functional." It is beneficial to request consultation from a speech or occupational therapist to discuss various strategies for working with a particular rider. They can be great resources for working with persons with cognitive disabilities or problems.

Resources

Allen, C.K., Earhart, C.A., & Blue, T. (1992). Occupational Therapy Treatment Goals for the Physically and Cognitively Disabled. American Occupational Therapy Association, Inc. Rockville, MD.

Hopkins, H.L., & Smith, H.D. (1983). Willard and Spackman's Occupational Therapy, Sixth Edition. J.B. Lippincott Company, Philadelphia, PA.

Introduction to Classic Hippotherapy. (1993) American Hippotherapy Association, Section of North American Riding for the Handicapped Association, Denver, CO.

Reed, K.L., (1991). Quick Reference Guide to Occupational Therapy. Aspen Publishers, Inc. Gaithersburg, MD.

Kathryn L. Splinter, MOT, OTR/L
University of Kentucky
Lexington, Kentucky

DRESSAGE AS A MODALITY FOR SENSORY INTEGRATION AND NEUROLOGICAL DYSFUNCTIONS

Barbara T. Engel, M.Ed., OTR

The use of dressage as addressed in this paper, is used as a treatment modality. The synchronization of control is developed through the systematic processes entailed in the classic art of riding or dressage. *Dressage refers to the gymnastic development of the horse and rider.* These processes are in many respects similar to aspects of development and the facilitation techniques used in habilitation or rehabilitation.

The goals using dressage as a modality for intervention as a treatment may include:
1. Development of a secure base of support - a prerequisite for upper body mobility, crossing midline and independent limb function.
2. Development of the ability to "feel" and motor plan to coordinate movement actions.
3. Coordination of head, body & limb movements with selective control during an activity.
4. To understand, sequence and execute instructions.
5. To respond appropriately to the perceptual stimulus of one's environment.
6. To be involved in a purposeful activity that "requires and elicits coordination among the individual's sensory motor, cognitive and psychosocial systems" (AOTA position paper 1993).

These goals can be extended, for example in a treatment plan, to meet other needs of a client such as developing focusing skills, modulation of vestibular disorders, develop upper body extension and stability of the shoulder girdle or, development of the selective fine motor control or expanding short term and or long term memory skills. Let us see how the above goals translate into the process of classic dressage.

THE GOALS OF DRESSAGE AS A MODALITY

Development of a secure base of support	A secure seat is primary to all levels of dressage. It is necessary for the rider to use effective hand, leg and weight aids. In riding, one often hears the phrase No seat, No hands. The "seat" is developed through centering and balance, a straight but relaxed back, relaxation and stretching of the thigh/seat muscles, softness and separation of upper and lower trunk to allow the pelvis to follow the movements of the horse.
Development of the ability of the rider to "feel" or motor plan to coordinate movement actions	Receiving the stimulation from the horse, focusing on this stimulation and learning to respond to the stimuli.
Coordination of head, body & limb movements	As one learns to first give basic subtle commands, then increasingly more difficult commands to the horse in the execution of maneuvers.
To understand, to sequence and to execute instructions.	Learning to listen to instructions as one combine sequential movement patterns in a coordinated manner.

To respond appropriately to the perceptual stimulus of one's environment	To maneuver and control the horse in specific patterns within an arena To spatially oriented oneself to the arena and dressage letters. To following the directions given by the instructor or the therapist as one focuses on ones own sensory, perceptual, & motor abilities.
To be involved in a purposeful activity that "requires and elicits coordination among the individual's sensory motor, cognitive and psychosocial systems.	Dressage is an acceptable activity with purpose and goals, which allows both choice and control. It can be broken down into simple steps but can progress to increasingly more difficult procedures requiring fine tuning of an individual's sensory motor, cognitive and psychosocial abilities. The client can focus his or her attention on the outcome of his or her skills allowing for the feeling of success.

How does the use of dressage relate to the conceptual framework of occupational therapy? Two major components of occupational therapy are adaption and purposeful activity. "The unique contribution of occupational therapy is facilitation of purposeful activities to be adapted by the person for acquisition of performance skills. Performance includes work, self-care, play, recreation and leisure skills"(Gilfoyle, Grady, Moore). The assumption of sensory integration theory is that the active participation in a self-directed activity promotes adaption and in turn causes sensory integration. It is believed that the adaptive process is driven by the engagement in activities. The adaptive response in occupational functioning requires the client to create the response in order for an adaptive response to occur. The client must make a choice and be in control.

Dressage requires the client to be in control for, even if the individual is given instruction he or she is the only one that can execute the command. Dressage is a purposeful activity and is self-directed with the client making the choices. Dressage is a performance skill whereby one can immediately see either success or failure of each action one takes. It requires sequential development, for, without conquering one movement, you cannot move onto the next. For example: If you are not able to maintain a balance upright position but fall forward, even slightly, with the movement of the horse, you cannot use affective seat aids. The commands are exact and the feedback by the horse is quick and without judgement - *I understand what you want of me and I will turn left -- or -- I am not sure what you are asking so I am just drifting and going slower -- no I'm not disobedient - I do not understand what you ask of me.* The horse thinks in black or white - **it is or it is not**.

We are referring to riding in the context of classic dressage where the horse is guided and manipulated through subtle body movements ---- not a rider who casually sits on his horse and steers the horse with the reins. Commands to the horse must not only be exact but must be exactly same each time. This requires the client to control the movement and repeat it each time he or she want this action. To do this one must produce a quick recall and learn to "feel" the action. For an individual with sensory processing problems, this is a BIG challenge and a great reward when you get it right!

Dr. Ingrid Strauss reminds us that living means movement. We see this clearly shown by children as they develop their motor, adaptive and cognitive skills - they are always practicing moving skills or always moving.. Suzanne von Dietz emphasizes that without movement there is no balance. Ayres' treatment methodology, which involves movement activities, strives to create a balance of the functions of the central nervous system that results in sensory integration. In classic dressage movement and balance are primary principles without which no progress can occur.

Why should we not use hippotherapy for treating of this population? Classic hippotherapy is a neurophysiological-based treatment method. The client is manipulated by a horse and a therapist. The client is a passenger on the horse but the automatic neurological systems are elicited and facilitated. The movement of the horse at a walk facilitates equilibrium and balance. The proprioceptive/vestibular and sensorimotor systems are stimulated which aid in the improvement of posture and strength. The rotational movements of the horse's back are transmitted to the rider's spine resulting in the opposing pelvis and shoulder positions - the pelvis and the shoulders of the rider parallel the pelvis and shoulders of the horse. According to Strauss this function of the spine in righting the trunk for walking is the aim of hippotherapy. One can see that classic hippotherapy does not provide for the interaction of the client with the horse on a functional bases. Choice, control and purposeful activity which addresses the sensory motor, cognitive and psychosocial abilities are not an option in hippotherapy. Classic hippotherapy treats specific neuromotor dysfunctions on a primary level. While dressage, as a treatment modality also address neuromotor dysfunctions, address a population with different therapy goals.

Sensory integrative intervention is also a neurophysiological based treatment method based on the principals of occupational therapy. Here the therapist initiates and manipulates the treatment process but the client selects and controls the type of activities and degrees of stimulation or movements desired. It is an active and functionally oriented treatment. Many of the components involved in sensory integration are also involved in dressage. The client is actively involved in a purposeful activity. He or she is in control and makes the choices as the instructor helps the client to carry out a maneuver by directing the client in how specific body motions should be made. Movement is a major medium of both methods.

The goal of dressage is not to teach "tricks" or perform an obstacle course but to maintain, cultivate and improve the horse's natural movements under the weight of the rider. Dressage is a process which requires the systematic development of the rider so that he or she can selectively control and execute subtle skilled movements. A movement can be the contraction of a muscle or it can be a combination of five or more actions coordinated into one command. These actions are developed one by one, then you add another until one can coordinate specific movements with each part of ones body. This involves the fine tuning of selective muscle control of all upper and lower body movements.

Dressage is also the systematic and gymnastic development of a horse. We will focus on the client with the assumption that we are working with a horse who has been developed to a point of self-carriage which allows the rider to be balanced between the hind and fore legs. The horse must be well disciplined and completely submissive since using dressage as a treatment method, the client rides independently in the presence of the therapist and instructor. Submission is also required for the horse to except the rider's aids willingly.

Dressage requires one to adapt one's responses as a method of communication with the horse and to refine one's coordination in order to allow the horse to move freely upon the rider's request. This requires the rider to rid him or herself of tension and resistance but to flow with the rhythm of the horse. The rider must learn to apply the aids in a very precise and consistent way in order for the horse to understand the command.

The horse does not reason --- *she turned but did not weight shift-- was that a leg aid? ---did she forget to weight shift and I should go ahead a turn left* --- No the horse thinks -- *I wish she would stop wobbling on my back!*

This process requires the client to develop increasingly subtle and selective body movements and a cognitive understanding of the process involved. An acute focus is gained as one develops a keen sense of "feeling" - both of oneself and of the horse. As new skills and movements are learned one always returns to the basics to allow for reorganization and integration. Because there are so many actions involved, dressage allows the instructor or therapist to work on small areas which do not overwhelm the client physically, mentally or cognitively such as learning to stretch the leg down and use the calf to cue the horse.

The processing operation involved in development, dressage, and rehabilitation that allows an individual to progress in function are:
1. Stability to mobility: stability yet relaxing the pelvis on the saddle and separation of the upper and lower the pelvis to move with the horse.
2. Separation of the left from the right allowing the independent use of the right and/or left aids.
3. Stability of the body to allow independent use of limbs. Independent action of the arms and legs allowing aids to be used without disturbing the balance of the torso.
4. Stability of the distal joints to allow movement of the proximal joints. The hand/wrist remain quiet, holding the reins, while the elbow/shoulders flex and extend following the movement of the horse's head/mouth.
5. Increased fine movements of the distal joints. Squeeze-release of the fingers to relax the jaw; to encourage the neck to stretch; to accept contact of the bit; or to gain attention.

The aids include the seat, legs and hand aids. In dressage, each of these aids are used in a variety of ways to give different commands. For example:
a) To go - with pelvic forward motion.
b) To stop - no motion
c) Momentary bracing - to re-balance or reorganize the horse.
d) Shifting the weight back on the inside hip/thigh - to turn.
e) Briefly stiffening of the seat and torso - to slow down the motion of the horse.

Various aids are used together to give specific commands. For example, the turning aid may consists of a squeeze of the inside hand (to pay attention), tapping of the inside calf/leg, turning of the spine in the direction of the turn and maintaining the outside rein. As one develops the sensation and control of one's body and begins to fine tune one's movements, the aids become more specific and the movements more complicated.

One must learn how certain postures interfere with what we are asking of the horse and then we must learn to avoid such postures and to replace them with a relaxed and flowing body. Stiffening the body stiffens the horse; or tipping the head forward, causing the chest to collapse and brings the body weight forward - causing the horse to go on the forehand. Bring the head up over the spine allows the weight to flow down the spine into the seat - creating a balanced seat on the three points of the pelvis. These are a few examples of the intrinsic processes involved.

The visual, oral, auditory, tactile, proprioception, vestibular and nurturing systems are all systematically stimulated within a controlled environment. Integration of learning, conceptual formation, appropriate behavioral responses, and neuromotor learning are all accomplished through an activity that has function and meaning. It allows the client to direct the activity to obtain the desired results and allows for experimentation.

These elements have been found to enhance the learning process and allows for carryover into the client's normal activities of daily living.

In this treatment setting, the therapist must carefully observe all of the client's reactions and guide the instructor so that the client is not overwhelmed, yet is challenged, and the dressage training continues, though at a slow pace. A focus is always maintained on the areas of disintegration and on the therapy goals. The client may provide on-going feedback to both the instructor and therapist on his or her ability to function. This helps the client to develop an inward focus on his or her perceptual-motor abilities.

No one in our profession is expected to be so physically perfect and have the total dedication to achieve perfection in dressage as it appears to be the requirement of the Masters of Equestrian Art of the 17th and 18th Centuries. After all, this was their profession. Certainly our clients would not qualify for their instruction. But nevertheless we will follow the <u>development of the dressage rider as described by the Old Masters</u> since they <u>parallel development and the neuro physiologically based treatments</u> used in treating persons with subtle or moderate neurological type disorders.

THE TREATMENT TEAM:

The team is comprised of a horse, the therapist, the instructor and the client/rider. An assistant may be used during the early stages of treatment when balance at a walk is a major focus. The therapist and assistant would become sidewalkers for facilitation purposes. The team must have a very good understand of each others views and work in harmony. This is a true *Team* venture.

THE THERAPY HORSE

The dressage treatment horse must be balanced, supple, rhythmic and at least in self-carriage, a training level skill, preferably in collections at second level. A horse in self-carriage is relaxed, rhythmic, forward and has begun to develop the strength in the hindquarters enough to begin to bring the hind legs under him in order to carry the weight of the rider. This allows the rider to be balanced between the hind and fore legs. The horse should have been trained in leg yielding, shoulder-in and lengthening strides in the trot at the first level. Ideally he should be collected so that he can perform haunches-in and collected strides. The horse must be submissive and alert. A horse who is not completely alert to the communication of the rider will not teach sensory processing or be perceptive to the aids. He must respond accurately and timely to the rider's communication. The horse must be forgiving to in-coordination and be able to distinguish fumbling from specific commands.

A horse is naturally very sensitive, feeling the slightest movements of the client and it is this sensitivity that is so necessary in this therapy process. This does not mean we want a hyper horse or one that cannot tolerate mistakes. We want a smart horse who is understanding of his job, is in full attention to his task and enjoys his work. The horse should be in harmony with the rhythm of the rider. Some riders cannot tolerate a horse with long strides, others cannot tolerate horses with a short stride or those with quick movements. Since dressage develops a union between rider and horse their must be a harmony between them.

This horse will require regular riding by the dressage instructor and preferably some local competition during the year to vary his interests and tune-up his skills. He should be rewarded with a trail ride evey so often to relax his mind, muscles and change his focus. Only arena work can make a horse sour.

THE THERAPIST

The therapist cannot understand the processes involved in dressage without basic dressage experience. He or she must experience the subtleness of communication, the body movements required to help the horse in carrying out requests and the depth of concentration required. Without this experience the treatment would be ineffective. The therapist must be able to perform all training level skills preferably with the dressage treatment horse. He or she must also understand the central nervous system's functions and be skilled in sensory integration methodology.

He or she must be able to identify subtle problems the client might be having and to intervene when the client cannot perform due to processing problems. Knowledge of the biomechanics of the rider and the horse is important. Patience is required since treatment in such areas as vestibular disorders or the lack of sensory processing do not subside quickly.

THE INSTRUCTOR

The dressage instructor must be knowledgeable - well read in the theory of classic dressage or the art of equitation. Understanding the building blocks in the art of equitation is essential if one is to use it as a modality. Working step-by-step is the focus - not being able to complete a test. Understanding the biomechanics of the rider and the horse is also important. The instructor should be able to see the problem the client is having by the reaction of the horse. He or she must be well trained in dressage at the second or higher level. Two very important characteristics that the instructor will need are a fine-tuned ability to observe and a great deal of patience. Normally dressage is a enduring process. Working with a client who has many problems beyond the normal rider takes a great deal of tolerance for, not only does one develop the coordination and skill but one must deal with repressing or correcting the problem involved in the disabilities. A highly skilled dressage instructor can accomplish a great deal with clients with minimal brain damage and sensory integrative dysfunction but may not understand or resolve the clinical problems without the therapist.

THE CLIENT

The client is a person who has the basic gross motor skills needed to sit on a horse independently. Cognitive skills are grossly normal or have the potential of developing to normal range since understanding the what and how are very important. He or she may have various forms of learning disability. There maybe poor sensory processing skills, lack coordination, poor endurance, and communication difficulties. The client needs to be an active part of the team in that he or she needs to provide feedback or guide the instructor/therapist team regarding relevant issues - "I am getting dizzy, I cannot feel that leg" or "I can only process one thing at a time".

One can use this technique with more physically involved clients. This requires much more patience and progress will be slow. For example, working with an adolescent client with cerebral palsy, it may take two to three months for this client to develop the "feel" of his or her legs to use it as an aid. One may also need to work on the leg extension first before the balanced seat can be developed. The rewards are great with the serious effort that client, instructor and therapist must put forth.

THE TREATMENT ENVIRONMENT

An arena with adequate fencing is required. During the early phase of therapy an arena with little or no distraction is desired since distraction will hinder the learning process. An indoor arena is preferable. The arena activity should be limited to the treatment team only. The environment will allow the client to focus on self, the horse, and the instructor/therapist only.

EQUIPMENT

An English saddle with a saddle pad are required, either a dressage saddle or a multipurpose saddle in good condition. The dressage saddle is preferred since it provides for a deeper seat and encourages better placement of the legs. The saddle must fit the horse well and be comfortable for the client. One must be aware that the male pelvis is different from the female pelvis and therefore the same saddle may not be appropriate for both clients. Dressage saddles can have a narrow twist or a wider twist. The seats can vary from shallow to quite deep. The male client may prefer a saddle with a shallow seat while the female may find more security with a deep seat. The comfort of the saddle is an important element in the execution of precise movements and communication with the horse. A saddle that does not fit the physical structure of the client will hinder the development of a secure seat and the communication with the horse.

One might come to the conclusion at this point that this is an unreachable treatment situation. The best of everything is required. Though this technique requires knowledge and skill, it is not unreachable. A therapist would be interested in becoming a GOOD rider. This requires a well trained instructor and a GOOD horse. A horse trained to first or second level maybe more difficult to find at a price one can afford but a horse who is sensitive, intelligent and responds well to good training can be used and trained by the instructor as the process moves on. He must be in self-carriage, be relaxed and supple, rhythmic and forward with the rider astride. Since the aids are developed from the horse's natural responses, the horse will respond to them when they are correctly applied. An alternative for obtaining a horse which has worked well, is to find a dressage rider (preferably a student of your instructor) with a 1st or 2nd level horse, borrow the horse for a couple hours a week. The horse would profit from the change in his normal routine and the owner would welcome the additional exercise the horse receives provided he is being handled by a knowledgeable dressage instructor.

Lets us now look at a treatment situation and how dressage works.

TREATMENT OF A MIDDLE AGED WOMAN WITH PROCESSING PROBLEMS SINCE INFANCY.

The evaluation determined the major problems that could be addressed during therapy in this setting. In this case, the lack of equilibrium was addressed first, since this caused the client to have a feeling of insecurity. The second major problem was a poor tolerance to movement.

The initial goal was to gain in the client the equilibrium which comes from the balance of the body's weight on the center of the moving horse. The client had to find her true center---not where she felt her center was to the left--- balance her head above her shoulders and relax her shoulders above her hips. With the shoulders forward, she would not be seated properly, and could not effectively communicate with the horse. The major communication with the horse comes through the seat bones or buttocks. A deeper seat was developed as she relaxed, sat back, gained abduction of hips and extension of the thighs.

At this point the "FEELING" of centering her body, the sensation of her head balance a straight back with an expanded chest, with the shoulders above her hips were developing at a walk. The client felt more in control and less fearful of movement once this was accomplished. She no longer sat in a forward flexed position which tended to raise her out of the saddle while trotting.

The next step involved maintaining the balanced riding position, while holding the reins and encouraging light contact with the horse, as she changes gaits from a walk to trot to walk and halt. As she felt more secure on the horse - decreasing her fear of movement - simple sequencing was added. This was accomplished by change of gait, change of directions, using schooling figures, adding the canter; increasing time and speed in each gait and focusing on "feelings". We focused on relaxation, developing a deeper seat and 'moving with the horse' instead of inhibiting the horse's movement by stiffening her body. This was a major challenge since she stiffened any time movement became over bearing. Could she tell when this was happening? We began to focus on her associated reactions which reoccurred with each new skill.

As her fear of movement decreased, sequencing actions and motor planning became more complex. Beginning with simple verbal commands such as halting the horse squarely,-- could you feel if he is square? and turning on the forehand. As these were mastered, leg yielding and shoulder-in were added. These action require separate motor-planning of each limb, the pelvis, and the spine. We always maintained the fundamental principles of correct positions, soft contact with the horse, and simple schooling exercises. We often had to return to the basics. She slowly began to understand that "soft-contact" meant the horse must hold his own head and not lean on the reins---rather then hold the reins lightly.

We discussed the feedback that the horse was giving the client, since he provided immediate feedback to the correct or incorrect action of the client. This helped to reinforce the client's sensory awareness and helped to fine tune her movements.

With the advance of movement control, memory skills were practiced which led to basic dressage tests. As the client gained more sensory awareness, motor control, and skill, all her accomplishments were brought to a new height during a schooling show. (A schooling show can be a show given by a local stable or club. They are 'practice shows' with less pressures then the AHSA approved shows.) Why would we include a schooling show in a treatment plan? We wanted to see any regression that occurred under social pressure. Would these areas need stronger intervention for maximum functioning or could the client continue to gain her skills under an instructor alone? After the show, the client felt good about herself. She was able to stay calm and relaxed. Her sensory feedback was somewhat dull but she could communicate with her horse. She was able to remember her test and performed with a fairly good score.

Because of the schooling show, the therapist could see areas that needed further intervention. The client became stiff when she had to canter and lost her ability to fine tune her horse due to her vestibular dysfunction. She also lost her ability to do three to five step coordination skills during the last part of her test showing that stress did interfere with her ability to function. The client gained insight into her ability and where she lost control of her ability to function.

A new treatment plan was developed by the therapist-instructor-client. Treatment intervals were decreased. The client now had one lesson with the instructor between each treatment session. We used two different horse increase the challenge to her vestibular system. She was asked to increase the time she worked on her own to decrease her dependency on her instructor and make her more aware of self..

THE TREATMENT RESULTS:

INITIAL EVALUATION OF PATIENT	BEGINNING OF YEAR	AFTER 12 MONTHS
Vestibular/proprioception problems: * Equilibrium - postural swaying .... ⇒ * Difficulty modulating muscle tone ..... ⇒ * Hyper-sensitivity to movement .... ⇒	Leans to left .... ⇒ Tense 95 % of time .... ⇒ No canter tolerance-fair trot tolerance-2 minutes .... ⇒	Can "feel" & stay centered Stays relaxed 30 % of time Canters 10-20 minutes
Lateralization * Right-left discrimination difficulty ..... ⇒ * Tendencies toward reversals .... ⇒ * Tendency to disassociated at midline .... ⇒	Minimal discrimination without focus . ⇒ 2 reversals during dressage test ...... ⇒ Going Lf to Rt forgets instruction .... ⇒	50% improved None during tests Can turn Rt or Lf with no focus
Poor tactile/proprioceptive processing * Hypersensitive to touch .... ⇒ * Difficulty in identification of body parts- Poor initiation of specific movements without direct attention .... ⇒	Shirt sleeve irritation interfere with ability to focus on instructor .... ⇒ Need to focus on limb to process given instruction delayed response to requested move .... ⇒	No longer bothered Only when stressed
Dyspraxia Impaired tactile sensation and proprioception * Difficulty in determining a sequential pattern of action .... ⇒	Delayed processing of 2 simple sequential actions .... ⇒	Processes 4/5 actions with difficulty
Auditory language dysfunctions * In sequencing words & information & 3 step directions .... ⇒ * In processing all words in a sentence........................ ⇒ * In recall instructions .... ⇒ * In visual tracking/reading causes dizzy . ⇒ * Poor vertical/horizontal alinement of eyes⇒	Mixes up given directions-can sequence one step .... ⇒ Misses 1 in 6 words .... ⇒ Recalls only simple instructions ..... ⇒ Becomes dizzy tracking while trotting ⇒ Vertical off 1 cm; horizontal off 1 cm . ⇒	Only under stress-can sequence 3 or more Misses 1 in 8 words Recalls a series of instructions Can trot & canter without dizziness without pressure Vertical off .½ cm; horizontal off ½ cm

References:
Albrecht, K. Brigadier General. (1993). *Principals of Dressage.* London: J.A. Allen. Translated from 1981 edition.
American Occupational Therapy Assoc. Inc. Position Paper: Purposeful Activity. *AJOT:* 47, 12, 1081-1082. USA.
Belasik, P. (1994). *Exploring Dressage Technique: Journeys into the Art of Classic Riding.* London: J.A. Allen.
Blixen-Finecke, Baron H. von. (1993). *The Art of Riding.* MD: Half Halt Press. USA Translated from 1977 edition.

Blixen-Finecke, Baron H. von. (1993). *The Art of Riding.* MD: Half Halt Press. USA Translated from 1977 edition.

Decarpentry, General. 1987. *Academic Equitation.* Translated by N. Bartle into English from 1949 French writing London: J.A. Allen.

Denoix, JM; Pailloux JP. (1996). *Physical Therapy and Massage for the Horse.* Vermont: Trafalgar Square Farm Books. USA.

Dietze, S. von. (1993). *Balance in der Bewegung: Der Sitz des Reiters.* FN-Verlag der Deutschen Reiterlichen Vereinigung GmbH, Warendorf, Germany. (Will be available in English from J.A. Allen in 1997/98).

Fisher, A.G., Murray, E.A., Bundy, A.C. (1991). *Sensory Integration Theory and Practice.* (pp 4,77,) Philadelphia FA Davis Co.

Froissard, J. (1988). *Classic Horsemanship for Our Times.* MD: Half Halt Press. USA

Gilfoyle, EM; Grady, AP; Moore, JC. (1981). *Children Adapt.* Thorofare, NJ: Charles B. Black.

de la Guérinière, FR. (1994). *School of Horsemanship.* London: J.A. Allen. (translated into English of Ecloe de Cavalerie 1733)

Harris, S. (1993). *Horse Gaits, Balance and Movement.* New York: Howell Book House, Macmillan Publishing Company. Hedlund G. (1988). *This is Riding.* Maryland: Half-Halt Press.

Harrtis, S. (199). *USPC Manual of Horsemanship:* New York: Howell Equestrian Library

Harris, S. (1995). *USPC Intermediate Horsemanship*: New York: Howell Equestrian Library

Harris, S. (1996). *USPC Advanced Horsemanship*: New York: Howell Equestrian Library.

Knopfhart A. (1990) *Fundamentals of Dressage.* London: J.A. Allen. (translated into English of 1979 edition).

de Kunffy, C. (1984). *Training Strategies for Dressage Riders.* NY: Howell Book House USA.

de Kunffy, C. (1994). *The Ethics and Passions of Dressage.* NY: Howell Book House USA.

Lewwewnz, T.L., Schaaf, R.C. (1996). Sensory Processing in At-Risk Infants. *Sensory Integration Special Interest Section Newsletter*, Vol 19, Number 1, pg 1-2, March 1996. American Occupational Therapy Assoc SA. Inc.

Li jsen, H.J; Stanier, S. (1993). *Classic Circus Equitation.* London: J.A. Allen. From a 1956 edition.

Ljunguist, B. (1976). *Practical Dressage Manual.* MD: Half Halt Press. USA

Loch, S. (1994). *The Clasic Seat.* (video). Vermont: Trafalgar Square Farm Books. USA.

Mosey, AC. (1986). *Psychosocial Components of Occupational Therapy.* NY: Raven Press U References

Nelson, N. (1992). *Francois Baucher The Man and His Methods.* London: J.A. Allen.

Oliveira, N. (1976) *Reflections on Equestrian Art.* London: J.A. Allen.

Oliveira, N. (1986) *From an Old Master Trainer to Young Trainers.* Australia: Howley & Russell.

Oliveira, N. (1988) *Horses and Their Riders.* Australia: Howley & Russell.

Podhajsky, P. (1967) *The Complete Training of Horse and Rider.* NY: Doubleday & Co. Inc.

Racinet, JC. (1991). *Another Horsemanship.* Cleveland OH: Xenophon Press, USA.

Schusdziarra, H; Schusdziarra V. (1985). *An Anatomy of Riding.* NY: Breakthrough Publications.

Steinbecht, G. (1995). *The Gymnasium of the Horse.* Cleveland OH: Xenophon Press, USA.

Strauss, I.(1996). *Hippotherapy: A Neurophysiological Therapy on the Horse.* Translated into English and vailable from OnTRA, 19 Alcaine Court, Ontario, Canada L3T 2G8.

Swift, S. (1985). *Centered Riding.* Vermont: Trafalgar Square Farm Books. USA.

Watjen, R. (1979). *Dressage Riding.* J.A. Allen, London.

Wood, W. (1996). *Legitimizing Occupational Therapy's Knowledge.* AJOT, 50, 8 626-634.

Ziegner, K. A. von. *The Basics.* Cleveland OH: Xenophon Press, USA.

HIPPOTHERAPY AND EQUINE-ASSISTED OCCUPATIONAL THERAPY WITH AN ADULT CLIENT WITH CEREBRAL PALSY

Barbara T. Engel, M.Ed, OTR

Joe is a twenty-five year-old man born with athetoid quadriplegia, severe spasms and associated pathological reflex reactions. He has moderate scoliosis which remains flexible in the upper trunk and static in the hip area. Joe has received intensive neurodevelopmental (NDT) treatment since he was six months old. He has participated in *Conductive Education* treatment technique for the last few years which is carried out by his mother daily.

Joe began riding when he was about twelve years old with a social riding group. He needed a great deal of support from side-helpers and a horse leader. He was learning how to direct the horse using one hand.

At nineteen years, Joe began in-home occupational therapy to increase functional living skills. When he was first seen at home, Joe was able to feed himself, type with one finger and walk with maximum support using scissoring gait. He was unable to roll over in bed, come to sitting position or help with his dressing. He could not sit without back and side supports. Generally, his sensory registration of touch or position sense (the ability to sense where his limbs were) was poor to lacking.

After six months of in-home therapy, the occupational therapist visited a new riding program Joe had joined. She began visiting the center once a week to advise the riding instructor in positioning techniques and skills to enhance Joe's riding. Coordination of the home program and the riding program began. At the end of eighteen months of in-home therapy, Joe was sitting independently on a bench, moving independently in bed, was able to come to sitting position and assist in dressing and bathing. He learned to use the phone, to sign his name, and to make a sandwich. In the riding program, Joe was using a Western saddle and could sit with minimal support from two sidehelpers or moderate support using a bareback pad and a surcingle. His movements were interconnected - reining with one hand caused body flexion and face and mouth reactions. Therapy at home was discontinued at that time due to funding (Figure 1).

At age of 24, Joe began hippotherapy one time a week. He sat fairly well on a saddle pad holding onto a vaulting girth surcingle handle but he needed support from the two sidehelpers for balance in turns and transitions at a walk. He controlled the horse using ladder reins only. He could not use his legs or seat aids and sat flexed forward with limbs flexed. Hippotherapy was used to facilitate relaxation, balance, equilibrium reactions, develop a deeper seat, trunk extension and sitting in an upright position. Initially this involved 80% of the session but was reduced to 20% within four months (Figure 2).

Equine-assisted occupational therapy uses purposeful activities to regain function. Joe's posture has improved and his increased relaxed state now allows him to ride independently for a period of time with a near normal posture and use of limbs without associated reactions of other limbs. He practices speech through repeating the dressage exercises and counting poles or turns and sometimes singing to help him relax.

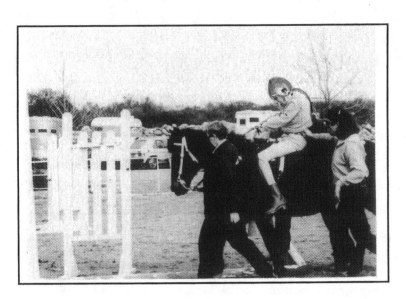

Figure 1.
JOE IS WORKING WITH HIS INSTRUCTOR DURING A RIDING LESSON
Before hippotherapy was started

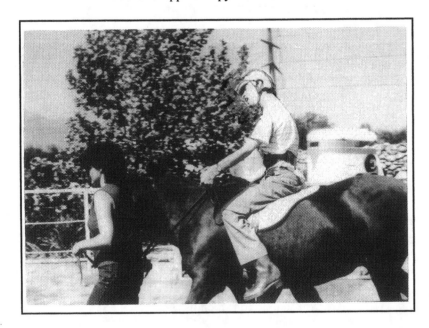

Figure 2.
AFTER JOE HAD COMPLETED HIPPOTHERAPY AND WAS BEGINNING THE RIDING PART OF THE SESSION

Joe feels good when he can control his horse and perform challenging exercises. He is motivated to improve his riding skills and work toward completing a dressage test. The exercises are kept at a level that does not stress his physical system nor decrease his postural control. Schooling figures challenge him mentally and increase hands quiet. Therapy techniques are constantly used to facilitate his functional movements. Riding continues as long as Joe's posture and functional movements remain coordinated or until he asks to stop.

Joe's riding experience involves hippotherapy and equine-assisted therapy, followed by a short session of sports riding. Hippotherapy and equine-assisted therapy are directed by the therapist with the riding instructor supervising the horse. The sports riding is directed by the instructor with the therapist providing assistance regarding his physical mobility. For example, Joe was working on performing a correct circle. After making two circles, he began to collapse, falling in at the waist. The therapist directed the instructor to change the direction of the circle and to circle at each end of the arena. This allowed Joe to rotate to each direction yet allowed him to regain the trunk straightness on the long side of the arena between circles.

Summary:
Joe's riding experiences have provided him with therapy which directly affected his functional living skills in an activity which he could use independently with pride. Joe is now riding in a dressage saddle. He rides without support from the sidehelpers or any assistance from the horse handler. He learned a dressage test which he can perform without a reader (a person reading the dressage test during a performance). He is beginning to sit to the trot for several strides at a time and maintaining good head control. Joe is also gaining more control over his posture and arm movements. By using `sport riding' within equine-assisted therapy/hippotherapy, Joe could gain a feeling of accomplishment which carried over to the knowledge that he was capable - capable to master other skills. His speech has improved so that others can understand basic words. As a result of generally improved function Joe is able to hold a part-time paid computer job at a local hospital and gain a feeling of independence which he never had.

CHAPTER 21

OCCUPATIONAL THERAPY/SPEECH AND LANGUAGE PATHOLOGY

USE OF SENSORY INTEGRATION TREATMENT STRATEGIES IN THE HIPPOTHERAPY SETTING

Ann Viviano, OTR/CCC/SLP

BACKGROUND INFORMATION

Specially trained occupational therapists, physical therapists, and speech-language therapists are using hippotherapy, treatment with the help of a horse, as an adjuctive modality or preferred modality for clients with a wide variety of neuromusculoskelatal and/or sensory motor disorders. Depending upon their professional expertise and client population, therapists are using several theoretical models of treatment during hippotherapy sessions. One of the models of treatment which has been incorporated during hippotherapy is sensory integration therapy (American Hippotherapy Association [AHA], 1996).

Sensory integration principles, based on a neuro-behavioral theory, were originally developed by Dr. A.J.Ayres to assist children with learning deficits. Sensory integration treatment is based on a child's neurologic and developmental needs. The goal of therapy is to improve the way a child's brain receives, processes, and organizes sensations. Treatment usually involves movement that provides tactile, vestibular, and proprioceptive stimulation. Integration and competence are achieved through the child's interactions within a carefully structured environment. During therapy, the child directs his or her own actions and the therapist moderates sensory input and environmental factors, depending upon the child's needs and responses during the session (Ayres, 1972, 1979).

Children with sensory integrative disorders may exhibit a wide variety of symptoms, such as:
(1) over-sensitivity to touch, movement, sights, or sound
(2) under-reactions to sensory stimulation
(3) high, low, or extreme fluctuations and activity level
(4) motor coordination problems
(5) delays in speech, language, motor skills, or academic achievement
(6) poor organization of behavior with impulsivity, distractibility, and lack of planning
(7) poor self-concept.

A qualified therapist can assess a child's sensory integration skills through an evaluation which may include standardized testing, such as the *Sensory Integration and Praxis Tests* and clinical observation of the child's responses to sensory stimulation, posture, balance, coordination, and eye movements. Several areas of sensory integration include sensory processing, particularly in the areas of touch, proprioceptive, and vestibular systems; visual perception, eye-hand coordination, and motor planning skills (Sensory Integration International, [SII], 1991).

SENSORY INTEGRATION TREATMENT DURING HIPPOTHERAPY

Very little has been published concerning the use of sensory integration practice during hippotherapy. Standquist (1992) provided an outline of sensory integration development during the sensory motor phase (0-12 months), the perceptual motor phase (1-5 years), and the learning phase. Lawton-Shirley (1990) discussed the sensory integrative value of therapeutic riding and noted improvements children made in the following areas: balance, equilibrium and postural responses, muscle strength and coordination, range of motion, socialization skills, self-esteem and self-confidence, eye-hand and visual-spatial skill development, bilateral motor coordination, and body awareness. Biery and Kauffman (1989) demonstrated increased standing and quadruped balance skills of eight individuals with mental retardation who participated in a therapeutic horseback riding program. MacKinnon, Noh, Laliberte, Lariviere and Allan (1995) completed a review of eleven data based studies analyzing the physical and psychosocial variables influenced by therapeutic horseback riding.

The following discussion will highlight six areas of specific disorders; sensory discrimination, sensory modulation, postural-ocular movement, motor planning, visual perception and eye-hand coordination, and auditory-language problems. The areas and treatment guidelines were adapted from the book, *Sensory Integration Theory and Practice* (Fisher, Murray, Bundey, 1991), and conference notes from Treatment of Sensory Integration Dysfunction (Koomar, Oetter, Spector, 1995), sponsored by SII, unless otherwise specified. The activities presented are suggestions and will vary depending upon the rider's particular needs, responses, and stage of therapy. Keep in mind the movement of the horse is the primary treatment modality during hippotherapy and must be appropriately graded for each rider.

SENSORY DISCRIMINATION PROBLEMS:

A rider with sensory discrimination problems may have decreased ability to discriminate sensory input in all modalities involving tactile, vestibular, visual, auditory, gustatory, and olfactory senses. In the area of tactile processing, a rider may have difficulty determining if and how he or she is holding the reins, if his or her body is being touched, and what type of touch is present (hard, soft, sharp, dull, deep, light). The rider may have poor ability to judge information about the position of his or her head and body in space. He or she may have difficulty understanding direction words, such as "up/down, back/forward" The rider may not discriminate speed, tempo, and changes in the horse's movement. The rider's performance may be slowed due to his or her increased reliance on cognitive strategies rather than an internal sense of body awareness. He or she may have poor force modulation and difficulty grading his or her arm and hand movements to control the reins.

Treatment Guidelines:
1. Provide opportunities for the rider to experience a variety of vestibular inputs involving angular and linear movement in different planes and directions.
2. Provide deep touch pressure and co-contraction around joints followed by a variety of tactile activities.
3. Begin with strong generalized input in any sensory area and move to activities involving discrimination abilities.
4. Provide compensation strategies for a decreased discrimination in a sensory system by using other sensory systems as possible. For example, if a rider has difficulty telling if his or her saddle pad is rubbing him or her, help the rider learn to perform a visual check of his or her body.

Example - Hippotherapy Activities:

1. Use different textured sponges to wash parts of the horse. Have the rider reach into a bucket of oats to find hay cubes to feed the horse.
2. Tack the horse with different textures of saddle pads for the rider to sit on when he or she is wearing shorts to provide intense tactile input.
3. Have the rider place sun screen and lotion on him or herself prior to mounting.
4. Wrap the reins or surcingle handles with different textures, such as rough tape, soft foam, or spongy packing material to give his or her hands different inputs.
5. Have rider complete upper extremity weight-bearing on the horse, sitting forwards and backwards, prior to having the rider work on hand skills with games or using the reins.
6. Use games with different textures of toys. For example: kush ball, rope baton, foam blocks, ribbon bracelets, cloth rings, and plastic frisbees.
7. Play "red light, green light" where the horse frequently accelerates and decelerates so the rider has to make frequent adjustments to the horse's speed.
8. Have the horse turn in different size curves and angles to enhance vestibular and proprioceptive information provided to the rider as the rider assumes various positions on the horse (prone over the barrel, prone prop on arms while laying backwards, side sitting).
9. Have the rider reach into a covered box to manipulate a toy animal which he or she must match or name by using his or her tactile, not visual, sense.

SENSORY MODULATION

A rider with sensory modulation disorders may demonstrate over-response, under-response, or fluctuating responses in regard to sensory input. The rider may be defensive to touch, demonstrate defensive reactions to movement, be insecure when his or her feet are off the ground, or dislike changing position This rider may be sensitive to auditory and visual input. The therapist must remember to respect the rider's level of discomfort, always grade sensory input, and structure the environment to meet the rider's need. When the rider has decreased responses to sensory input, he or she may lack appropriate arousal responses and show few responses to movement and activities.

Treatment Guidelines:

1. For a rider who demonstrates fluctuating responses to sensory input, provide input that brings the rider to a place of homeostasis. Activities may involve proprioceptive and deep touch input while working in midline and working in symmetrical patterns. It may be necessary to provide a horse with an even, rhythmical gait.
2. For the rider who is over-aroused by input, provide slow movement, deep touch, and reduced stimulation. Give the rider a wider and more stable base of support on the horse. Use a horse with consistent gait patterns.
3. For the rider who is under-aroused by sensory input, provide alerting activities which may involve pulling, pushing, bouncing, irregular movements, and heavy work against gravity. Trotting provides more intense input then walking. Long reining may be more effective to increase the impulsion of the horse, compared to leading the horse.

Example - Hippotherapy Activities:

1. If a rider is oversensitive to light, provide a helmet with a brim, use sunglasses, or ride in a darker indoor arena.
2. If a rider is oversensitive to touch, the rider may want to dress in longer pants, wear gloves, and wear high top shoes or boots; use a saddle pad that is less abrasive for that particular rider in regard to texture.
3. If a rider is oversensitive to sound, have the rider wear headphones to dampen environmental sounds, play calming music, or use a softer voice.
4. If the rider is fearful, have the rider complete ground activities (brushing and leading the horse, walking up and down the mounting ramp, walking around the arena) to help the rider feel more secure in the environment.
5. If the rider is fearful at the height of the horse or aversive to movement, start the rider out on a vaulting barrel that is lower to the ground; once the rider is mounted, provide for more linear movements without the rider varying his or her head movement.
6. For an under-stimulated rider provide a trail course of varied terrains, sights, and sounds.
7. For a rider that is under-stimulated by sensory input, provide pushing and pulling activities, such as having the rider carry out his or her own tack; use a pitchfork, shovel, or broom; carry a bucket of water to his or her horse; or push a wheelbarrow.
8. For a non-alert rider; provide frequent drinks of water or a cool washcloth to increase an alerting response.
9. For a rider who has fluctuating responses, it may be helpful for him or her to wear a weighted vest, neoprene vest, or spandex clothes to provide deep input in the proximal area. Remember, some riders prefer loose fitting clothes and may not tolerate a vest.
10. If the rider is oversensitive to smells, do not use fly spray, liniment, or hoof dressing on the horse. The sidewalkers should not wear perfume or scented lotions. The arena should be free of manure.

POSTURAL-OCULAR MOVEMENT PROBLEMS

A rider with postural-ocular movement disorders generally have reduced ability to process vestibular and proprioceptive input which can result in poor balance and equilibrium reactions, poor modulation of force and grading of movements, diminished awareness of body position and movements, difficulty assuming and maintaining postures against gravity, and difficulty developing proximal control. The rider's responses to sensory input do not usually vary and are not at the extreme ranges of responses. A rider's ocular movement and respiration development may be affected by decreased postural control.

Treatment Guidelines:

1. Develop an automatic and postural base of support
2. Achieve tonic muscle patterns in flexion extension.
3. Develop rotation patterns.
4. Treat bilateral motor coordination problems.
5. Improve ocular control.
6. Improve respiratory control.

Example - Hippotherapy Activities:

1. Provide vestibular input in a variety of head positions in all three planes of movement involving sitting, supine, and prone positions as the horse is completing circle, figure eight, and serpentine figures.

2. Vary the speed of the horse, size and angles of turns, and terrain going up and down hill.
3. Vary the base of support from a wide to a narrower base as treatment progresses so the rider is more challenged to develop balance reactions.
4. Develop sequences for rotation and reaching across midline by way of exercises, holding front and back of saddle pad, reaching across midline to place rings on pegs or balls in baskets.
4. Complete developmental sequences on the horse which involve joint compression and more heavy input against gravity going prone on elbows, prone to extended elbows, quadruped and kneeling positions.
6. Achieve and maintain two-point position with the rider's feet in the stirrups with and without weight bearing on hands.
7. Organize the oral area by blowing whistles, harmonicas, and bubbles; making animal noises; or drinking water with crushed ice from a straw.
8. Track a moving target visually and throw a ball at the moving target.
9. Complete basic upper extremity theraband activities as the horse is completing patterns and turns.
10. Have the rider wear different colored wrist bands to help him determine "left" and "right" directions.

MOTOR PLANNING PROBLEMS

A rider with motor planning difficulties will have problems planning and executing skilled or non-habitual motor tasks. Typically, when a new skill is learned, much conscious effort or motor planning is required before movement and sequences come more easily. A rider with motor planning problems needs to practice using his or her body in a wide variety of activities.

Treatment Guidelines:
1. Provide tactile, vestibular, and proprioceptive input to form a basis for a strong motor response.
2. Involve many varied activities so the rider learns how to plan movements depending upon environmental demands.
3. Provide opportunities for the rider to increase ideation and sequencing of steps.

Example - Hippotherapy Activities:
1   Vary reaching patterns, such as having the rider hold a ball on a cone; transfer the ball and cone from hand to hand; or pass the ball on a cone back and forth to his sidewalkers.
2. Use activities with rings, such as asking the rider to place a ring on one arm, both arms arm and leg on same side, or arm and leg on opposite sides.
3. Play "Simon Says" with visual and auditory cues and have rider depend on visual cues and fade out the auditory cues.
4   Have rider imitate a sequence of exercises, then have the rider vary the pattern by one or two movements.
5. Play follow the leader and have rider initiate different sequences of movement.
6. Complete the following three-part activity; have the rider build and traverse (walk, jump, hop) an obstacle course of ground poles and cavelletti; ride the course; and draw a map of the course.
7. Have the rider fold horse blankets, roll up leg bandages, and roll up velcro leg wraps.
8. Clap in time to the horse's stride and have the rider clap with and without the therapist's model.

9. Have the rider look at a picture of a rider on a horse and imitate the position in the picture on his or her own horse.

10. Have the rider guide the horse through a maze of ground poles. Give the rider a starting and an ending point.

VISUAL PERCEPTION AND EYE-HAND COORDINATION PROBLEMS

A rider with visual perception difficulties will have difficulty with rotation of shapes in space, use of eyes to determine relevant stimuli from a background of stimuli, and combining eyes and hands for functional tasks. Eye-hand or fine motor coordination involves several factors, such as visual perception, motor coordination, muscle tone, the ability of the trunk and shoulder to provide stabilizing control for the hands to work, and tactile discrimination skills in the hands.

Treatment Guidelines:

1. Give the rider a sense of his or her body in environmental space and set visual boundaries. The rider may benefit from visual cues, such as painting a red stripe on the mounting ramp, discouraging the rider from stepping out into space at the top of the ramp.
2. Give the rider a sense of objects in relationship to space, such as counting horse strides between two objects.
3. Provide object manipulation games.

Example - Hippotherapy Activities;

I. Provide eye-hand manipulation activities, such as fastening buckles on helmets, picking the horse's hooves, clipping clothes-pins to the horse's mane or the edge of a bucket, using a spray bottle to wash the horse, brushing on hoof dressing, or using a leather punch.
2. Provide spatial activities, such as having the rider follow a map of where to ride or follow a trail of ribbons to find a treasure.
3. Have the rider ride to different cutout shapes and then match the shapes; or ride to different dressage letters and write a word that starts with that letter.
4. Have the rider look at a picture of a grooming item and then pick out that piece of equipment from a box filled with grooming supplies.
5. Show the rider a picture of his or her horse and have the rider identify his or her horse from several horses.
6. Play the "I see_____" game using colors or shapes.
7. Play target games with varied sized targets such as basketball, ring toss, and horseshoes.
8. Have the rider write and connect a dot-to-dot pattern that spells his or her horse's name.
9. Make a tic-tac-toc grid in the arena footing. Have the rider throw bean bags, taking turns with therapist, to play tic-tac-toe.
10. Tie a magnet to a piece of baling twine. Have the rider "rope" a picture of a cow that has a metal paper clip.

AUDITORY AND LANGUAGE PROBLEMS

A rider with auditory-language problems may not be able to follow directions given verbally, understand what is said to him or her, or have difficulty expressing his or her wants and needs on the horse. The relationship of auditory-language development and sensory integration or motor development has been expressed in several

<u>**Treatment Guidelines**</u>:
1. Provide basis of somatosensory and vestibular and proprioceptive input.
2. Allow the rider an adaptive motor response to auditory input.
3. Give the rider language models that include sequencing words (first, second, third), label words (nouns), action words (verbs), location words (back, front, beside), temporal words (before, after), inclusion exclusion words (not, except, either, or all, all but one), and descriptive words (color, shape, size, number).
4. Teach conventional greetings and social phrases.

<u>**Examples - Hippotherapy Activities**</u>:
1. Supplement auditory directions with another modality involving gestures, signs, pictures, or written words. Use a picture schedule board to sequence the session.
2. Teach vocabulary words specific to the hippotherapy setting using labels paired with objects, pictures, and/or written words. Example worksheets are printed in Aspects and Answers. (Joswick, Kittredge, McCowan, McParland, Woods, 1986)
3. Give the rider several choices of activities which he must verbalize to his sidewalkers.
4. Gradually extend the number of directions the rider is expected to remember at one time, having the rider direct the horse to different locations in the arena
5. Have the rider repeat directions to his sidewalker that the therapist gives him.
6. Play twenty questions. Tell the rider what category (food, clothes, animals) your word is in. The rider asks" yes/no" questions until he or she can guess your word.
7. Play musical cones in which the rider listens for music that is on/off or loud/soft, and stays by the cone when the music is off or soft.
8. Play "Simon Says" with visual and auditory cues and then fade the visual cues, using auditory cues alone.
9. Enhance auditory vocalization skills by having the rider direct the horse to a hidden "beeper" ball.
10. To increase auditory discrimination, play "red light/green light." If the therapist says two words that are the same, the rider holds up a green card and can go. If the therapist says two words that are different, the rider holds up a red card and must stop.

<u>**CASE EXAMPLE**</u>:
J.B. has a history of developmental delays including a two year delay in speech, language, and motor skill development. He has sensory integration dysfunction characterized by sensory defensiveness, fluctuating responses to sensory input, gravitational insecurity with an under-responsive vestibular system, reduced ability to motor plan and sequence activities, difficulty handling transitions, and frequent withdrawal from adults and peers. J.B. was responsive to proprioceptive input and would calm and increase his attention when given deep pressure, heavy work activities, or a weighted vest.

Due to a contract between Memorial Hospital and Pikes Peak Therapeutic Riding Center in Colorado Springs, J.B received periodic hippotherapy sessions in addition to his speech-language and occupational therapy pediatric rehabilitation program. From April to October, 1995, J.B. attended a total of eleven forty-five minute hippotherapy sessions. J.B. was three years, nine months of age in April of 1995.

His long-term goals were as follows:
1. Increase social interaction and play skills.
2. Increase balance and motor planning.
3. Increase expressive language skills.
4. Increase receptive language skills.
5. Increase muscle tone and strength.
6. Increase upper extremity function.

Short-Term Goals (April 25 - May 30, 1995)

	Goals Met	Goals in Progress
(1) Follow one-step directions in 4 out of 5 trials.	✓	
(2) Produce 5 spontaneous verbalizations in one session.	✓	
(3) Produce three word responses 5 times in one session.		✓
(4) Independendently change position from backward to forward when the horse is standing still.		✓
(5) Repeat names of instructor	✓	
(6) Maintain sitting at midline as horse is walking a figure eight pattern		✓

Summary: J.B. responded positively to riding the horse. He consistently gestured for the horse to walk and he occasionally said "go". He waved and smiled at people when he was on the horse. He maintained midline 80% of the time when making a straight line. He readjusted and righted himself to midline 50% of the time during turns. He pointed to pictures to request activities, such as balls or rings, during the session.

Short Term Goals: (September 5 to October 24, 1995)

	Goal Met	Goal in Progress
(1) Engage in three different turn-taking games.	✓	
(2) Produce four-to-eight word sentences.	✓	
(3) Keep trunk centered at midline as horse walks up and down hills.		✓
(4) Independently change position from back to front when the horse is standing still.		✓
(5) Assume four different positions on the horse.		✓
(6) Complete three modified sit-ups and push-ups as the horse is walking.		✓

Summary:

J.B. made excellent progress during his hippotherapy sessions. In the area of language skills, he verbally expressed choices, formulated several eight-to-ten word sentences, and connected three or four successive sentences to express an idea. In the area of balance, he maintained midline 75% of the time as the horse walked up and down hills and made a figure eight pattern. He was very motivated to learn to direct the horse with the reins. He followed several two-step directions. J.B.'s parents noted an improvement in back extension, balance, verbalizations, self-confidence and willingness to try new activities as his hippotherapy sessions progressed.

CONCLUSIONS

The results of using sensory integration techniques during J.B.'s hippotherapy sessions were measured by improvements he made on his individual goals and objectives. The effectiveness of sensory integration procedures has been summarized by Clark and Pierce (1988) and Ostrow, Lawlor, and Joe (1988). The effectiveness of combining sensory integration procedures and hippotherapy techniques needs to be studied further. Single subject and group designs could provide objective data for appropriate, efficient treatment plans and justification for treatment to consumers and third party payers.

REFERENCES:

American Hippotherapy Association Task Force. (1996, Sumner). **AHA Creates Position Paper on Hippotherapv.** *AHA NEWS.*

Ayres, A. J. (1972). *Sensory Integration and Learning Disorders.* Los Angeles: Western Psychological Services.

Ayres, A. J. (1 979). *Sensory Integration and the Child.* Los Angeles: Western Psychological Services.

Ayres, A.J., & Mailloux, Z. (1981). **Influences of Sensory Integration Procedures on Language Development.** *American n Journal of Occupational Therapy,* 35, 383-390.

Biery, M.J., & Kauffman, N. (1989). **The Effects of Therapeutic Horseback Riding on Balance.** *Adaptive Physical Activity Quarterly,* 6, 221-229.

Cermak, S.A., Ward, E.A., & Ward, L.M. (1986). **The Relationship Between Articulation Disorders and Motor Coordination in Children.** *American Journal of Occupational Therapy,* 40, 546-550.

Clark, F.A., & Pierce, D. (1988), Sumner). **Synopsis of Pediatric Occupational Therapy Effectiveness.** *Sensory Integration News.*

Clark, F.A., & Steingold, L. (1982). **A Potential Relationship Between Occupational Therapy and Language Acquisition.** *American Journal of Occupational Therapy,* 36, 42-44.

Fisher, AG., Murray, E.A., & Bundy; A.C. (1991). *Sensorv Integration Theory and Practice.* Philadelphia: F. A. Davis.

Joswick, F., Kittredge, M., McCowan, L. McParland, C., & Woods, S. (1986). *Aspects and Answers.* Augusta, Michigan: Cheff Center.

Koomar, J., Oetter, P., & Spector, K. (I 995, September). *Treatment of Sensory Integration Dysfunction.* Torrance, CA: Sensory Integration International.

Lawton-Shirley, N. (199, June). **The Sensory Integrative Value of Horseback Riding Therapy.** *Sensory Integration Special Interest Section Newsletter,* American Occupational Therapy Association.

MacKinnon, JR., Nob, S., Laliberte, D., Larkiviere, J., & Allan, D.E. (1995). **Therapeutic Horseback Riding: A Review of the Literature**. *Physical & Occupational Therapy in Pediatrics*, 15(1), 1-15.

Ostrow, P.C., Lawlor, M.C., & Joe, B.E. (1988). **Research Supports Efficacy of Sensory Integration Procedures Efficacy Date Brief**, 3(5). *American Occupational Therapy Association.*

A Parent's Guide to Understanding Sensory Integration. (1991). Torrance, CA. Sensory Integration International.

Standquist, J. (1992). **Sensory Integration Development**. In B. Engel (Ed.), *Therapeutic Riding Programs: Instruction and Rehabilitation.* (p.205). Durango, CO; Barbara Engel Therapy Services.

Windeck, S.L., & Laurel, 1-1. (1989, March) **THEORETICAL Framework Combining Speech-Language Therapy with Sensory** Integration Treatment. Sensory Integration special Interest Section Newsletter, American Occupational Therapy Association.

CHAPTER 22

SPEECH AND LANGUAGE PATHOLOGY

SPEECH-LANGUAGE PATHOLOGY ADDRESSED IN THE RIDING SETTING

Ruth Dismuke-Blakely, MS/CCC-SLP

The speech-language pathologist is constantly challenged to find treatment settings and activities that will allow maximum integration of the various components of speech and language in meaningful fashion. Language is simply a set of symbols used to represent reality. We tend to present language as being made up of grammatical or syntactic structures that have semantic meaning and that are used for a variety of communicative functions. Speech is one tool by which one conveys our language symbols to another. Written words as well as sign language would be other tools by which communication is conveyed to others.

Current treatment models used with speech and language disorders are oriented toward the provision of services using real experiences and activities. Such activities allow the therapist to include various physiological and perceptual forms of input. These models are described as being placed in pragmatically loaded, experientially based settings.

Riding therapy offers a ready-made pragmatically loaded, experientially-based setting for addressing speech and language disability. The speech-language pathologist can develop a highly integrated and highly specialized treatment program through careful consultation with physical and occupational therapists. The activities of riding and those related to it offer a motivating and meaningful context in which to address the broad realm of communicative disabilities. The three dimensional movement of the horse offers controlled stimulation to the neural pathways involved in speech and language functioning. The strong neurological/perceptual components of riding can be manipulated by the speech pathologist in consultation with the occupational therapist to provide a more integrated treatment plan. The stimulation provided by the movement of the horse appears to provide vestibular and other perceptual types of input that in effect can be used to facilitate the client's receptiveness to therapy. Arousal states, and subsequently, attentional focus can be brought to a more normal level, making the time spent in treatment more productive. The postural elements of riding can be used for enhancement of basic speech processes (respiratory control, phonation, intensity, pitch, and articulation). The activities of riding and learning horsemanship skills offer natural communicative opportunities between client and therapist. In short, riding therapy provides a flexible yet dynamic setting for speech and language intervention.

Barring medical contraindication, a broad range of clients with all manner of cognitive, communicative, motoric, perceptual, and behavioral deficits is able to receive productive speech and language therapy in the riding therapy setting. Age groups served may range from infants requiring an intensive early stimulation/intervention through school-age children and adults. Both developmentally disabled and trauma clients are seen. The format and content of therapy will depend entirely upon the treatment needs of each particular client. All therapy services must be provided by a licensed, ASHA certified speech-language pathologist. It should be remembered that speech and language therapy "on horseback" uses treatment goals, criteria for reaching goals, and remediation procedures that are standard to the field of speech and language pathology.

Developing the Therapy Session

Prior to the initiation of speech and language therapy in the riding setting, the speech-language pathologist will have evaluated the client with regard to deficit areas using standard assessment tools. The written treatment plan should parallel that written for more traditional treatment settings. An example goal for a child with language disability might read, "Ben will reduce discourse errors to fewer than 20% occurring in a 150 utterance conversational language sample." One for a client with a voice disorder might read, "Susan will demonstrate sustained phonation in two-word phrases at a level of 90% accuracy over 10 trials." The riding setting is simply the context in which these goals will be addressed. Therefore, it is not professionally appropriate to write treatment goals that reflect the acquisition of specific riding skills any more than it would be appropriate to write goals that reflect specific achievements on other therapy activities (say skills involved in the use of baking cookies as a language experience).

As the speech-language pathologist writes the treatment plan, it is appropriate to discuss the manner in which therapy is to be provided. A paragraph detailing that "...Tom's therapy will be administered in the context of a structured riding therapy setting using a variety of intervention techniques...these techniques will include..." is fine. Often, the therapist will need to refer to how the three dimensional movement of the horse will be manipulated to address a specific goal. However, the therapist need not go into extreme detail. It is not the case that a speech-language pathologist puts down on paper every therapy activity and/or stimulus that he or she might use in the course of a client's treatment.

Once treatment goals have been established, the speech-language pathologist is charged with the task of analyzing how those goals might be addressed in the riding therapy setting. There are many different modes of handling clients in this setting. The theme of horses and riding offers a dynamic and flexible content area for facilitation of more efficient communication skills, whatever the cognitive, motoric, behavioral, perceptual and communicative levels a client might demonstrate. Due to the powerful physiological components of riding, it is important that the speech-language pathologist be in close communication with the occupational and physical therapists involved with his or her clients. Because of the tremendous sophistication of the riding setting itself, the speech-language pathologist also needs to maintain consultation with the horse professional on the staff as well.

As therapy is established, clients are typically seen either individually or in very small groups. Sessions will last from thirty minutes to ninety minutes, with a one hour session being the average. The ideal therapy situation involves the speech-language clinician and from one to three therapy aides depending on the physical problems of the client and the nature of the therapy setting. These therapy aides should have professional horse knowledge in order to provide safety constraints, especially if the therapist is not a horse person. The number of aides will depend upon the physical needs of the individual clients and the nature of the riding setting itself. The type of riding equipment used will be mandated by the cognitive, perceptual, motor, and behavioral needs of the client. The choice of the horse will also be mandated by these needs.

Once the proper equipment and horse have been selected, the client can be managed in a number of ways, depending upon treatment goals. Possibilities include being lead from the ground with side aides, having a back rider, having a side rider, or riding independently with monitoring. Many times it is appropriate to use alternative positions for the client on horseback (side sitting, back sitting, lying prone over the horse, or other positions) to facilitate certain physiological effects for more efficient speech and language production (back sitting to stimulate thoracic/abdominal muscle tone for a client with low tone and poor respiratory function, for example). Teaching riding skills is not the primary emphasis, but rather the remediation of the communicative disability. Therefore the communication needs of the client will dictate the nature of the session. Each client's therapy management should be designed to address not only the speech-language goals, but the goals established by any other therapists on the team as well. The riding session is thus designed to reflect a true interdisciplinary treatment plan for the client. Each therapist on the team becomes a good "technician" for the other therapists involved.

The speech-language pathologist should do a task analysis of the various opportunities present in the riding setting for targeting the treatment goals of his or her client. He or she then carefully integrates his or her remediation strategies and techniques into the setting. Tasks such as identifying and catching the horse, grooming, tacking and untacking, discussing the physical attributes of the horse, learning the basic elements of maneuvering the horse, carrying out designated patterns and movements on horseback, learning to care for the horse, and problem solving of naturally arising issues, are but a few of the activities available.

The riding setting can be designed to reflect as little or as much content structure as is deemed appropriate for any given client. Many well conducted speech-language therapy sessions on horseback have the appearance of nothing more than a very detailed riding lesson. The linguistically based processes required to "listen and repeat" the steps involved in tacking up the horse, for example, offer a naturally occurring, but easily manipulated stimulus activity for the clinician to use in addressing auditory processing deficits or language production breakdowns. The planning of a three step obstacle course can be used to target sequencing difficulties while training some verbal rehearsal strategies ("Ride over two logs, go around a yellow cone, and stop by a black square.").

The speech-language pathologist is able to address deficits in all of the structural aspects of speech and language (phonology, syntax, semantics), the pragmatics of language, language for problem- solving, conceptual development, processing breakdown, and general linguistic organization and efficiency. Secondary language concerns (reading, writing) can be successfully integrated into the riding setting, as can the use of augmentative or alternative communication modalities.

One of the more valuable aspects of speech and language therapy in the riding setting lies in the continuity of the stimulus material. As the client is introduced to the riding setting, tasks will be at a very basic level. The speech-language pathologist expands upon the theme of horsemanship as the client is able to demonstrate some basic horse knowledge, always building upon the same reference point. As more sophisticated horse skills are acquired, the speech-language clinician can address more subtle and more abstract elements of cognitive-linguistic functioning. Because there are ever- expanding levels of horse knowledge, the clinician does not easily run out of stimulus material. In addition, the client does not have to re-orient to a new therapy activity each session.

Documentation of the client's progress in the riding therapy setting is done much as in a clinical setting. Session-by-session notes are often required, with formal assessments done periodically. Of particular value is the use of trained and untrained probe measures designed to tap into specific areas of ability or disability. They should be consistent in design for pre - and post - evaluation purposes. The use of video or audio taping of therapy sessions is invaluable for reviewing client functioning and treatment effectiveness. As treatment data is generated, progress summaries are written up in standard report fashion.

Specific Treatment Strategies

It is beyond the scope of this discussion to detail all of the speech and language therapy options available in the riding setting. What follows is a short description of some client management strategies to stimulate ideas for speech-language pathologists interested in the use of riding therapy for their clients.

Populations with Severe and Profound Problems

It is often difficult to find a salient stimulus activity for clients functioning in the severe and profound range of intellectual ability. Effective stimulation for the low functioning client is very accessible in the riding setting. Such clients are typically motivated by the movement of the horse, and are thus more readily focused. A basic requisite for communication lies in demonstration of "communicative intent" or the need to represent something through use of a symbol--be it vocal, gestural, pictorial. Using a gross gesture and/or vocalization to indicate "horse go" can generate a motivating and successful activity for the severe/profound client. As he or she discovers that he or she is able to "control" the horse using a communication symbol, the foundation for a more broad-based communication system is laid. Simultaneously, the movement patterns of the horse provide powerful vestibular stimulation that typically arouses the client to a level of increased spontaneous vocalization. The speech-language pathologist then has more vocal output to work with and is able to generate a more accurate idea of the client's potential in expressive and receptive areas of communicative functioning.

Clients With Language Processing Deficits

Clients who demonstrate any of a broad range of linguistically-based processing deficits benefit dramatically from the strong neurological and psychological elements of the riding setting. The activity of riding provides an ideal situation in which to create a meaningful learning environment. As the client learns to move the horse through various maneuvers, he or she is involved in the coordination and organization of a number of cognitive, perceptual, motor, and linguistic elements. Consider, for example what is involved in retaining and executing the following directive: "Walk around in a circle and over the log before you stop your horse." Using a small group format, with clients alternately instructing each other, maximizes the opportunity for addressing both expressive and receptive deficits. Showing the client the natural consequences of being vague or nonspecific can be achieved by having a therapy aide carry out the client's instructions in literal fashion. For example, with the client stating "Put it on", the saddle blanket might be placed on the horse's neck. The patient did not specify where the blanket was to go. Another excellent technique is to use flow charts for mapping out various activities and maneuvers in the riding setting, to facilitate better organization and retention skills. The riding setting offers a virtually unlimited variety of processing tasks that can be manipulated by the speech-language pathologist.

Integration of Speech-Language Therapy with Occupational Therapy * (See illustration on the this page)

* THE SENSORY INTEGRATION- COGNITIVE/LINGUISTIC CONNECTION

THE SENSORY INTEGRATION - COGNITIVE/LINGUISTIC CONNECTION

Sensory Input To The Individual ⇓		Linguistic Message Is Conveyed ⇑
Reception By System Through Sensory Receptors ⇓	I N P U T	Production Of The Verbal Thought Through Voice, Graphics, Gesture ⇑
Perception And The Decoding Of Sensory Input ⇓		Formulation Into A Verbal Thought To Be Communicated ⇑
Interpretation And Integration Of Sensory Input At The CNS Level ⇓	**COGNITIVE PROCESSING**	Selective/Analysis Of Information For Verbalization ⇑

Storage In CNS- Short And Long Term Processes ⇒	Integration Of The Information Into Conceptual Knowledge ⇒	Organization Of Stored Information Together With Previous Knowledge ⇒	Retrieval Of The Information From Storage Of Knowledge In The Mind

©

377

Combining speech-language therapy with occupational therapy in the riding setting greatly facilitates the effectiveness of both. Speech and language are a higher level cortical function in the human brain, and are greatly influenced by how the client's neurological system is functioning at other levels. Using a team approach within the same session, each therapist is able to make assessments and/or alterations to treatment in a "hands-on" fashion. Most of the clients seen in therapeutic riding have multiple handicaps, and the constant monitoring by both the speech-language pathologist and the occupational therapist enables the professionals to better serve the client. In the case of a person with sensory-integrative dysfunction, for example, the occupational therapist can supervise the optimal degree of vestibular input, the levels of arousal, perceptual defensiveness, and subtleties of functioning that might impact speech and language. The speech-language pathologist can provide strategies for facilitating more efficient communication functioning. In addition, working together, therapists are able to generate a comprehensive diagnosis of the client's deficits.

Summary Statement

The provision of speech and language therapy services through the manipulation of the riding therapy setting offers a highly flexible and powerful approach to the habilitation/rehabilitation of persons with all manner of communication disabilities. The examples of therapy application previously discussed are but a few of the ways in which the riding setting can be used in this application. It is important to recognize that treatment of communication disabilities is a very complex and sophisticated science. The use of therapeutic riding is also a very complex and sophisticated science. When implemented together by licensed speech-language therapists and trained horse professionals, the scope of the services available in the riding setting is limited only by the creativity of the individual speech-language pathologist involved.

Sensory input is provided from auditory, visual, tactile, vestibular, proprioceptive, gustatory, and olfactory channels. Disorders in sensory processing and sensory integration can occur at any level or at several levels. These breakdowns result in the individual trying to deal with his environment based on faulty information. Incorrect incoming information leads to the formulation of faulty knowledge and conceptualization. Difficulties in sensory processing and/or integration can create severe disorganization in the individual. Deficits in the filtering and regulating of incoming sensory information can block the individual's ability to engage in effective and/or efficient communication on both receptive and expressive levels. The application of knowledge and communicating by using that knowledge is made ineffective by breakdowns in sensory integration.

Ruth Dusmuke-Blakely,MS/CCC-SLP
Albuquerque, New Mexico

LESSON PLANS AND TREATMENT SESSIONS
SPEECH AND LANGUAGE THERAPY UTILIZING THE HORSE

Peggy McClure, MS, MBA, CCC/SLP

A. LESSON ONE

DESCRIPTION OF CLIENT/RIDER TYPE:
Severe/Profound Mental Retardation.
Communication was by making sounds that convey feelings and for play (vocalizations).
Does not use words.
Does not initiate interaction.
Moves about independently (ambulatory).
Horseback riding is one of the few activities this adult person prefers.

LONG TERM GOALS:
Client/Rider will indicate intent. _____ will tell/show his or her friends what he or she wants.

ACTIVITY:
Environment: Communication aids (see the following note) will be placed near each task. Position the communication aid for "Lets's Ride" near the mounting area, the "Water" communication aid at the water jug and the "Walk on" communication aid with the therapist. (The communication aid for "Walk on" can be made portable so as not to compromise any safety considerations.)

Using the communication aid most suitable for the rider, the therapist will encourage him or her to indicate the need to start the ride by mounting, move forward at the walk and take a drink of water.

Over the course of many riding treatment sessions the client/rider will be introduced to each communication aid and then is encouraged to touch, press or look at the aid by being cued through pausing, pointing, modeling or by verbal direction by the therapist until he or she moves to an independent use of the communication aid.

During a riding treatment session the "Water" and Walk-on" expressions can be used much more often in a natural and meaningful way than the first request, "Let's ride." "Let's ride" can only be used at the beginning of each session, unless one has a rider that will happily mount and dismount many times during a session.

NOTES:
1. Riding is never withheld. It is not conditional upon communication response. If, after a few minutes there is no response, use an appropriate level of prompt/cue.
2. Communication aids can be pictures, drawn symbols, concrete objects, tangible symbols, a voice output communication aid (VOCA).
3. The use of communication aids can be cumbersome and inconvenient. Staff needs to be willing to try aids, modify aids and practice using them in order to develop those aids that permit the smoothest method of communication, teaching and riding.

4. Repetition of communication is important but "nagging" and interfering with the joy of riding is to be avoided.

5. If the clients' diet, their safety and one's treatment philosophy permit, using a small food reward can be more enticing and focus attention quickly to the efficacy of the communication needs of the client/rider.

6. The messages and vocabulary used by the staff will be determined by the natural conversation that exists among the group and the communication needs of the client/rider.

7. The level of response for an individual may not ever be independent. An appropriate goal may be to use the communication aid with a verbal prompt.

B. LESSON TWO

DESCRIPTION OF CLIENT/RIDER TYPE:
Adult, Developmentally Disabled (Moderate Mental Retardation) Ambulatory, Verbal, Social. Client uses questions, relatively lengthy sentences, does some critical thinking, has a relatively good basic vocabulary, recognizes objects represented by photographs or line drawings.

Long Range Goals
Improve linguistic fluency (decrease word finding problems)
Improve intelligibility
Increase attention to complex tasks

Lesson Objectives
Client will use target vocabulary of lesson to describe a sequenced riding task,

Rationale
Use of visual prompts, pictures, aids in retrieval of words,

Materials
A variety of games and riding equipment such as barrels, cones, mounting block
Pictures of individual pieces of equipment, directions, and moves (Halt, Walk On)
Portable picture boards or some system on which to display pictures in sequence

Assumptions
Prior to the specific language objectives the normal routine of a lesson would include greetings, physical exercise before mounting, grooming, tacking up, riding- warm up time and skill building for riding.

Lesson
1. Rehearse names of equipment, moves and directions with client using pictures
2. Therapist describes task. Example: start at the orange cone, walk on to pole, walk over pole, turn right and pass the blue barrel, halt at the red bucket.
3. Client performs the task.
4. Client describes the riding task using pictures.
5. Repeat (Steps 1 thru 4) with same and/or different tasks.

C. LESSON THREE

DESCRIPTION OF CLIENT/RIDER TYPE
This is a lesson that could be used with a school group, not enrolled in a therapeutic riding program ,but has horse backriding scheduled as a field trip (Community Based Instruction).

Clients
High School, learning disabled with communication disorders of language

Long Range Goals
Each individual would most likely have goals such as improving interaction with peers and adults, following complex directions, vocabulary development, organizing language for giving information, word retrieval, etc.

Objective
'The students will:
1. Complete a written closure activity based on the target vocabulary.
2. Name five (5) jobs/careers related to horses.
3. Write an essay or give a class presentation about the horse backriding experience.

Rationale
Labeling objects and discussing the sequence of activities prior to the experience aids in language development. Relating this experience to their current "World of Work" class connects the material and experience to the academic curriculum.

Possible Vocabulary
Rural, river, valley, trail, wrangler, horse, mane, hoof, corral, stable, saddle, saddle blanket, stirrups, bridle, reins, fee, mount, bit, halter, lead rope, wildlife.

Materials
Objects, photographs, drawings, books, slides, video; any material that illustrates vocabulary, sequence, concepts.

Activity
Pre-Horse backriding
Depending on level of student
1. Present word list or word cards.
2. Play "Hangman" with words.
3. Match words with pictures and objects.
4. Discuss function or attributes of each object or word.
5. Using materials, brainstorm and create a list of 20 jobs that are necessary to the horse industry.

Follow the next classroom lesson or immediately following the field trip complete:
1.   A closure worksheet (ex: when riding, the rider usually sits in a ----------.
2.   A list of 5 jobs related to horses, and
3.   Describe the experience in an essay or class presentation.

CHAPTER 23

EQUINE-ASSISTED PSYCHOTHERAPY

THE HUMAN-HORSE BOND

Elizabeth Atwood Lawrence, VMD, PhD.

> *"He who has seen the tree-tops bend before the wind or a*
> *horse move knows all there is to be known about dancing."*
> (Porter, 1989)

The vital role that the horse can play in human healing--both physical and mental--is a contemporary dimension of the equine animal's capacity to serve as an indispensable partner throughout the history of civilization. During the centuries following its domestication, no animal has been more closely intertwined with human life and culture. Wherever the horse's strength was utilized to confer power and mobility, it transformed people's way of life and contributed in countless ways to the improvement of human welfare.

Associated with the equine capacity for providing traction and transport have always been the horse's extreme sensitivity and an unusual potentiality for fine-tuned communication with people. In its role as a living vehicle, carrying human beings forward into space, the horse has provided new dimensions of experience and sensation. Also, by means of shared kinetic processes--the physical and mental merging of rider and mount--this has awakened the human spirit to fresh aspects of perception through its special qualities of pace and rhythm. The horse affords satisfaction for our species' profound fascination with motion, and has near-universal appeal to the human senses of sight, sound, and touch.

The fact that there are said to be more horses in America now, when their use is almost entirely restricted to pleasure, than there were during the age when the animals were the essential means of transportation demonstrates the appreciation that the present society has for horses. Part of their appeal is that horses confer a feeling of heightened self-worth that is reflected in the behavior and perceptions of people who interact with them. Throughout much of human social history it has been the general rule that horses, both in a literal and symbolic sense, elevate the status of those who ride and use them. As Walter Prescott Webb wrote,

> *"The horse has always exerted a peculiar emotional effect on both the rider and the*
> *observer: he has raised the rider above himself, has increased his power and sense of*
> *power, and has aroused a sense of inferiority and envy in the humble pedestrian...*
> *Through long ages the horse has been the symbol of superiority, of victory and triumph."*

The historian goes on to point out that *"A good rider on a good horse is as much above himself and others as the world can make him."* (Webb, 1936)

A survey of horse-owning cultures of the world reveals a pervasive theme of high regard for the horse, which is almost universally recognized as the aristocrat among domestic animals, often identified with luxury, leisure, and power (Barclay, 1980). Evidence indicates that from earliest times, human relationships with horses have been especially meaningful. From the dawn of human consciousness, the horse has been a source of inspiration. Its beauty and strength were first immortalized in Paleolithic cave paintings. The admiration that all equestrian societies throughout history have felt for horses persists into modern times, for the aura of equine grandeur remains to grace the machine age. The term most frequently applied to horses is "noble." Again and again people reiterate the concept of the horse as the noblest of animals. Somehow the horse's traits--dignity and refinement, grace, beauty, and power--are felt to be transmitted to its human associates, for the equine animal seems to confer self-esteem and even ennoblement.

As a huge and powerful animal, the horse represents a paradox, for its strength can be guided and controlled according to human bidding. That mounts respond to people with such gentleness and dependability seems miraculous. Even more remarkable is the plasticity demonstrated by horses that allows them to adapt their behavior to the particular rider and situation at hand. Differences in interaction with one rider as compared to another show the horse's capability for discrimination and individual experience. The sensation of riding, as described by one keen horseman who spent the early part of his life in the saddle each day from dawn to dusk, means that a horse is "not a mere cunningly fashioned machine" which *sustains us; but a something with life and thought, like ourselves, that feels what we feel, understands us, and keenly participates in our pleasures. Take, for example, the horse on which some quiet old country gentleman is accustomed to travel; how soberly and evenly he jogs along, picking his way over the ground. But let him fall into the hands of a lively youngster, and how soon he picks up a frisky spirit! (Hudson, 1903).*

Although the extraordinary intercommunication that takes place between people and horses has not been adequately explained, it continues to amaze those who observe it and experience it for pleasure and for healing. Today, though mechanization has made the historic utility of horses for transportation and work virtually obsolete, and societies no longer revolve around them, contemporary people still turn to their traditional equine partner for important functions. Horses are companions of a different order than most other domestic species, for they provide an experience of motion that defies machinery. Equestrians can merge their own being with the rhythm and power of their mounts, bonding with a living creature in a participatory rather than a passive way. Communication between horse and rider is both physical and mental. The grace of movement of the horse somehow becomes possessed by the rider.

In our highly industrialized, mechanized age, horses have the unique role of leading us back to nature, back to our roots, back to the elemental rhythms and cycles of life. To ride a horse is to leave the cares of the mundane world behind and to become fused with the movements of a splendid creature that still belongs to the realm of nature, though it lends itself so willingly to humankind. The image of the centaur is deeply embedded in the human psyche, for it expresses the universal dream of unity with the animal world. And no other creature elicits or fulfills a deeper desire for that merging, that oneness with the elemental forces of nature, than the horse.

So wondrous is the bond between people and horses that it can never be definitively defined or wholly explained. Its richness and complexity give many facets to this age-old affective relationship. Mounted on a horse, the rider feels exhilarated in body and spirit. The animal not only provides an elevated position, but confers a heightened awareness that is an essential component of any type of healing process. The unbridled horse is a symbol of freedom, yet the equestrian, for a time, can direct the animal's path and share its swift flight, partaking of a marvelous adventure. But the benefits that horses bring to human life do not depend only on being ridden. Even the sound of equine hoof beats may afford comfort and tranquility (Lawrence, 1985). The feel of a horse's velvet-soft muzzle, the warm curves of its neck and flanks, the sight of its flowing mane and tail that blow in the wind, the sweet smell of its hay-scented breath--all these give solace to the horse lover that is like no other. In modern society, the horse has a role as healer--both for those who are weary of life's stresses and for those who have mental or physical handicaps to overcome. In some remarkable way, whatever quality an individual may lack, whether it is confidence, serenity, courage, or coordination, or whether it is health of mind or body, the horse willingly helps to evoke that quality so that it becomes the person's own possession. It is this complementarily that so endears the horse to human beings and cements the bond between them. An old adage states that "there is something about the outside of a horse that is good for the inside of a person." Folklore, which even many modern physicians believe, though they cannot explain it, holds that association with horses brings good health that leads to longevity. The extremely beneficial results that are being obtained through therapeutic horseback riding programs are evidence of the great effectiveness of healing through horses. Such programs demonstrate the adaptability of the horse in lending its many unique and wonderful attributes to the improvement of the quality of human life. The dramatically favorable results obtained from therapy using horses to promote human well-being depend upon and give testament to the enduring strength and power of the special bond between people and horses.

References
Barclay, H.B. (1980). *The Role of the Horse in Man's Culture*. London: J.A. Allen Co. 396-70.
Hudson, W.H. (1903). *The Naturalist in La Plata*. New York: E.P. Dutton & Co. 352.
Lawrence, E.A. (1985). *Hoofbeats and Society: Studies of Human-Horse Interactions*. Bloomington:Indiana Univ. Press. 145-46, 180-81.
Porter, V. (1989). *Horse Tails*. London: Guiness Publishing Ltd. 109.
Webb, W.P. (1936). *The Great Plains*. Boston: Houghton and Mifflin. 493.

Elizabeth Atwood Lawrence, VMD, PH.D
Tufts University School of Veterinary Medicine, USA

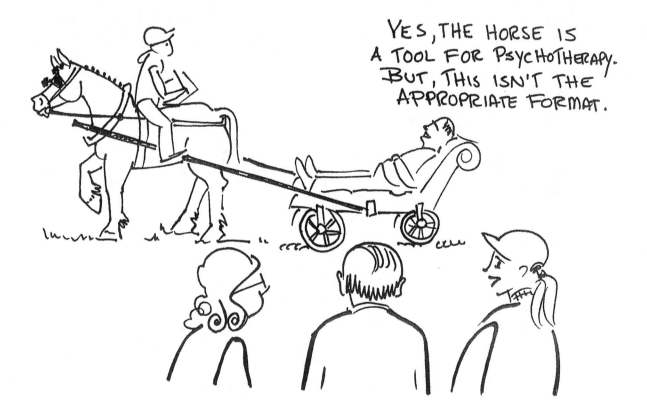

HORSES IN PSYCHOTHERAPY
A KINESTHETIC METAPHOR

Joanne Henry Moses, PhD

While horses have been assisting physically challenged people in therapeutic riding programs here and in Europe for about thirty years, they have only recently begun to help those suffering from often hidden but very real temporary and permanent psychiatric problems. TAAPA (Tucson Animal Assisted Psychotherapy Associates) has worked exclusively in mental health and personal growth since it was organized in 1990.

Equestrian psychotherapy, TAATA's primary focus, is the use of horseback riding to facilitate emotional healing and personal growth. An experiential approach, it requires simultaneous integration of body, mind, emotions, and spirit. The rider has to merge stimuli to sight, hearing, smell, and touch while maintaining balance astride a thinking, moving animal.

In addition to being an acronym for a long but meaningful name, TAAPA holds a rich meaning in the Sioux language. Literally, it means ball, or roundness, wholesome, peace, fullness of life. The Sioux acknowledge their relatedness to all of nature, perceiving animal therapists, and staff, in an atmosphere of hospitality. Suggesting that they acknowledge their relatedness to al of nature opens for clients a new and broader sense of family. To keep staff and clients cognizant of this significance, horses bred by TAAPA are named in Sioux.

Advantage of Equestrian Psychotherapy
Riding a horse affects posture, balance, mobility, and function. Change these factors also alters attitude. The motion of the horse at a walk promotes relaxation of the entire central nervous system, both voluntary and autonomic. The repetitive movement of the horse at a walk can lull the person into a deeply relaxed state. On the other hand, a brisk trot can energize someone with dulled affect.

Horseback riding also demands clear thinking to direct the horse and make correct and reasonable responses to its input. At the same time, the rider can savor a deep communion with nature. This synthesis of sensation, reasoning, and spirituality merges these stimuli into a unique healing encounter.

Merely sitting on a horse gives the client visual perspective unlike ordinary perception. Things look different with the eye four or five feet higher than when one is walking or riding in a car. Using this contrast can help a person to alter his or her perspective on problems. A rider can also gain increased self-awareness by having to balance and coordinate the body in a new way. Trying something new or revisiting a familiar skill evokes the whole pattern of emotional responses that the individual experiences in coping with life's challenges.

Equestrian psychotherapy gives the person a chance to get away from the clinical setting for a time. Being out side takes advantage of both the horses movement and naturally occurring unexpected events. How the person deals with challenging situations becomes readily apparent and provides rich material for debriefing after the ride. These occurrences present a metaphor of the individual's approach to life. Recognizing and describing demeanor can crystallize unsatisfactory coping mechanisms and offer the rider an opportunity to practice new behaviors.

The equestrian approach can be a deeply meditative experience, particularly for people who have ridden previously. Once the purpose of the session has been discussed, very little talking needs occur until debriefing. Even when a group of people share this activity, each participant spends much of the time on horseback alone more in communication with the horse than with the other riders. Group sharing after this reflective individual involvement, like nominal group process, has a more powerful impact than a purely verbal modality.

A Typical Session

At the beginning of a typical session, therapist, riding instructor, and client take a moment to set goals for the session, taking into account the long range treatment plan as well as the person's immediate need. They proceed to the rituals of calling, haltering, leading, and grooming the horse. In a society largely deprived of its rituals, this time spent in following established patterns in set sequence relaxes both horse and rider. Each knows what comes next.

The therapist observing this process can gauge the mood of both horse and rider. However, the person's "alone time" with the animal needs to be respected. TAAPA clients are encouraged to share their feelings, hopes, and expectations with their equine therapist.

Unlike individual talking therapy in which the client focuses solely on self, riders in equestrian therapy spend considerable time attending to the needs and feelings of another living being. For many this is good practice for living.

After the client has mastered the grooming ritual (usually around the second or third session) the riding experience begins. With the horse readied and the goal for the session determined, the rider and the team proceed to the mounting block.

Keeping the horses as willing participants in this sensitive process requires some special considerations. TAAPA riders do not use reins at first. Instead, they learn to communicate with their horse through turning their heads, settling their weight, using their voice, and communicating with the legs. Only after they have ridden the horse along the rail three times around the arena in each direction, guide the horse through a figure eight, and reversed directions using these subtle body signals are they allowed to use reins. The therapist or a volunteer guide holds the horse's lead rope during this initial phase and follows the horse's nose. It is the rider's responsibility to control the horse. If the rider directs the horse into the fence, into the fence they go. If the command to stop is ineffective, they keep going. The therapist/horse handler's task is not to guide the horse, but to be there to insure the rider's safety.

While this technique started as a way to protect the horses' mouths, it proved to be a valuable therapeutic tool. The rider has to focus on what he or she wants and communicate that intention clearly. Awareness of one's body becomes unavoidable with no reins to clutch in order to maintain balance. Trust issues become evident immediately. So does passive behavior. But in contrast with a strictly verbal modality, the client has to do something about these problems on the spot. As a result, self-confidence grows quickly.

Should emotionally charged issues arise, the team stops and deals with the feelings on the spot. The therapist makes the judgement whether to take the rider off the horse or to let the animal take part in the process. During a self-improvement workshop, a women who had been riding for over thirty-five years became overwhelmed by sudden surge of emotion over how harshly her family had taught her to deal with horses. As she experienced the willing responsiveness of her horse, she burst into gut-wrenching sobs of grief. The therapist and a nurse participating in the workshop invited her to lie down and clasp her arms around the horse's neck. Her sobbing continued unabated for twenty minutes as the therapist and nurse gently massaged her. Suddenly Wacin (her mount), who had stood silent and unmoving through the entire episode, put her nose on the women's left knee and nickered to her just as she did to her new-born foals. The rider bolted upright and asked, "Is she ok?" "Yes. She's just comforting you," the therapist assured her. With that she plopped back down on Wacin's neck and continued sobbing. Wacin then tenderly placed her nose on the woman's right knee and continued to nicker.

Once they had mastered basic riding skills and are relatively stable emotionally, clients may choose to go out on trail. Usually these riders proceed in silence for three reasons. First, the client has already decided on the emotional work to be done during the ride and need quiet to experience the horse, nature, and inner self. Secondly, talking can evoke highly charged emotional issues and memories. A person cannot be overwhelmed with intense feelings and still be expected to maintain control of the horse. Finally, idle chatter diverts the client from attending to feelings and doing the needed emotional work.

After the ride, the client dismounts, removes the helmet, and takes the bridle off the horse. Usually the client and team debrief at that point. Staff give the person positive feedback about the session and invite him or her to identify strengths exercised during the ride. While self criticism comes easily to most clients, speaking well of oneself takes concerted effort. Therapist and client evaluate how effectively goals for the session were met. The key question often is, "How does this behavior show up in the larger issues of your life?"

Usually the answer reveals what TAAPA therapists call the kinesthetic metaphor. In a kinesthetic metaphor, problems in coping and dysfunctional behaviors manifest themselves in the rider's gestalt of body and behavior on the horse. Usually the person recognizes the pattern and may have been dealing with it verbally for years. But astride the horse, the rider has both the occasion and the need to practice new and more effective ways of coping.

While equestrian psychotherapy unlocks a powerful new tool for people in emotional pain, it is not for everyone. It is most effective with people not responding to traditional therapy, perhaps because the metaphors this modality presents are so clear. A number of TAAPA's clients have been in the mental health system for many years. Struggling for so long with their chronic condition often leaves them hopeless and discouraged. They have been talking about their problems most of their lives. While equestrian psychotherapy will never cure their underlying condition, its emphasis on practicing new behavior impacts the quality of their lives directly. And the pleasure they get from the relationship with the animal as well as the endorphin stimulation resulting from the horse's movement brings motivation and excitement into the treatment process. Utilized as an adjunct to traditional treatment, equestrian psychotherapy speeds up and enhances the therapeutic process. Employing the human-animal bond in this way is one small step in developing a simple, humane, as well as environmentally and scientifically sound approach to achieving mental health.

THERAPEUTIC HORSEBACK RIDING WITHIN PSYCHIATRY *
Thoughts about Contents and Relevance

Dr. med. Dr. med. dent. Michaela Scheidhacker

Contents:
   Psychiatric illnesses
   Therapeutic aspects
   Treatment methods
   Indications and contraindications
   Training and credentials
   Billing of costs [in Germany *tr.*]

[The discipline of *tr.*]therapeutic riding within psychiatry is practiced in many places but only in the last few years has it received widespread recognition. Psychiatry, as a discipline for healing the mind, soul or spirit ["Seelenheilkunde"], is a main branch of medicine. Nevertheless, it touches the fields of psychology, psychotherapy, education and philosophy ("the striving of the human spirit to recognize the nature of being and its authentic values.") Psychiatric illnesses include a wide range of different disabilities and impairments that are to be taken into account if intervention and treatment with therapeutic riding is undertaken.

Psychiatric illnesses

A mental disability can arise through genetic [deformity] or accidental damage to the brain (e.g. birth trauma, accident, tumor, poisoning). In these cases, healing is usually not possible. It results in a permanent state of decreased mental capacity of more or less extreme degree. The goal in treating these people is to make it possible for them to lead a dignified life in some kind of community in spite of their disabilities and, to prevent medical complications from arising.

Substance addicted people do not show brain damage early on in their addiction. Body damage shows up only after continued consumption of the poisonous material over a longer period of time. These people are usually unstable, unsure of themselves and lonely. Their only partner in life is the addictive substance which brings on their ruin.

In contrast to the above conditions are those psychiatric illnesses which offer no demonstrable changes to the brain. In psychoses, there is a loss, temporary or permanent, of the ability to orient oneself in one's environment. The patients hallucinate, i.e. they see and hear things that do not really exist. People who tend toward having psychoses are often weak but also oversensitive, intelligent and even creative; nevertheless they still either have difficulty meeting the demands of everyday life or they fail completely to do so. For this reason, some of them can live only in the protected environment of an institution. Borderline patients (those on the borderline between psychosis and neurosis) often demonstrate superior abilities in their work and social lives.

Their illness is not noticeable to untrained people. However, they tend to divide people into the categories of either all good or all bad, they cannot maintain relationships with other people over time and they are plagued

Translated by Eberhard Walter Teichmann

by deep loneliness and emptiness in their inner life. Neuroses are caused by mental or spiritual crises that result in "a disturbance of equilibrium" that leads in turn to mental or somatic
symptoms. Everyone may have neurotic characteristics, either continuously or from time to time, without being substantially disabled by them. Neuroses take on the character of illness only through the suffering that arises from constant inner conflict. In that form they restrict a person's development and influence their quality of life and their capacity to produce.

Psychosomatic illnesses arise from a repetitive mental conflict which causes a neurovegetative disturbance of function in a particular organ, at first without physical illness. In fixations, organic illness (e.g. stomach ulcer, bronchial asthma, eczema) can result. The people with these problems often have substantial problems experiencing their own body and their feelings in a positive way.

Common to all psychiatric illnesses is a disturbance, which varies in extent from case to case, in the patient's ability to form and maintain human relationships. At this point the horse becomes useful.

Therapeutic aspects

Horses are especially suited for therapeutic intervention because of their nature as herd animals. Being domesticated, they have included humans in their herd sense. And, the rider maintains close bodily contact with the horse when they are riding. Learning to ride is peripheral to this (therapeutic) process. The main thing is [for the patient] to get acquainted with his or her abilities in a playful and stress free manner. In the course of this activity, the person is touched in various ways: in his or her sense of body and bodily movement, in his or her perceptual ability and sensibility, in his or her relational and discriminatory capacity as well as in his or her responsibility for self and others and his or her reality based self assessment. The therapeutic points of departure start with body- and movement therapy perspectives (similar to hippotherapy), continue through education and training (remedial riding and vaulting) viewpoints and finally include behavioral therapy, depth psychology and analytic treatment methods. The latter approaches can be brought together under the concept of "psychotherapeutic riding." Mental equilibrium can also positively influence athletic riding, with its contact between horse and rider, and its goal of increasing physical ability.

The interactions between horse and rider proceed nonverbally in analogic communication. Language is relegated to the background. Gestures, emotional intention and the authenticity of the relationship are what are essential in the mutual experience of horse and rider and are decisive in the therapeutic work. The immediate reactions of the horse can be experienced as mirroring unconscious states brought on by the discovery of individual biographical connections. Happiness and the joy of living can appear naturally, physical effort and resulting tiredness have content and meaning, and the frustration and disappointment over not achieving a freely chosen goal don't necessarily mean interruption and loss. Instead, having the living horse as a partner turns these events into experiences of insight, change and strengthening.

Treatment methods

The large variety of therapeutic possibilities available with horses can be used with different psychiatric illnesses, taking into account the different methods, courses, and goals of treatment that are appropriate to the particular needs and deficiencies of a particular patient. Therapy can be conducted in groups or with individuals. Children, adolescents, and adults with a psychiatric illness can benefit equally; the form of treatment is tailored to fit the appropriate developmental stage of the individual patient.

a) [Observing *tr.*] the horses running freely and interacting competitively in their status hierarchy can make natural, limiting, and aggressive disputes as well as loving attraction evident [to patients *tr.*] and make group phenomena more conscious and understandable [to them *tr.*]. The horses, being curious, can spontaneously involve the people and make the first contacts between them easier.

b) The care and proper grooming and saddling of the horse [also *tr.*] serves [the purpose of *tr.*] making contact with it, getting to know its peculiarities and natural reactions, and dismantling the fear of contact with it.

c) Being longed on an unsaddled horse, equipped with only a vaulting girth, allows one to feel the movements of the horse's back. Being "carried and rocked" by a living being and being in close, direct contact with it at the same time allows one to become intensely conscious of one's own body and emotions. Using horses of different colors and sizes with various gaits and temperaments encourages one's experience of different visual, acoustic, olfactory and tactile stimuli. A positive body sense can develop. Longeing is a setting in which regression may be encouraged; this must be taken into account especially with regressive patients in order to not encourage unwanted, increased regression in them. But in other patients, the regressive quality of this setting has special therapeutic utility.

d) The path to riding on one's own goes through being longed while sitting in the saddle, then being led by the reins, riding behind another rider and finally, truly being in charge of the horse as a rider. Horses that are trained and also are patient and good natured help make these therapeutic developmental steps toward assertiveness, self-consciousness, and independence easier. The goals of the treatment are ego strengthening and discovery of an identity. Riding on one's own is a progressive process in which the degree of symptoms of illness must be taken into account.

Indications and Contraindications

Mental illnesses are much more difficult to grasp than are most physical illnesses. For this reason, the question of indications and contraindications is complex and must be answered on an individual bases dependent on the training of the therapist and the involvement of the client.

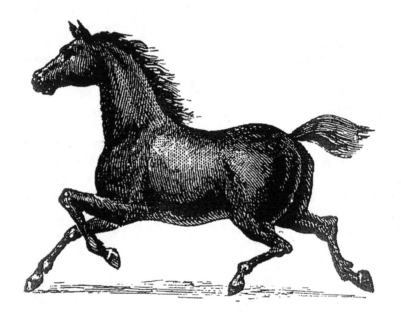

WINDOWS OF OPPORTUNITY
Psychological Principles Present in Therapeutic Riding Sessions

Barbara Kathleen Rector, MA

The purpose of this paper is to set out some examples of psychological principles that commonly operate during a therapeutic riding session. Becoming aware of these dynamics enables staff, volunteers, and ultimately students to take control of their own inner reality. The process of validating our personal reality and choosing to appropriately express it allows us to integrate our inner personal truth (reality as experienced by us) with the surrounding consensus reality of the therapeutic riding session environment. This individuation and integration work is the task of every human being. The equine facilitated experiential process work serves as a metaphoric bridge to the world of everyday life.

Some of what I say here will feel unfamiliar and alien. That's OK. It may not be your truth. I suggest you check inside your body as you listen or read my words. Most of us recognize our truth from a deep feeling response deep within our center: the internal "aha." My own personal test for truth is to ask myself, "Is this particular belief or idea going to improve the quality of my life experience?" Will practice, adoption, or work with this idea noticeably improve my feelings about me and my life experience?

During a therapeutic riding session, the equine facilitated experiential process is operating at every level of consciousness for every individual present. No one is excluded. Individuals are unaware of this dynamic are oblivious to its function according to the degree of habitual, rote, mechanical movements and thoughts present in their consciousness. The more conscious, aware and focused in the present a person is, the more expanded the choices for experiencing reality.

I believe the experiences of working in the therapeutic riding session setting allow every individual participating (volunteer, staff, student) an opportunity to access more knowledge about self. One may working as part of a treatment team as either horse handler, side walker-safety aid, one on one communicator, therapeutic instructor and therapist. All are roles in an interactive experience of horses as compassionate teachers. Exercising the spirit is as important as exercising the body/mind. While the horse provides a unique vehicle for these essentials, participation as part of a group treatment team is a significant contributing factor.

The group clustered around a hippotherapy horse is a unit - a team. The awareness and focus of everyone present contributes to the group's consciousness. One of the first "rules" of counseling is: The identified patient is not the source of the problem. They are a "container" having absorbed unconsciously unresolved issues originating in the family of origin, current life situation or environment, and culture.

The next time you are a part of such a group, make a conscious choice to **both** notice your feelings felt internally while continuing to focus on the task at hand. Simultaneously focus inward and do a feelings scan of your body, noticing any pain or stiffness and its location. Make no judgements. Just notice. At the same time continue to remain alert to the group's activity. Again, simultaneously, consciously acknowledge to yourself the truth of your feelings. I believe that this meditative practice of mindfulness allows one to perceive more clearly the truth for yourself. This awareness of your feelings fully felt in the moment is a GIFT. You now experience the opportunity to choose to feel differently. Freedom of choice is a gift; an opportunity to alter your personal experience of reality.

Quantum physics is revealing the plasticity of reality. Indeed, the energy of our feelings and the focus of intention in their expression contributes to designing the reality we experience. The very fabric of our lives is woven from the warp and weft of our conscious and unconscious feelings influenced by our unconscious thoughts and beliefs. The field of somatic psychology maps the cartography of our bodies as developed through our unconscious, habitual emotional responses. (Stanley Keleman's Emotional Anatomy, 1985)

It is my belief that we humans are here in earth school in our specifically designed space suits (our bodies and minds) for a purpose. We have some lessons to learn, wisdom to acquire, feelings to feel and gifts to share before we complete our lives and are ready to "graduate" to other planes of existence. Life is designed as a group experience. We do our best learning in relationship: relationship to self, to others, to family, friends, community, culture, country, and planet.

These experiences of "other" mirror for us aspects of ourselves with which we are unfamiliar; through the sacred compassionate experience of each other, we befriend those unknown parts of our self. In recognizing, validating and appropriately expressing these "splintered aspects of self", we become whole. Everyone qualifies for this work. No diagnosis is necessary. The life experience is designed so that all of us develop as we mature through the growing process in our individual cultures with certain coping mechanisms and survival skills. We come equipped (in personality theories of character-temperament; typologies) with certain underdeveloped functions that demand recognition or else we act out unconsciously through the disease process or physical accidents or traumatic experiences of chaotic situations.

In the situation of the full treatment team, you've done your feelings check and you notice that you really do have difficulty with one of the other team members, or maybe it's the horse or the student. For whatever reason you are aware that as you practice this mindful noticing of inward feelings, there are certain individuals or situations that truly give you uncomfortable or resistant or negative feelings. The therapeutic instructor, or the program coordinator has probably coached you to make them aware of intense levels of discomfort if you are assigned to work with particular people, horses, or students.

Projection is at work. Projection is defined as the act of attributing to another person, animal, or object the qualities, feelings, or intentions that (unconsciously) originate in one's self. The critical variable in projection is that we do not see in ourselves what seems vivid and obvious in another.

"Whenever we characterize something "out there" as evil, dangerous, perverted, and so forth, without acknowledging (consciously) that these characteristics might also be true for us, we are probably projecting. It is equally true that when we see others as being powerful, attractive, capable, and so forth, without appreciating (consciously) the same qualities in ourselves, we are also projecting." (Frager-Fadiman, 1984)

Let's look closely at the associated schematic. It is my personal effort to draw a pictorial representation of psyche that fits easily within the framework of a multitude of belief systems: psychological schools of thought (Freudian, Jungian, Adlerian, Behaviorist, Transpersonal, etc.) or religious beliefs. The drawing is an attempt to illuminate the basic function of the psyche in such a fashion as to make it compatible or complete with what ever system of beliefs are operating for an individual.

This is my rendering of my current understanding and experience of how psyche functions. I recognize that my thoughts are colored by my personal filter; my perceptual sense is distorted or is a product of my current state of personal integration and individuation. The sum total of my life experiences, influenced by my current mind/body/spiritual alignment, affect my ability to experience reality.

Studying the works and teachings of Carl Gustav Jung serves to influence my continuing fascination with the interplay of psychology, philosophy, quantum physics and spirituality. One of Jung's central concepts is **individuation**, his term for a process of personal development that involves making a conscious connection between the personality self's ego and the core self. In Jung's cartography of psyche, the ego is the center of consciousness and the self is the center of total psyche, including both consciousness and the unconscious. Jung believed there is constant interplay between consciousness and the unconscious. They are two aspects of a single system. Individuation is a process of developing wholeness through integrating all the various parts of the psyche.

The mechanism of projection is a tool for recognizing those aspects of self with which we are unfamiliar. For me, a key to recognizing whether or not I'm projecting is to notice the intensity of the energy generated feeling my feelings while being critical of another's behavior or in the company of someone I'm experiencing as difficult. This can be a positive experience too. I may be feeling deeply appreciative of another's gifts or discovering how much I admire certain qualities in another. With expanded awareness and growing consciousness I'm literally looking in a mirror.

Consider another "rule" from basic counseling courses. Remember the first one: The identified patient is not the source of the problem? The second "rule" is that the person doing the most finger pointing with the most heated energy is really talking about self. Another way of expressing this concept is that I can only know another or help another to the extent that I first know and help myself. It is impossible to give that which I don't have. Without personal intimate knowledge of self, true, deep intimacy with another isn't possible.

The first half of our lives is generally devoted to the developmental stages of growth: childhood, adolescent, young adult. The concerns are one of mastery of life skills in the outer world. Physical, mental, and emotional development is tied to relationships as experienced in family, schools, church, peers, community, education, and career development. It is usually in the phase of our life where our own children are leaving the nest that we become aware of further growth available to us on the inner planes. The last frontier for exploration lies within self - within psyche. Postscript: I believe the technological advances of our culture are creating a speeded up necessity for our young people, even children, to do this work in an earlier phase of their development (crack babies, kids having kids, children who are HIV positive, fetal alcohol syndrome).

I believe that the therapeutic riding session offers a unique opportunity for the study, practice and processes of this psychotherapeutic exploration of ourselves and each other. Self determined psychotherapeutic work, done consciously, allows the safety of the surrounding group working with large and powerful horses and ponies to act as a "container" for the full development of **feelings fully felt and appropriately expressed.** I use the term "container" in the Jungian sense of setting - of a template. The design of the stable yard ritual of work with horses, the disciplined steps to horse training as characterized by classical dressage and the acknowledgment and practice of the NARHA guidelines provide for a safe structure to work with, around, and on horses.

A conscious agreement in the collective reality of therapeutic riding sessions operated under NARHA guidelines for safety around horses is: a horse is always a horse first. The horse's basic psychology is ruled by the fight or flight syndrome when startled or in fear. The horse has limited vision and is easily startled by sudden movement or loud and unusual noises. A horse always knows when you are feeling afraid; even when you are not conscious of feeling afraid. A horse seems to know the axiom that our feelings are the vital currents that energize our thoughts and actions.

In a letter to me in 1992, a beloved friend, Bazy Tankersley, founder of Al-Marah Arabians in Tucson, Arizona, wrote the following words describing our human relationship to horses.

"A beguiling thing about horse is that such a large, strong creature should be so dependent for elemental care -- (not just from weather). Basically, horse wants nothing more from us but kindness and consistency. The horse is not very smart and I must communicate with him simply and in a manner that admits no apprehension. Because he is so big, I forget he's timid. It is difficult for the horse to communicate with me so I must be very perceptive and must learn horse language. We can both reach a wonderful thing if I can make clear to horse what I want him to do to make me happy and I must treat him with the understanding and skill acquired to bring him to the frame of mind necessary for him to accept my requests, act on them and feel satisfaction in accomplishing what I want. He needs to be taught about praise and gratitude so he will be glad he pleased me and will look forward to doing it again. Rewarding him will be as great a pleasure to me as the enjoyment of having him respond to my requests.

No love is perfect so there will be times that I will be mad at him either because he does something nasty -- anything from nipping me to avoiding being caught -- or he is stubborn about doing something I think I have taught him (or even something he knows full well) or I may even be mad at him because he stepped on my big toe by mistake. I sincerely hope I will not react badly in any of these situations. If he nips at me I should only flick him on the nose and that only if I do it fast enough so he knows why I did it. If he doesn't want to be caught, I need to work on our relationship and not chase him about yelling at him. If he steps on me, it's my own stupidity and I hope my anger will be at myself, or better still, that I will laugh after I've said, "Damn!". If my temper gets the best of me and I smack him unjustly (I'm entitled to smack him on the butt if he won't go in his stall), I must quickly make peace with him and try to erase the memory of my little injustice.

Sometimes he'll have a bad day and be mad at me and not want to do what I want him to. I'm smarter so it's up to me to let him do something easy and then let him alone for today. The teaching-learning modality is an intellectual experience. But horse will give me other types of experiences appealing to other senses than my brain. There will be many that are beautiful with horse, from the "moss" in his eyes to the poses he strikes grazing, gazing, etc. He is good to feel. I can't keep from stroking him and when my stroking finds a spot on his withers or forehead which he likes, this appeals to another of my senses. I enjoy the way he smells.

I want horse to feel this way about me. I don't know what is his conception of beauty. Perhaps I can develop a body language that will appeal to him. I know he likes to feel my fingers on his shoulder when

I have just taken off the bridle and let him rub his head on me or respond when he pokes his face in my hand. Sometimes he like to smell me too. I think he likes to sniff the sun screen on my cheeks, and if I am quiet and welcoming in his stall or in a big field, he will come up to me and linger around me because he likes my companionship.

I think I do more for him than he does for me, what with feeding, grooming, stall cleaning, etc. I do it because I love him. He probably thinks <u>he</u> does more for <u>me</u> because that's generally the way love is."

When we are unaware of how we are really feeling (and most of us work earnestly to suppress our feelings all the time through keeping busy, and practicing addictive and compulsive behaviors or thought patterns) then the horse knows there is potential for trouble. A Jungian would say that is the moment when the Trickster Energy Archetype surfaces. Some event or situation will serve as a wake-up call to increased awareness and expanded consciousness.

Occasionally people who have been repeatedly traumatized physically, emotionally or psychically use the defense mechanism of disassociation. The pain of allowing feelings to be felt is both consciously and unconsciously is so threatening to the personality ego's sense of survival that the personality consciousness seems to leave the body/mind and goes elsewhere. You may have had the experience of driving day after day over the same familiar route. Occasionally you seem to "snap" to and be further along the route than you thought. Where were "you" ? Daydreaming -- fantasizing? You were not conscious and focused, aligned and attuned with mind, body, and spirit fully present to self.

What riding instructor hasn't patiently talked through a run-away, the sudden leap into canter by an unbalanced student. But there is no student to hear the coaching. They are not present in their body on the horse in their fright. The instructor talks to the horse. With voice, focused mind, and intensity of heart energy, the horse is brought back to the instructor and into a halt. You can almost see the student re-enter their body. Indeed, most instructors find themselves saying, "Breathe. Breathe. It's OK."

The problem is one of reconciliation of opposites. How to deal with the existence of good and evil, right and wrong, negative and positive, health and disease. I quote from Jung in his commentary on "The Secret of the Golden Flower".

"Out of evil, much good has come to me. By keeping quiet, repressing nothing, remaining attentive, and by accepting reality - taking things as they are, and not as I wanted them to be - by doing all this, unusual knowledge has come to me, and unusual powers as well, such as I could never have imagined before. I always thought that when we accepted things they overpowered us in some way or other. (Twelve Step program's concept of surrender.) This turns out not to be true at all, and it is only by accepting them that one can assume an attitude towards them. So now I intend to play the game of life, being receptive to whatever comes to me, good and bad, sun and shadow forever alternating, and in this way also accepting my own nature with its positive and negative sides. Thus everything becomes more alive to me. What a fool I was! How I tried to force everything to go according to the way I thought it ought to!"

Anthony Storr comments that Jung called such an attitude "religious" although the person who achieves it may not subscribe to any of the recognized creeds. By sacrificing the ego's mundane goals, and accepting what comes, the individual is acknowledging dependence on something beyond the ego, which lives in and through him or her. In Twelve Step programs this self-regulating principle manifests as tough love, divine guidance, even in neurotic symptoms which force an individual to take notice of what is going on inside self. Storr believes this attitude of paying careful attention to whatever comes, and of acceptance, would be described by religious people as "waiting upon God."

It is my belief that the horse grows more and more uncomfortable when working with individuals unaware of their feelings. The horse doesn't care what we are feeling as in the instances of when one admits to feeling fear of working with or mounting a strange horse. The verbal expression of feeling afraid, immediately calms the horse. Horses require congruency (matching) of feelings felt inwardly and outwardly expressed and acknowledged. The horse will tell us when a student has disassociated. Its behavior will be aimless or unguided.

I believe horses have a powerful message for humans. When we first befriended the horse, a moment in time akin to the discovery of fire, or the planting of a seed our domestication of the horse radically altered the way we oriented our lives. We could now travel great distances, meet new people, discover and, conquer new worlds. Even today we speak of wealth or power in terms of possessions. He who had the best horses, won wars, or moved more goods and services had the most power. Today our engines are capacity rated in terms of "horsepower."

Now for some definitions. In the field of alternative experiential education "therapy" is defined as "moving towards beneficial change." "Psyche" is a Greek word for soul. Psychotherapy is the work of the soul moving towards beneficial change. Webster defines psychology as the study of the interactions of the biological organism, man, and its physical and social environment; the systematic knowledge gained through such study.

My own soul work is anchored in re-envisioning my right relationship to self, to others and to the planet. This work is illustrated by my emerging conscious work with horses and people. In developing the courage to grow more and more aware of my inner feelings, to feel them fully and appropriately express them, I 'm discovering more about the participant/observer principle. In order to observe or experience a particular situation, I have to name my intention to observe what I observe. In a sense, the old wives tale of self-fulfilling prophecy.

I'm growing more aware of my inner challenges to the current status quo of horse training. We dominate the horse using power tactics to get him to submit to the will of the rider. I am recognizing that the idea of dominance through human control as an operative in my belief system is no longer comfortable. It's time for me to replace it with a more mutually empowering belief. I prefer the heart energy surrounding an attitude of joining with, asking for cooperation, designing win/win situations and relationships. Conscious effort of working together for the mutual benefit of both or all concerned.

Horses are large animals with huge hearts and major sensory systems throughout their body/mind. While anatomically their brain is relatively small for their enormous body size, the mind is present in every cell of their body as it is in ours. It's easy to find a horse person with a story or two of how horses think, survive, and help their human caretakers through some rough spots or tough times. Horses are helpful for depression because they are survivors. No matter how man adapts their living environment, horses surrender and accommodate. We humans create eating disorders in horses with thoughtless training techniques and ignorant stable management. The emotional sensitivity of a horse is unfathomable to most humans. They know us, and our energy; they are intuitively connected to our spirits. They experience easy access to the collective unconscious.

Horses are always reading our spirits. They know our inner thoughts in the sense of how they direct our usually unconscious feelings. When developing a relationship with a horse, the human is afforded a unique opportunity to learn, to practice, and to validate the principle: OUR THOUGHTS CREATE OUR REALITY. Unconscious mental processes are allowed expression when working in a round pen doing free longe work with a horse. Even in the activity of a traditional mounted skills development, stable management practicum, or vaulting lesson, an individual's habitual mode of processing new information is revealed.

Often people report that their horse, or their dog, cat, or bird seems to understand English - the spoken word. Of course! Giving voice to our conscious intention (with focused mind fueled with the heart energy of desire) aligns mental, emotional, physical and spiritual energy. This alignment of focus produces an energy field manifesting the reality. This particular principle of energy is generally experienced unconsciously by most people as life and events happening to them. For those people who doubt the truth of this energy principle, personal work in the round pen, or observation of the unfolding equine facilitated expressive play (psychodrama) between horse and human serves as first hand validation. An individual personal experience of a particular reality is a powerful motivator for expanding awareness of the different levels of consciousness (hence, realities) available to us all.

I'll close with a story. At the hospital our medical director was taking a visiting dignitary, a nationally known and respected psychiatrist famous for his research protocols on a tour of the facility. They visited the barn and this distinguished guest demanded I explain equine facilitated psychotherapy in three sentences or less.

The three of us were propped against the arena fence observing the therapy horses turned out as a herd. We had been enjoying the antics of one particular bay horse in his efforts to keep the flirtatious red mare from enjoying the attentions of the other geldings. "Well, which of these horses are you feeling drawn to and why?" I asked him.

"Oh, that handsome bay! He's so charismatic and vibrant! While he's not having much luck keeping the mare away from the other guys, he's sure willing to prance and dance for her attention. In fact now that I really notice him, he doesn't seem real confident off by himself. He wants that mare in attendance with her attention and affections only on him." "And how much have you told me about yourself?", I inquired of him. A moment of blank stare. Pregnant pause. His face suffused with emotion and his eyes became moist. "Why I've told you more about me just now, than I've told my analyst."

Barbara Kathleen Rector, MA
Assistant Executive Director
Co-founder of TROT (Therapeutic Riding of Tucson)

THE RESIDENTIAL FARM SCHOOL APPROACH

Samuel B. Ross, Jr., Ph.D.

Imagine a tough, troubled young teen from the mean streets of New York City patiently soothing a frightened pheasant or gingerly setting a rabbit's broken foot. Watch another child work with a gentle team of Percherons or drive a young Haflinger gelding as part of the horse's schooling. These are some of the many small daily miracles at Green Chimneys' farm and wildlife center where animals help troubled urban youngsters heal and blossom.

Near Brewster, New York, on 150 acres purchased in 1947 by the Ross Family, Green Chimneys, a residential treatment center with a special education school, has become home to 102 inner-city youngsters who share its rolling campus with a host of rare and common barnyard animals. Here for the past 49
years staff have pioneered the use of the healing power of human-animal interaction as the cornerstone of our work with youngsters.

Many of the Green Chimneys children arrive with histories of neglect or sexual, physical or emotional abuse. Many are also learning disabled and have never experienced success at school. They have had a rocky existence at home, in school and in the community. They come defeated because they have failed in those things by which children get judged. They must learn that there never has been an animal which asked a child his achievement test score. Children here learn self-worth. They begin to excel and are given a chance to share their new found skills with others.

Green Chimneys has inspired child care specialists and others here and abroad. Unlike many programs for children with special needs that become magnets for community protest, Green Chimneys attracts local residents to a broad range of recreational and educational activities. On any given day the young residents join visitors for classes in nature, horticulture and horse care as well as riding lessons. The rewards are great. The funds acquired through programs offered to the community help to support the entire agency.

Certified by the state and federal government as a "disabled wildlife rehabilitation center", the barn and pens now shelter mending turkeys, geese, owls and falcons. A wildlife rescue station has been opened on the grounds of a Green Chimney's group home in Bedford, N.Y. Here again the community becomes tied in to the children and the program.

Thanks to a special interest of the farm staff, modern breeds graze alongside rare breeds. Under the leadership of the farm director, Green Chimneys residents and local visitors learn to care for these and the hundreds of other animals on the grounds. On evenings and weekends, Green Chimneys' youngsters gently help community children out of their wheelchairs onto horses as part of the farm's therapeutic riding program.

Taking year-round care of animals, including over 20 horses, donkeys, and ponies, teaches children responsibility. Caring for animals can be the first step in developing the human ethic: a concern for other people that comes from the opportunity to love and be loved. The farm draws the children who are upset, sullen, depressed and frustrated. The animals serve as catalysts--linking child to child, child to staff, child to family.

The following letter, written from one student to another whose horse had died, illustrates what the horse care program means:

> *Dear R.D.,*
>
> *I am sorry about Jagger. He was a special horse. We all loved him.*
> *If there is anything I can do to make you feel better, I will do it because*
> *I know how you feel. I am upset myself. I know you will miss him for I will miss him too.*
> > *Your Friend,*
> > *M.P.*

Jagger's death was an emotional time for many children. Many had family or friends who had died or were killed. It gave them a chance to mourn old friends and ask many questions, along with coming together to support one another. For children who might have trouble expressing themselves in verbal therapy in an office, animal-assisted therapy becomes a vital link in the child's treatment.

The program was originally founded to house a private school where children could interact with farm animals. From the very beginning ponies and horses were the biggest attraction. Seemingly, they reduced the anxiety of being away from home. The school, which is in session year-round--223 days per year, evolved into specializing in the care of children with special needs, and in 1974 expanded its scope and became a social service agency. The agency now serves children with handicapping conditions as well as local children and adults from New York City, Westchester, Putnam and Fairfield (CT) Counties who participate in the variety of programs being offered.

Therapeutic riding instructors provide classes indoors and out for 102 residents and 30 day students and 35 mentally retarded and/or physically disabled youth, a summer riding clinic, the agency's 200 day campers and 50 year-round pre-school children, as well as hunt seat lessons for children and adults in the community. The program is staffed throughout each day--seven days a week. The children in residence serve as aides for the instructors. The main emphasis remains the 102 resident children and is designed to provide an opportunity for social, emotional, academic and physical growth and progression through the medium of therapeutic riding and horse care. This is achieved through a variety of equine events including 4-H, Learn and Earn, "adopt a horse" program, various contests, skill team, vaulting team, field trips, trail rides, horse shows and, of course, riding during program time.

Each child at Green Chimneys adopts a horse as a project. The child may ride the horse during the program times and during special programs. The student is responsible for care of the horse, with supervision in event of injury to or sickness of the horse. Some children are reluctant to ride but are still involved in horse care and equine studies. Children can be found at the farm throughout the day. Top riders within each class are united into a team that performs patterns and maneuvers. Teams perform for Green Chimneys events including times when families are on campus and for the public.

An extensive Learn and Earn program is provided. A number of hours are regularly scheduled for residents to learn the responsibilities of holding and keeping a job. The students are able to earn some money which, in turn, they bank in a savings account. Other residents have experience working at the Horse Center. During an average week, in addition to riding, 30 residents work at the Horse Center. Job experiences range from:

- Unsupervised morning student workers who arrive at 7:15 A.M., measure and feed the correct types and amounts of feed to the horses
- Supervised barn management where students sweep, hay, water, lead horses, mucks stalls and do whatever is necessary to maintain the barn and a healthy herd
- Advanced riders work as one-on-one peer tutors with new or young students teaching them horse science grooming techniques and walking beside them to insure their safety

Young students get first job experiences as part of a clean-up team, one-on-one, with an instructor. They learn to put equipment away, rake, sweep or do within their ability whatever is needed. Emphasis is on learning and job responsibility.

Residents are trained to work with riders with disabling conditions either as a therapeutic riding leader or sidewalker. Children learn to care for others and become more service-oriented as a result of this experience.

Some residents are selected to join the vaulting team because of ability or need. They learn cooperation and team work as they work in pairs to do "tricks" and gymnastic exercises atop a moving horse. It is a great confidence builder. Teams perform at many annual events. Students create written and visual reports of these activities. All of this is considered part of the student's school program. An extensive 4-H program overlaps with the adopt-a-horse program. Children participate in the Putnam County 4-H Fair Horse Show. Well over 50 residents earned the honor of representing Green Chimneys. 4-H members enter the local record book contest. The 4-H quiz bowl team competes in the NY State Regional Horse Bowl. Children learn to ride English, Western and bareback. They participate in vaulting, learn to harness and drive the pony cart and draft team.

College students of many majors (psychology, agriculture, science (pre-med), animal behavior, liberal arts) are recruited and assigned to the Horse Center. They spend at least four months in residence as interns. They expand the program by doing special projects related to their fields, with the animals and children. One instructor is assigned responsibility for training, supervision and evaluation of college students. Courses are offered for Mercy College, Dobbs ferry, N.Y. The farm is the site for the college's Vet tech course work in large animals.

The Farm Center also includes a staff person who serves as a liaison to the treatment teams and who represents the program at all reviews of a child's progress. The availability of such a person has increased the effectiveness of the program. Everything the child does is included in the child's academic program and documentation is absolutely essential. Specific skill cards have been designed for every activity.

Many people have spent their lifetimes searching for means for humans to better understand and accept the responsibility of environmental stewardship. Green Chimneys sees itself as part of that effort. When one learns to nurture, he or she is able to accept responsibility and learn to be patient; then he or she has the attributes which will serve him or her well for years to come. These are some of the major goals of the program at Green Chimneys.

Children are our future. Every child therefore is important. Children need to be able to take their places in society and society has to be prepared to let them.

Samuel B. Ross, Jr., Ph.D
Executive Director
Green Chimneys Children's Services
Brewster, NY 10509

THE RIDING PROGRAM

Eva Pheleps

Here at Green Chimneys we use the therapeutic riding program as therapy utilizing a multi-sensory approach to developing and facilitating psychomotor, language, math, social and emotional skills. Being responsible for care for another living creature is an essential part in developing a healthier and happier "SELF".

The therapeutic riding at Green Chimneys has demonstrated its effectiveness in inducing a positive change in the child's attitude toward self and peers, and his or her own ability, which has promoted a sense of accomplishment and increased self confidence. The children have become confident in their ability to master and control themselves and their environment and also to have the confidence in others who can help them master skills.

The therapeutic riding program is divided into two equally important components:
1. The care of the horses (which involves practical instruction in grooming and feeding and time for bonding).
2. Riding, with an emphasis on the development of those physical and psychological skills and strengths required to be free and in control of one's horse and oneself.

There are certain essential things in life that most children seem to take for granted, such as running, walking and controlling their bodies with strength. There are those other children who can never seem to do these things from the beginning. Learning to handle a thousand pound animal is perhaps one of the most easily understood lessons in honor and self-esteem. On the back of a horse, nothing is taken for granted. The child has earned the privilege to feel special in a very normal way. Bonding between child and horse has extended itself to the ultimate objective of the program. Charles Appeistein,* who has written on the subject of the usefulness of therapeutic riding for emotionally disturbed children, states: "If a troubled child can develop a special bond with a horse, it becomes easier for that child to generalize such feeling into the human world. Additionally, because other relationships with the horse are so gratifying and fulfilling, the people who work with the horse(s), the instructors, become symbols of the good feeling, the children experience. In psychological terms, the riding staff becomes what are called transitional objects. The riding staff remind the children of something that feels special, and they can talk to and counsel the children. Because of their association with the horses, the riding staff almost immediately get "a foot in the door" with respect to counseling, guiding, and impacting these very troubled and mistrustful children.

Due to numerous factors, including underlying depression, emotionally disturbed children often have a hard time delaying gratification. Such children typically find it difficult to save money, practice an instrument, control sexual impulses, and manage their food intake. They seem to need immediate "payoffs" to help soothe their torment. However, to succeed in life, a troubled child must eventually learn to delay his or her gratification (no pain, no gain). (1990, p2.)*

* The author did not provide references.

Before a child can ride the horse, he or she must first learn how to take care of it. Grooming cleaning and feeding are not always glamorous tasks. But the child learns and internalizes the idea that the gratification in riding comes only in response to the preparation.

Several therapeutic riding manuals point to major concepts and skills learned through therapeutic riding. Children learn basic skills through planned interactional experience with the horse. Some of the major concepts and skills developed during the physical interactional experiences between the child and the horse are:

BODY LOCALIZATION: Child develops the ability to locate and identify parts of the horse's body. This activity aids in developing an awareness and understanding of one's own body.

HEALTH & HYGIENE: Child develops an understanding of the principles of health and hygiene. In caring for the horses, students are led to understand and utilize good habits.

BALANCE & RHYTHM: Child develops the ability to maintain gross and fine motor balance and to move rhythmically with the horse. Child is continuously involved in interpreting and reacting to the horse.

DIRECTIONALITY & LATERALITY: Child develops the ability to know and respond to right, left, up, down, forward, backward, and directional orientation. Activities focusing on directing the horse in a specific direction are used to aid the child in developing sensitivity to directionality of his body and space.

TIME ORIENTATION: Child develops an awareness of determining feeding time, exercise time, and resting time for the horse. Students develop an awareness of the appropriate horseback riding activities due to weather and seasonal change.

ANTICIPATORY RESPONSE: Child develops the ability to anticipate the probable outcome of his or her behavior with the horse. If the child yells or kicks the horse, the child knows the horse will probably become frightened or run. This aids the child in predicting the consequences of his or her own behavior and that of others in a given situation.

COMPREHENSION: Child develops the ability to use judgment and reasoning in riding and working the horse. This enhances his or her ability to use judgment and reasoning when interacting with other forces in his or her environment,

VOCATIONAL BENEFITS: Child develops skills learning barn management and grooming as well as advanced riding. All that provides helpful job training for young people and adults.

PERCEPTUAL & COGNITIVE: Child develops and is stimulated through training in spatial orientation, body image, hand-eye coordination, motor planning and timing, improved attention span, memory and concentration.

PHYSICAL: Child develops physically which influences muscular strength and tone.

Much of what Appelstein has observed with his children in therapeutic riding we have also seen here at Green Chimneys. The bonding that occurs between the children and the horses and staff, gives the them a sense of security from which to take risks and learn. I have observed children who have never experienced a sense of power and control in their lives get onto a 1,000 pound horse and the look on their face tells me this is a life changing experience for them.

Story of "W"

"W" carne to the farm particularly frightened of horses. Over the last two years I worked with "W" on a one to one basis as much as possible during class time. We began by not touching the horse and learning only about equipment needed for riding. I gave him much positive reinforcement as he performed horse related jobs. As "W" gained confidence and saw that the daily comings and goings of the horses were not personally threatening to him, he began to take more risks. For several weeks we had him sit on a horse and from there walk with me leading him. I constantly gave him positive reinforcement as he began to trust me and the gentle movement of his special horse, Pongo. Over the next several months "W" was able to ride on his own as well as learn how to trot and do a posting trot. This was very rewarding for both of us.

Story of "M"

"M", a completely out of control, hyperactive child who seemingly responds well to medication is especially difficult to handle between 4:00 AM - 7:00 AM when the effect of his last dosage is practically nil.

We scheduled "M" for a "learn and earn" job in the horse barn during the early morning chores. At first his behavior continued to be out of control (due to his not having taken his medication as well as the rigid structure of his job routine.) As he learned that there was some flexibility within the structure and a lot of positive reinforcement from his staff worker his behavior improved. It was found that his being able to move around and help with some physical chores relieved him of some of his anxiety and hyperactiveness. He really loves to work with the horses and has developed a wonderful partnership with many of the horses. Today "M" runs to get his medication first thing in the morning and that helps him have another enjoyable work time in the horse barn.

Misty

We had the students create a symbol for alerting others to Misty's blindness, such as a blue ribbon around her tail, or a sign on her stall door. Included in this were questions about how the environment can help us learn to work with our strengths and weaknesses. For example, how does Green Chimneys help you with your strengths and weaknesses?

All of the riding students were involved in the project. When Misty became totally blind, she was returned to her original owners who wanted to create a home for her to live out her days. Her former owners were unaware of her sight problems because Misty was a horse who always went "the extra mile". She was a wonderful horse. The children learned a great deal from her.

James Harris, DMV, states that, "The death of a companion animal provides a unique opportunity for children to practice and prepare for the future losses they will inevitably face throughout life." What Harris speaks of occurs from time to time at Green Chimneys. One of our two farm and wildlife conservation center's treatment coordinators reported in one of the campus bulletins in 1991 "The farm is sad to report the sudden illness of one of our most loved and hard working horses. Squire, a 25 year-old buckskin gelding who has been an integral part of the horseback riding program here since 1986 had a stoke on May 5. Although Squire's stroke was not fatal, he is no longer a safe mount for our program. He will be leaving Green Chimneys by the end of this week." Squire had been ridden almost every weekday by residents. Several students had a particular attachment toward him. Eight students considered Squire their project horse. All of the residents had to be told about Squire's retirement. The residents, it was felt, might have a hard time with his departure. To create such an environment requires a variety of actions, some of which will require little, if any, funds to establish. Answers to any questions or concerns had to be handled by the farm staff.

Eva Phelps
Certified Therapeutic Riding Instructor
Green Chimneys
Brewster, New York

MISTY, A HORSE WITH CHALLENGES

Eva Phelps

Green Chimneys became the owners of an Appaloosa horse, "Misty", who had been diagnosed with cataracts. Misty was blind in her left eye and it was anticipated that she would eventually become totally blind. After several weeks of evaluating Misty's talents and challenges, the staff found her appropriate for the riding program.

The riding instructor and our farm clinical coordinator took her challenges one step further and developed therapeutic activities. These activities included the students' understanding of Misty's special qualities as well as increasing the students' awareness of their own strengths and weaknesses. This project became part of the regular riding hours. Some of the activities included:

1. What is an Appaloosa horse?
2. How do we use our senses?
3. Relationships
4. Maximizing our strengths
5. The process of change
6. Saying "good-bye".

Our main objective was to involve the students in sharing Misty's current challenge regarding her blindness. This naturally included discussions with the children for better understanding of their own personal challenges. The interns at the farm were asked to attend these classes as a learning activity. Part of their participation was to document the session with a GLAS (Green Chimneys' Longitudinal Assessment Score), as well as to include any anecdotal information that was pertinent.

An example of the form that was used is included here.

MISTY THE HORSE   Student's Name:
Lower barn Project   Class and Time:
Scores For Documentation   Date:

1. Staying with the group
2. Attention to task
3. Interest in activity
4. Able to contribute to discussion
5. Examples of discussion

OTHER:

A brief outline of the proposed activities are as follows:

Activity I. General Overview of Misty's History
    A. A description of the Appaloosa breed

Activity II How Do We Use Our Senses?
    A. Since Misty cannot use both her eyes to see, what does she use to move about her world and have her needs met?

    B. If one of our senses can not be used, how would we negotiate our world?
        1. Staff and students together. We take turns blindfolding students' left eyes.
            a. Walk in stall
            b. Walk in pasture
            c. Walk over a puddle
            d. Walk to stall to find food

Questions to ask:
1. Which of your other senses did you use to help you find things?
2. How does a horse see?
3. What do you notice Misty does to help her see?
4. What are cataracts?

We planned and carried out similar exercises, games, with the children for each of the five senses.

The following questions were used to create discussions with the students:

Activity III. Relationships
What is a relationship? Who has them? Do animals have relationships? How do animals and people show they have a relationship? Does Misty have a relationship with us? With other horses? What is it about her behavior that tells us this? What do we need to have a good relationship (trust)? How does Misty show trust? How do we show trust?

Activity IV. Maximizing Our Strengths
We all have strengths and weaknesses. What are yours? How do we know we have strengths and weaknesses? Can weaknesses become resolved? Which ones can not? What conditions are necessary to maximize a strength? How does Green Chimneys help you? What does Misty need to maximize her strengths?

Activity V. The Process of Change
The process of change is the process of life. We all change.
Questions: What do you notice about changes in you? How will being blind affect changes Misty will go through? Are there little changes and big changes? What are some examples?

Activity VI: Saying "Good-bye"

Misty may have to be put down if she is unable to interact with her world in a safe way despite assistance from staff and students. How do we say good-bye to someone we care about? What feelings do we have about this experience? A good-bye ceremony in case of her death that encompasses hope and sadness. Ceremony was planned by students and staff.

Eva Phelps
Certified Therapeutic Riding Instructor
Green Chimneys
Brewster, New York

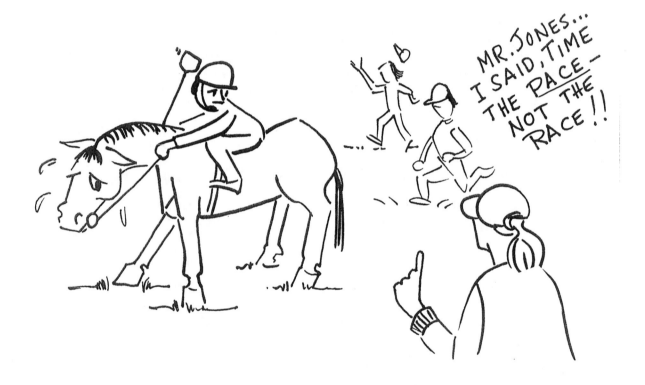

SPIRITUAL PSYCHOLOGY: AN APPROACH TO THERAPEUTIC RIDING

Barbara Kathleen Rector, MA

Sierra Tucson Adolescent Care is a private psychiatric hospital for severely emotionally disturbed adolescents who have substance, chemical or behavioral abuse problems. The treatment philosophy is of a traditional Western (cultural) medical model interfaced with emerging experiential therapeutic modalities, including wilderness experience, riding therapy, 18 foot wall climbing, ropes course, dance and the arts, all of which are oriented within the Twelve Steps of Recovery Framework.

Sierra Tucson's Integrated Riding Resource Program's (STIRRUP) purpose is to elevate the troubled adolescent's self-esteem through the therapeutic use of the horse and the horse experience. Carefully structured sessions provide safe nurturing opportunities to elicit an expanded awareness, develop multi-sensory integration and contribute to an increased capacity for individuation. Healthy, conscious choice-making is practiced and mastered. Relationship and skills are developed. Communication, interpersonal and intimacy skills are crafted and practiced.

The horse experience includes mounted skill lessons, TT.E.A.M work, basic stable management skills, farrier and minor veterinarian techniques in a comprehensive curriculum of cognitive learning and hands-on practicums. Riding activities develop self-awareness, build confidence, cultivate concentrations, and self-discipline. Posture, balance, coordination, strength and flexibility are improved. Riding is especially valuable for people who have impaired mobility and/or limited awareness of being "in their body." Exercising the spirit is as important as exercising the body. The horse provide a unique vehicle for both of these essentials. The horse opens previously closed doors for people with physical, mental and emotional disabilities.

EQUINE FACILITATED PSYCHOTHERAPY, A TWELVE STEP APPROACH

1. We admitted we were powerless over (alcohol, drugs, physical or emotional abuse)--that our lives had become unmanageable.
2. We came to believe that a Power greater than ourselves could restore us to sanity.
3. We made a decision to turn our will and our lives over to the care of God as we understood Him.
4. We made a search and fearless moral inventory of ourselves.
5. We admitted to God, to ourselves, and to another human being, the exact nature of our wrong doings.
6. We were entirely ready to have God remove all these defects of our character.
7. We humbly asked him to remove our shortcomings.
8. We made a list of all persons we had harmed, and became willing to make amends to them all.
9. We made direct amends to such people whenever possible, except when to do so would injure them or others.
10. We continued to take personal inventory and when we were wrong, promptly admitted it.

11.   We sought through prayer and meditation to improve our conscious contact with God as we understood Him, praying only for knowledge of His will for us and the power to carry that out.

12.   Having had a spiritual awakening as the result of these steps, we try to carry the message to persons who are (alcoholics, have drug, physical or emotional abuse problems), and each individual practice these principles in all our affairs.

Equine Facilitated Psychotherapy is an experiential treatment method utilizing horses to assist with access to the psyche's inner processes. The experience of the horse and the relational dynamics of human to horse brings forth to conscious awareness certain habitual patterns of thought within the client that serve to shape his experience of reality. A specific conceptual framework, a template (map) of a person's way of being in the world of matter, substance, and form, emerges in the close observation of the developing relationship between client and horse.

It is the nature of the horse's association with man to always be in the process of "being trained." Every interaction, each facet and nuance of communication between horse and human is a continuous learning and teaching situation. These human-animal (horse) interactions serve as conscious practice for developing personal choices about feelings and behavior that enhance the quality of life, in the stable as well as in the external world's ordinary experiences. The recovery process evokes conscious awareness of the rules by which one lives one's life. Working a Twelve Step Program makes possible an objective assessment of how helpful such behavior and thought patterns are to the creation of quality - life experience in the here and now.

Therapeutic riding instructors use the process of learning to ride as a tool for developing intimate relationship skills. They teach the art of joining with the horse in a partnership of communication to develop mutual rhythm, harmony, balance, and alignment: all helpful attitudes and postures for the process of living in "real" life. Therapeutic riding instructors teach these skills on all levels: mental, physical, emotional, and spiritual.

In the STIRRUP program, the most valuable aids are the focused mind filled with purposeful intent aligned with the big-hearted energy of desire and a "want to" attitude. Students are taught the skills of being fully present "in their own bodies" while attuning their energies to those of their horse. Beginning mounted work is done on the longe line with the horse wearing side-reins. The student becomes accustomed to accommodating his or her body to the horse's movements. Once independent, each student practices simple school figures on the circle, turn through the circle, transitions through walk, trot, and canter in a 60 foot longe pen. The experience of the horse's movement produces relaxation of tense rigid muscles. New sensory input is absorbed throughout the entire physiological system. The significant relationship of personal body language and the focused mind to the horse's response produced with the application of subtle classical "aids" is reinforced continuously through successful practice on a well-schooled therapy horse.

Mounted work is done on the longe with the instructor demonstrating the lesson skills to be "mastered." A "seasoned" client begins to practice these skills and when he feels confident and ready, he becomes the "teacher-coach" for the next client. The last client "teaches" the primary counselor or counselor aide. Generally there is time in the lesson for several "rounds" of teacher-student coaching; an ideal ratio is three clients and a counselor, with instructor and therapy horse. The process of experiencing the role of both student and teacher is a powerful anchoring technique for newly acquired information and skills.

Basic aids for the mounted work are framed within the Twelve Step Program language and tied to the concepts of the recovery process. Graduation to independent mounted work first in the longe pen and then the riding arena is generally dependent on the client's ability to align his or her mind and his or her body for the short duration of the practice work. Twenty minutes is about maximum time that these clients can work in this intensive energy processing environment. The STIRRUP program works weekly with the primary group therapy members (6 clients), their primary counselor, and their counselor aide. Initially these people are divided into two groups to learn basic barn safety, elementary grooming, tacking skills, and to attend a basic equine psychology lecture.

The **STIRRUP program barn** contains within its equine personalities the labeled dysfunctional family components of "identified client," co-dependent, acting-out scapegoat, hero/achiever, lost child and various combinations thereof. Clients are invited to walk through the barn and pick out the horse they notice most: the one horse that seems to call to them with its particular energy, appearance and behavioral characteristics. Invariably the client chooses a horse that represents to them their own role in the dysfunctional family. Over the course of treatment as the client reaches some insight and acceptance of self, his or her preference in horses shifts to reflect a particular treatment issue that has emerged in the course of the process.

One phase used to describe survival skill of disassociation, a defense mechanism first described by Freud to explain the process whereby a portion of the mind "travels" elsewhere while the body continues to function on "auto pilot." An example is while driving your car over a much traveled and familiar route, you suddenly snap to awareness that you're further along than you realized. Where were "you" or a portion of your mind while your body continued driving the car. The **ego** part of `you' had disassociated, i.e., a portion of your conscious mind split off in a daydream or fantasy trip from full conscious presence in the body.

Story of Elliott
One of the STIRRUP program horses, T.S. Elliott, has volunteered to serve as the challenging, acting-out, and behaviorally difficult adolescent of the barn herd. All barns include, within their equine group, exact duplicates of the human family constellation prevalent in local collective consciousness. So, our barn contains the labeled dysfunctional family components of "identified client," co-dependent, acting-out scapegoat, hero/achiever, lost child, and various combinations thereof. Elliott makes it difficult for you to like him. He pins his ears and bares his teeth when you enter his stall. He is mouthy and "lippy" as you halter him. If tied too loose for grooming, he will continually dive his nose to the butt of the person cleaning his hooves. Why is Elliott even in our program barn, you may ask. Why? He represents that scapegoat, acting-out, "bad" child within us all. He craves love. His life experience has taught him a distorted way of asking for and giving love, recognition, and attention. Our task in the barn for both clients and staff is to model for Elliott more healthy, helpful forms of asking for and receiving attention, recognition, and love.

The adolescent clients have designed a remedial treatment/training plan for Elliott. The plan mandates lots of "positive" response for appropriate behavior no matter how small - seeming or insignificant. Elliott is worked in the round pen with the John Lyons body language longe techniques. No equipment other than the handler (client) in the center holding a longe whip is used. The clients learn the significance of body language, personal boundaries (personal body space), and the power of the focused, attentive mind. Elliott is given lots of verbal praise.

In mounted work, Elliott is challenged by his riders to fit in and conform to the discipline of arena exercises. All are careful to ask Elliott to produce an effort he is capable of, while gently stretching his capacity for disciplined work. The other day, a significant gain was achieved when, without benefit of a lead rider, Elliott and a client produced a straight walk of regular cadence and harmony over the ground pole. Elliott was praised for his efforts. The client's warded him by dismounting, running up the stirrups, and loosening his girth.

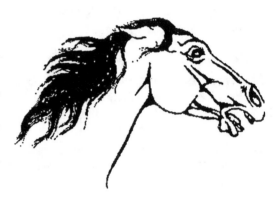

Clients have more than once been heard saying in the barn, "Elliott makes it hard to like him. He is like us. He needs treatment." Yes, and he is capable of change. He is capable of being remediated. And if for some reason he were experienced as an active danger to himself or others, he would, like the clients, be isolated and given a time-out until he stabilized. Then, he would be reassessed and evaluated for either re-admission to the STIRRUP Program or for a transfer to a more appropriate living situation to best meet his needs for optimum functioning in the life experience.

Story of Shasta: A spiritual Archetype

The STIRRUP program barn also contains, within its herd members, representatives for the various archetypical aspects of psyche. Carl Gustau Jung characterized psyche as an organizing locus for the myth-creating level of mind he called the collective unconscious. The collective unconscious is an unlimited reservoir of latent primordial images linking all humanity.

These innate behavior patterns are what Jung termed archetypes: an original model, a prototype of a behavioral matrix. Jung said, "Just as instincts compel man to conduct a life that is specifically human, so the archetypes compel intuition and apprehension to form specifically human patterns." The archetype image represents to consciousness an innate predisposition for responding to typical human situations or being in human relationships. Some major archetype images described by Jung are Persona, Shadow, Anima, Animus, Wise Old Man, Great Mother, Miraculous Child, Hero/Savior, and Self (these are represented among our herd).

The other day, in a budget discussion, a corporate executive invited me to justify "that little hay-burning pony." He was referring to Shasta, our aged (28 years) palomino Shetland pony who only occasionally pulls a jogging cart.

Currently, Shasta resembles the classic chubby "Thewell" pony wearing her blonde fluffy winter coat, body clipped with a large heart emblazoned on her rump and the shaggy, shaggy leggings of a mini-Clydesdale. She came to the STIRRUP program suffering from not being used or feeling useful in her work. Our clients created an individual treatment plan for her remediation which includes much love and appreciation. Love is demonstrated through frequent grooming, long slow walks on a leadline and cross country long reining practice. Most important of all (for Shasta, clients and staff) she is given complete freedom in the barn and stable yard.

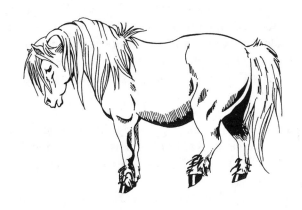

Complete freedom? Yes! She is allowed to mosey about, or run, or buck, or zip in and out of wherever she pleases. She has, however, one "off limits" activity. Apparently, there is always an "off limits" in every life. Shasta's is the <u>field of dreams</u>: the lush, green, irrigated playing field used by the recreational therapy department for its multi-purpose outdoor games. It is located just adjacent to our STIRRUP program barn area. On rare occasions, usually when that same executive is about, Shasta forgets herself. She will wander over to the tempting lushness of the green, green field. The field has a very expensive underground irrigation system that is not designed to tolerate pony prints.

A fairly sharp shout in her direction from the barn staff or an alert client sends her zipping back to the stable yard at a rapid clip. Shasta is most frequently seen on a lead line between an adolescent client and primary counselor who are "walking her out" as part of her remedial conditioning program. Some valuable one-on-one psychotherapy is also occurring as client and counselor join efforts in helping Shasta with her rehabilitation regimen. There is also the added element of mutual support as the trio is astonished by the therapeutic instructor to take no "guff" from the maintenance and grounds personnel who are fond of providing jesting remarks centered around the theme of "walking that funny dog."

Archetypically, Shasta represents that precious perfect core element of us all. She is. She is love energy. You feel, see, sense, and know love with Shasta. She represents that core aspect of our inner self that needs no justification for being. Being is enough. She is precious. She is perfect.

Spiritually, Shasta anchors for us our inner knowing of ourselves as essential elements, integral to humanity's function. Our being is enough. No justification is needed. No activity or achievement is required. Our essential energy is vital and important to the functioning totality of our collective experience. We are enough. And Shasta's very presence reminds us of this truth. She represents the healing in our shame. She is perfect just the way she is. Core energy. Love.

Post Session Processing
A recent post session processing group revealed some significant connections and insights gained by the clients during a typical primary group experience. A young fourteen year old girl severely depresses with active suicide ideation accessed some deeply buried rage in her frustrated attempts to use one rein in each hand. (She was only comfortable with neck reining.) Her deeply felt shame at not being able to achieve success while trying something new was blocking her ability to even function. Staff urged her to use this frustration energy to make clear to the horse her wishes (to have the horse stay on the rail of the 60 feet round pen and not cut into the middle of the circle). She became more and more awkward and disjointed as her frustration level elevated. Finally, in tears she stopped and heaved out.

"I can't do this. I'm no good. I can't do anything right. I'm worthless. I give up." "And isn't that exactly your attitude facing life?" suggests staff gently. "What? Well, yes I guess it is." Her tears are flowing openly. "And that's why you're here in our hospital; to acquire tools for changing your attitude."

As the tears stopped, she was willing to take several deep breaths and to listen intently to the instructor/therapist who coached her in precisely how to take her horse back out to the rail, one rein in each hand with a focused, intentional mind. She told her inner critic out loud to "take a break" while she suspended all judgement about her feelings of awkwardness and allowed her body-mind to follow the coaching directions. Shortly, the client and her horse achieved unity and a semblance of harmony with walk-trot transitions. Eventually, a lovely sitting trot was produced by the team (the client, horse, and therapeutic instructor also functioning as therapist).

Post session processing ties together the awkward frustration feelings of those new to recovery and the use of the Twelve Steps as healing tools for improving the quality of one's daily experience of life. It begins by letting go of "control" and admitting to needing help.

The group closes by standing to form a circle, arms linked about waists and repeating out loud the Serenity Prayer--

"God, grant me serenity
to accept the things I cannot change,
the courage to change the things I can,
and the wisdom to know the difference."

Reference
O'Connor, P. (1985). *Understanding Jung, Understanding Yourself.* New York: Paulist Press.
Frager, R., Fadiman, J. (1984). *Personality and Personal Growth.* New York: Harper and Row.
Alcoholics Anonymous. (1976). Alcoholics Anonymous Word Services, Inc. New York, N.Y.
Zlukau, G. (1990). *The Seat of the Soul.* Simon and Schuster, Inc.

EXPERIENCE OF SOCIAL INTEGRATION
A Residential and Educational Farm Service

Miquel Gallardo

INTRODUCTION

Sac Xirio is a residential center that provides educational services in the rural farm setting in the hills above Barcelona, Spain. The farm provides a neutering environment that allows for caring and bonding between human and animals. Sac means welcome and it is open to those who have difficult needs. Xiroi means that which is happy and pleasing. The two together signifie the unique experience of the center.

Sac Xiroi is a nonprofit, accredited institution classified as a residential center for educational services. It is established on the following principals:

1. It is a residential center for eighteen boys and girls from four to eighteen years old that provides a nurturing environment. Children with physical, social, psychological, and educational problems are provided both material security and moral support.
2. The residential center serves the student's needs by providing essential education, strengthening their emotional and physical health, and fostering each student's personal development.
3. The philosophy is based on socially accepted rehabilitation concepts and aspects of the program are modeled after Green Chimney of New York.
4. The dimensions of Sac Xiroi allow the center to reproduce the ordinary living conditions of a big family because of the small numbers of residents and a large staff. This allows the staff to focus on the major goals for each student in a causal way.
5. Sac Xirio is a totally open center integrated with its environment and its community of el Barri de les Cases Noves de la Riera, a Castellvi de Ia Marca corporation. It participates in community activities, especially with the annual program with the Educational Farms Association of France.
6. Students from France intern at the center that helps provide staff and provides the residents with young and enthusiastic leadership who can devote individual time to students.

The Sac Xiroi teaching farm is coordinated by a team of professionals that include social workers, family therapists, and educators. This group lives at the center. The professional team is responsible for adapting the educational, family, and social setting to change the residents' behavior for reintegration back into society. Most residents are referred to the center through the justice system or through child welfare departments. This close knit professional group provides the necessary training that allows for rehabilitation and changes in the residents' social and emotional values.

The institution has achieved a 40% success rate with its residents in both the social and educational areas. This has been due to the talents and devotion of the young staff of educators. Credit for success must also be given to the therapeutic use of the horse: Riding Therapy. Equestrian therapy is a method used in France, Denmark and other European countries since 1965. In New York, Green Chimneys has used therapeutic riding since 1945 with seriously emotionally involved children. Green Chimneys is also a farm intervention program.

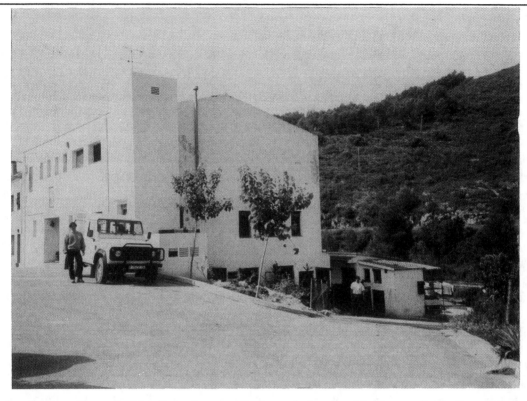

Equestrian therapy allows the blending of responsibility and pleasure. The horse allows the residents to bond and develop a rich emotional attachment. This helps them establish values before which they may never have developed.

Pets can help children and teenagers with social - emotional problems and can give educational support to extremely shy children. With Jose we will give an example that illustrates how our center might work.

Jose states "I was in a very bad situation. I was lost, I mean as if I were in a gully ready to drop into it. I was in a shelter of scum speaking like that. They sent me here...I had been in other schools but not in any like this one. The treatment is different. Here we see the animals, mainly horses......... I've cried with this horse next to me often. I've cried at the problems and all this, the girlfriend....I get angry and the horse doesn't listen to me but I know he'll be with me...with his ears and staring at me and then he'll push me. I've cried many times riding him, feeding him, or telling him things. He's the best friend. The dog and the horse are the best we can have on this planet."

Jose is a twelve-year-old who was motivated to learn to read and count with the help of a horse. The horse has also helped Jose develop personal and social skills to allow him to participate as a member of our small "family" and develop social skills that he will need to integrate into society out side of our center. He had a special attachment to "Hurricane" one of our horses. After five years, Hurricane's hair has become whiter and the relationship between the boy and the horse have become very strong.

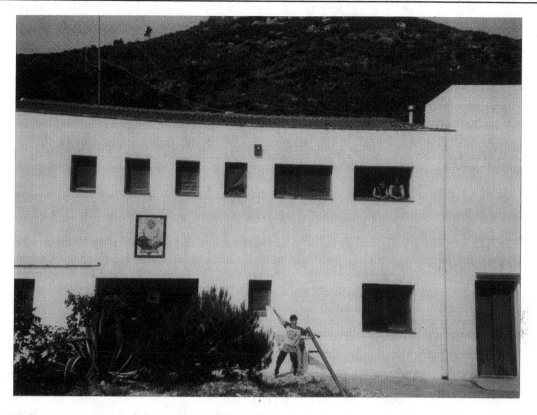

Jose will tell you that if you are nervous or anything like that and are with an animal, stroke it and the animal will push you away. When you are with the animal and forget everything - that you have a child or are married - what ever you are - you play with the animal and the animal responds to you.

When a child comes to our center, he or she may think that if these people take good care of animals they will also take good care of me. The children are told that they can also take care of the animals. The child may think "I am not as bad as people say I am if they let me take care of their animals." A boy who can control a horse thinks he can control himself. When he rides a horse, the difficulty of riding becomes the difficulty of life. He learns to ride and he learns to overcome the difficulties of life. If the boy can control the horse on a narrow path or way down a steep hill, it is like the paths of life that the boy must face. Gradually, the boy builds the confidence with the horse and with himself.

Last year Jose took a train from Vilafrance to l'Hospitalet every morning. He has finished the course for being a stable boy in the Agrarian and Equestrian training school. He has the School Certificate and now he wants to get the primary education qualification and his driver's license. Jose looks forward to a profession with a future related to the equestrian world that he discovered in Sac Xiroi.

"I would really like to work as a blacksmith, not as a stableboy. You are not working ten, fifteen, twenty hours in the same place. As blacksmith you can shoe in stables from Tarragona, BGN, Vilafranca, Sant Sadurni, and

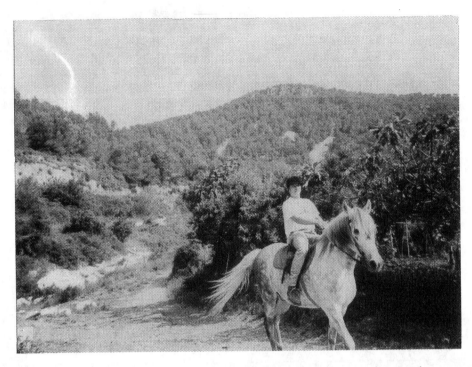

all the villages. You can come and go, and you are never shut up in the same place at the same time. You've got your phone, your car, somebody phones you and says "I need to shoe 6 horses" and you say "OK I'll come at midday"' and you go, then somebody else phones you and you say "OK I'll come tomorrow.." and you know you aren't forced to, you are your own boss and you don't take order from any body.

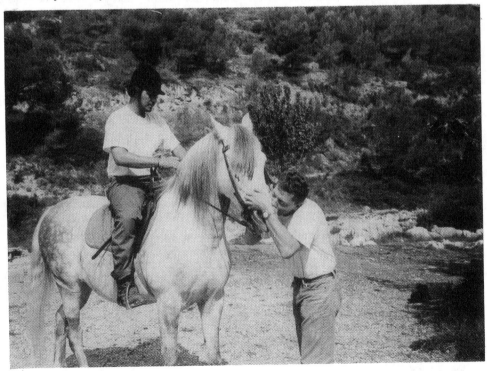

After doing the course for stable boy, Jose has gotten his first job in the school, a contract of employment for two months taking care of some horses that were confiscated. He was the stable boy and with this experience he hopes to be able to take the course to become a blacksmith. He has learned to control horses and to control himself.

It is difficult for these young people once they are out of the center. It is already difficult for any of us. We try to lengthen the umbilical cord as much as possible and cut it just when is absolutely necessary. For example, now we have opened a subsidized flat for Jose and all the others that gradually are going to leave our center. As things stand we really do not say goodbye to our sons and daughters just because they are eighteen. Just as with our real children we want them to fly, the higher the better but we never say good bye. Sac Xiroi is a very special large family. Trini, Miquel and his two sons are all educators and live with the children taken in. The doors are open. Sac Xiroi is a house in Penedès villiage, Castellvi de la Marca and it is at the same time a farm, allowing contact with the country and to be in contact with nature.

MiquelGallardo
Sac Xiroi
Castellvi de la Marca
Alt Penedes Barcelona
Spain

COMBINING CENTERED RIDING AND JUNGIAN THEORY TECHNIQUES IN PSYCHOTHERAPY

Anne P. Cole, M..S.,C.S.,R.N.

In this paper I will describe how I use *Centered Riding* techniques and horse symbolism in traditional psychotherapy and in horse-oriented psychotherapy, using clinical examples with details altered in order to protect client confidentiality. I will use myself as an example of how my own blend of Jungian theory, practice, and centered riding technique and theory helped me to come into my own energy, spirit, and power. I had not accomplished this in psychotherapy and analysis augmented by sonic bodywork.

I have worked in psychiatric nursing for twenty-two years, and as a psychotherapist for fifteen years. I first started riding when I was four but had no lessons of any kind until I was in my thirties. My initial riding lessons were taught by a woman who knew some *Centered Riding* techniques, and by 1987, I had come to use those techniques (though not horseback riding) in my psychotherapeutic practice. I had read Sally Swift's book, *Centered Riding,* and watched her videotapes. Horseback riding played an integral part in my own psychological process, and I began to think that it could have a beneficial effect for certain clients. In private practice I ran an outpatient program for adolescents at West Pines Hospital in Denver, Colorado, and wanted very much to share ideas from *Centered Riding* for psychotherapeutic purposes. I became certified as a centered riding instructor. I looked into and was inspired by a program run by Phil Tedeschi at an adolescent residential treatment center in Larkspur, Colorado. I was introduced to a program developed by Barbara Rector at Sierra Tucson in Arizona. I first taught a clinic on horse-oriented psychotherapy in 1992 at West Pines. I also developed a slide-illustrated lecture on horse symbolism and mythology that I began to integrate into my centered riding work. Since then I have taught centered riding techniques.

I used these techniques more for the sake of helping people with horseback riding than primarily for psychotherapeutic purposes. This was largely due to the cost and liability prohibitions in the public sector agencies where I have been working with HIV/AIDS patients for the last five years. However, the centering riding techniques and horse symbolism I have taught people have never failed to help them psychologically and with their riding skills and confidence. Even people who do not think about or have any interests in psychological processes invariably feel better and are more relaxed after learning *Centered Riding* techniques.

I grew up in a traditional Southern family in Texas in which women were assumed to be inferior to men in every way except mothering and nurturing and occasionally beauty (a category I did not fall into). Men were all-powerful. This idea was endorsed not only by family and society but also by religion with the idea of a patriarchal God . This was long before women's liberation found Texas. Unfortunately, my mother bought into these assumptions about women, heart and soul. It was only in my late teenage years that I discovered the underground and mostly unconscious phenomenon of the southern woman as an "iron butterfly". My grandmother embodied this so perfectly that I realized only in adulthood that in many ways she ran everything in the family, rather than my grandfather who was the grand patriarch. I probably would have been totally lost, as my mother was, if it had not been for the nurturing by the iron butterflies in my family. My father was more able to see me and love me as I was beneath the cultural dictates. Unfortunately, he was not around much when I was little. He had problems with depression that were never dealt with which made him only intermittently available to me.

As a teenager I aspired to be as unlike my mother as possible, but of course the mold had set long before; I had no confidence in myself and especially not in love relationships with men. I was totally helpless. Fortunately, I had never been physically or sexually abused, so that was not a problem I ever got into with men, despite being a prime target for letting me be controlled in other ways. Nevertheless, I also had a contrary, independent streak that made me the black sheep of the family and totally unsuited to the kind of marriage relationship and family life I was brought up to enter into. At the age of eighteen, I escaped into the budding world of women's liberation, hippy life, and academic pursuits, for none of which I had the slightest preparation. I eventually came apart at the seams and at that point began the long ongoing journey into reclaiming and growing into myself. I spent years in therapy and Jungian analysis trying to get back what had been suppressed or repressed. I gained insight during these years: that I projected all my strength and power onto men and then could be in touch with these attributes only by trying to be in relationship with a man. Despite periodic deep depressions and chronic Dysthymia, I got several degrees including a master's degree in psychiatric nursing, worked and supported myself financially, and eventually entered the Jung Institute of New York. I had already been in Jungian analysis for a number of years with Gertrud Ujhely who was not only an analyst but also a nurse and one of my first female mentors and role models. She helped me develop a strong yet porous observing ego, but still I did not have significant access to or connection to my basic life energy; it, rather, came and went as it pleased and sometimes ran away with me and got me into all kinds of trouble.

In Jungian training we learned about various mythological systems. Jung theorized that was what he called the collective unconscious, as opposed to the personal unconscious that Dr. Freud believed that the personal unconscious was the only unconscious; a receptacle for repressed, suppressed, and forgotten previously conscious material. The collective unconscious, Jung postulated, was a deeper part of the unconscious. It was shared in common by all and was in fact the psychic and physical bedrock and groundwater for all humanity and perhaps even for animals and everything in this world. Humans were blessed (and cursed) with a partial ability to access this deeper life energy level mentally through archetypal images that Jung thought to be reflections of this basic instinctual energy. Through symbolization, we try to understand our physical and psychic world, which Jung said at heart is one. Mythologies, whether modern or primitive, are attempts to explain our experience of the totality of the world, including ourselves, as perceived by our senses and our psychic faculties. The collective unconscious is inherent in all of us and is fed by universal energies into our genes, into the soul. At its most basic levels, it funds instincts with information. I remember once a friend asked me to come to get a rubber snake out of her children's room. She was quite embarrassed that she was afraid to pick up a rubber snake and could give no reason for this fear. However, she wanted this snake out of her house so I took it home with me, thinking my cats would like to play with it. I was a city dweller then, and my cats had never even been outdoors, much less crossed paths with a snake. This rubber snake was quite realistic looking. The cats loved to chase things around, pounce and bite toy mice, etc., but they, much to my surprise, were absolutely terrified of this snake and would not go anywhere near it.

Because the collective unconscious is common to all of us, similar images and motifs occur throughout the various mythologies, even when various cultures could have had no direct or indirect contact. Yet the way the motifs manifest themselves and the meanings that collect around them may vary somewhat from one ethnic or cultural energy field to another. The importance, meaning, and occurrence of certain images may even be inherited and carried by people into cultures other than their own. I had a patient who began having vivid dreams of an underground kingdom filled with strange symbolic drawings and objects that she could not identity but which felt familiar, even intimately connected to her. She had been brought up by Protestant parents with Anglo-Saxon names, but after several months of dreaming of this strange kingdom, her father revealed to her that he had been told by his parents that they were actually both Jewish. We were then able to identify her secret kingdom as filled with Jewish symbolic images. She instantly felt more grounded upon hearing this information, and the unidentified existential anxiety that had been with her all her life gradually ebbed away as she explored her Jewish roots.

One of the mythologies that we studied at the Jung Institute was Celtic mythology. I am mostly Irish but had never thought much about this until then. I was most intrigued with the Irish regional goddesses who were the opposites of the female ideal with which I had grown up; they were powerful, lusty, outspoken, and independent, and they all had horse attributes--they could run as fast as horses, could shape shafts into horses. All my life I had unconsciously connected horses with the masculine. My father was in the cavalry when I was conceived and born, played polo, and learned military dressage before the army got rid of its horses at the end of World War II. I associated horses with my father and my grandfather who always had a horse and first put me on one when I was four years old. The horses I rode as a child were as poorly trained as I was; I spent my childhood being bucked off and run away with. I was terrified by them and fascinated at the same time. It was not until analysis and studying Celtic mythology that I realized I associated horses with masculine power and even more unconsciously with my mother's repressed and, therefore crazy and unrecognized power. I began having horse dreams night after night. I began to study horse mythology and symbolism. At that point I went to Ireland for the first time, rode horses there, and began to take riding lessons. I realized that in order to ride without being terrified I would have to take back my projections of my own power and energy abandoned and run amok. The horses, I discovered, were more than happy to have me take all that back; it terrified them as much as me. I had to develop a partnership with each horse and its energy. To do that I had to develop a partnership with my own powerful energy. This caused me to reclaim it as my own, a scarier process than one might think. I was assisted in this by two Jungian analysts: Sylvia Perera, who introduced me to Celtic mythology and gave me another role model for the feminine, and Dan Young, whose steady presence and courage allowed me to withdraw my projections from the masculine (and descend into the black hole where my life energy had hidden) in order to reclaim that energy and bring it home with me. I was assisted and continue to be assisted by every horse I ride, and especially by Bonnie, my own horse for the past eight years. And by my clients, who face similar dilemmas.

Before Ireland and getting back into horseback riding, I had a lot of insight and a lot of intellectual understanding of how I became the way I was psychologically, and I could use that understanding to help in overcoming certain kinds of fears and difficulties. Nevertheless, my body still carried all the old stuff. I often felt weak and fragile physically. I walked around with my shoulders up around my ears, trying to use my shoulders to hold myself up. I felt spineless; I tired easily and got sick often. I inherited a predisposition for ankylosing spondylitis from my mother and grandfather and had terrible problems with my lower spine and sacroiliac joints. While I was at the Institute, I did some body work with an Alexander Technique teacher and learned I could still stand up even if I did not "scrunch" up my shoulders. In my hippie days I had learned Transcendental Meditation and, with it, the necessity for breathing as a way of relaxing and settling in. Then I took up yoga. Yoga gave me a sense of my relationship to gravity and an ability to meditate through movement. Nevertheless, I still did not have much sense of my own life energy on a cellular or spiritual level. Certainly I had no sense of it as something I could be in relationship with, much less rely upon. I could feel it in my sexual relationships with men, sometimes in meditation and yoga, when doing creative intellectual work, and always when working psychologically with others. Nevertheless, it was not anything that I could rely on in my own everyday physical life or in my psychological work on myself. Because of all the bareback riding I did as a child, I had something that an Irishman calls natural balance. Another Irishman, Willie Leahy, told me one day when I had first started riding again, "Well, ye don't know how to ride, but you're sure sticky!". That was a great mystery to me at the time and not anything I could count on until I learned effective methods from *Centered Riding*. Through the bodywork that is an initial part of learning the centered riding technique, and through the riding exercises, I found tension in my legs that I had never realized existed, and I was able (with much conscious work) to let go of that tension. I began to experience the energy of the horse I was riding without panicking, as well as experiencing my own energy. I learned use my own centering to help the horse relax, collect, and center himself.

When I started riding again using centered riding techniques, the horse became the metaphor for my own repressed, split off, and therefore wild, undomesticated energy. Bit by bit I withdrew the projections and learned to create a partnership with the horse. It was not a matter of control--nobody ever wins power struggles--it was a matter of convincing the horse to do what I wanted it to do, that it would be safe, not painful, and maybe fun. Through centering, I could stay with all that collective energy and quickly help the horse and myself re-center when faced with snow avalanches off the roof of the riding arena or horse-eating rocks on the trail, or soul-boggling encounters with my own demons. *Centered Riding* teaches the rider to be centered and relaxed in order to be more in touch with one's own experience and also with that of the horse. It teaches centeredness and therefore, balance as the key to riding the horse, rather than holding on and trying to control by force that invariably engenders panic and loss of centeredness in both the horse and the rider. Sally Swift's basics--soft eyes, breathing, centering, and balancing (or working with gravity)--break down the components of centering into manageable exercises. Her translation of half halts as "center and grow" brings together the components of centering into a momentary experience that cannot be held , but that which can be recreated again and again in the process of riding--and living. The emphasis in *Centered Riding* is on the rider, with the understanding that if the rider is centered, then the horse can also be centered and collected. If the rider is unfocused, unaware of his or her own body, mind, and spirit, it matters little how experienced and knowledgable the rider is. The horse is, by nature tuned, into the rider's physical, emotional, and spiritual state and will respond to that more strongly than to what the rider is consciously asking the horse to do. If the rider can sit in a balanced way and use seat, hands, and legs in a way that gives clear directions and does not interfere with the horse's movement, the rider has a much better chance of getting the horse to do what is asked. This can be accomplished only with a rider who can re-center and re-focus, again and again.

Through learning to center on horseback (my metaphor for my coming into relationship to the energy of the earth and my own body), I began to be able to center in every aspect of my life, even in the presence of patriarchal systems. I found myself using centered riding techniques in my psychotherapy practice. One day a young man with tremendous manic energy, at that moment totally given over to an erotic transference toward me, seemed to be taking over my own psychic space, sending my own energy into panic/flight mode. I found myself literally retreating, moving my chair back, which caused him to take over more space in panic that I was abandoning him. I found myself centering and growing, centering and growing which had an incredible calming effect on this young man without my ever having said a word. He was eventually able to modulate his own energy and to sense how it affected others. It was my own experience and awareness in those seminal moments that allowed this to happen quickly rather than taking months of analysis. I now teach Sally Swift's four basics of centering to psychotherapy clients who never go near a horse. I have found that the basics help them deal more effectively in the moment with problems, anger, loss of perspective, fear, tendencies to be or to feel victimized. They are more effective than pure meditation techniques, because they are intended to be used while in relation to another living being in order to be more engaged and in touch.

I also discovered in learning and teaching centered riding methods that the release of this energy when it has been long blocked and split off can be terrifying and traumatic. The first time I did bodywork on someone, the person wound up with a splitting headache, and there are frequent occurrences of people feeling dizzy or faint during or after bodywork. We all unconsciously hold tension in various parts of our bodies which blocks energy flow, and when those long-blocked energies are released, they can cause people to feel dizzy and even off-center, until the energy stabilizes. My centered riding certification instructors, Sally Haney and Susan Harris, taught us how to deal with these occurrences in ways that resolve the physical manifestations without being intrusive psychologically. And, I still use these techniques even when using riding for psychotherapy if the person is not yet ready to deal with that energy directly. Sometimes the person is able to feel and then look at and trace that energy block to past adaptations or trauma, which helps the person to be able to work on freeing up that energy for conscious use, as I had. I cannot stress enough the delicate nature of this work and the necessity of profound sensitivity and skill from the therapist in helping the person deal with the release of blocked energy in a way that does not cause trauma to reoccur. That energy was hidden away for good reasons. Its re-emergence is a moment of rebirth that can be joyfully rejuvenating or horribly traumatic, depending on the timing of its reappearance and how it is handled. I have had my greatest successes, but also made my greatest mistakes, in using this bodywork for teaching riding and for psychotherapy. With people who have been physically abused and often with children and adolescents, I do bodywork through imaging rather than a hands on technique. Even imaging can stimulate flashbacks to trauma. Working on ego strength must be done before bodywork of any kind in psychotherapy so that the person can manage the sometimes overwhelming energies and images that arise from dissolving energy blockages in the body. And even for those who are ready for these experiences, support and follow-up sessions are essential.

The centered riding technique of riding with the following seat is yet another metaphor for being sensitive to and going with the ebb and flow of the energy within us and throughout the universe. We cannot go against it; it is stronger than ego or will. I remember a chamber music demonstration in which someone in the audience asked the violinist how she knew when to signal the beginning of the music, and she said she listened for the rhythm of the earth and went with that. Similarly, we have to feel the rhythm and energy of the horse, go with it, and then ask for what we want. Similarly, we have to feel our own energies and rhythm, be able to follow them, and, to ask for alliance and cooperation. People learning centered riding techniques often say later that the exercises focusing on riding with the following seat are the turning point in their riding. There are many other techniques in *Centered Riding*, all of which can be used in psychotherapy. The above basics give you an idea of how they can be used.

We are, for all our intellectual and rational capacities, still instinctual beings, connected by our roots and genes to the collective nature of being. Staying in contact with these energetic depths gives us the strength, power, and collective knowledge to find our own paths and to become as wholly alive and effective as we can possibly be. The accomplishment of this, in my experience, comes only with the combination of physical, mental, psychological, and spiritual energies that are by necessity separated in our process of surviving, growing up, and becoming conscious beings. The task of maturity and human consciousness is then to bring what has become disparate back into centeredness, unity and wholeness, a thing that Jung called individuation. An important route to individuation can be utilizing the techniques in *Centered Riding*, for those whose symbolic processes embrace it.

EQUESTRIAN PSYCHOTHERAPY:
AN OVERVIEW

Joanne Henry Moses, PhD

Equestrian psychotherapy *is* an experiential modality requiring simultaneous integration or body, mind and spirit. Riding permeates the senses of sigh, hearing, smell, and touch all at the same tune. Proprioception, the mind's internal synthesizing of sensory input, integrates these sensations with the internal experience or balance.

Riding also demands clear thinking to direct the horse and make correct and reasonable responses to its input. At the same time the rider can savor a deep communion with nature. This synthesis of sensation proprioception reasoning, and spirituality merges these stimuli into a unique healing encounter.

Riding affect posture, balance, mobility, and function. Changing these factors also changes attitudes. The motion of the horse at a walk promotes relaxation of the entire central nervous system, both voluntary and autonomic. The repetitive movement of the horse at a walk can lull the person into a deeply relaxed state. On the other hand a brisk trot can energize someone with dulled affect.

Equestrian psychotherapy also requires the client to be out of doors and in contact with nature. .Here in Arizona we are surrounded by breathtaking beauty at nearly even turn of the trail. Merely sitting on a horse gives the patient a different visual perspective from the ordinary, This can be employed in helping clients alter their perspective on their problems.

Clients, especially passive women, also gain self-confidence and assertiveness in getting such a large animal to do their bidding. Abusive and domineering patients learn gentleness in dealing with a horse. The horse is too large to be forced and does not respond to bullying. For women with unresolved sexual issues, the horse symbolically represents male energy. How they deal with the horse will reflect their usual way of approaching men.

Equestrian psychotherapy gives the client a chance to get away from the clinical setting for a time. It can be a deeply meditative experience, particularly for the patient who has ridden previously. Once the purpose of the session has been discussed very little talking need occur until debriefing. Even when a group of patients share this activity each participant spends much of the time on horseback alone more in communication with the horse than with other riders. Group sharing after this reflective individual involvement, like nominal group process, has a more powerful input than a purely verbal modality.

Equestrian psychotherapy is not for everyone. It is most effective with people not responding to traditional therapy, perhaps because the metaphors this modality presents are so clear. Those having difficulty with relationships also benefit from this approach because riders learn to communicate effectively on several levels simultaneously. Utilized as an adjunct to traditional treatment, equestrian psychotherapy speeds up and enhances the therapeutic process.

CHAPTER 24

REMEDIAL AND SPECIAL EDUCATION

USING BEHAVIOR MODIFICATION IN THERAPEUTIC RIDING

Ronald Fischbach, Ph.D.
and Nora Fischbach

What is Behavior Modification?
Behavior modification is a method for teaching behaviors and skills through the careful manipulation of antecedents and the judicious application of rewards. All behavior is a product of what comes before it and what comes after it. For most children, the first sight of a beautiful horse will cause them to approach the animal. Depending upon the response of the horse, this child may forever want to be with horses, or may develop a strong reluctance to go near a horse.

The Foundations of Behavior Modification
Before you can teach anything, you must really understand it. Breaking a skill down into its teachable parts is called *task analysis*. Any new skill consists of a number of component parts. Mounting a horse may require knowing how to climb a mounting ramp, where and how to stand, how to put a foot in the stirrup and which foot to use, and how to swing your leg over the horse without losing your balance. To learn the skill of mounting, one must learn each of these component parts.

Teaching requires an understanding of what circumstances are most likely to be conducive to a child's learning. In addition, it requires an appreciation of what will motivate the child to learn. Responding in a punishing way to a child's behavior results in reluctance to behave in general. Nothing is learned without a reward. The more a behavior is rewarded, the more likely it is to be learned. In a teacher-student relationship there is always the opportunity to reward behavior. Unfortunately, sometimes a teacher may reward unwanted behaviors rather than wanted behaviors. For example, a child who has Attention Deficit Disorder is often rewarded for *not* paying attention by the teacher who requests that the child pay attention. In such a case, *not* attending is being rewarded by giving the child's inattentive behavior attention. The inattentive behavior is, therefore, more likely to occur with greater frequency. A more effective approach to teach attending would be for the teacher to reward with positive comments the times when the child *was* attending to task, while ignoring the inattention.

All teaching begins with the first step. The first step always involves the identification of one behavior or skill to be taught. Only after this first behavior is learned, is it advised to begin teaching a second behavior. Learning is the gradual acquisition of many individual behaviors.

Setting Up Goals and Objectives
A goal is a general direction that the teacher strives to attain. For example: *Jimmy shall improve his posture while on a horse*. Objectives are the measurable steps required to attain the goal. For example: *Jimmy shall sit in an 90 degree posture for 15 seconds*. A set of objectives adds up to the achievement of a goal. In order to set appropriate goals and objectives, it is necessary to assess a child's behavior against specified criteria. The chart below provides one example of such a measurement tool. Completion of an evaluation using such a tool provides the teacher with the starting point for the development of goals and objectives.

RIDER PERFORMANCE RECORD				
RIDER _____ INSTRUCTOR _____				
SKILL OR BEHAVIOR _____				

TASK ANALYSIS	CONDITIONS/CRITERIA FOR MASTERING	DATES OF SESSION	METHOD OF INSTRUCTION USED	DATE MASTERED

CODE   METHOD OF INSTRUCTION
PG = PHYSICAL GUIDANCE   PP= PHYSICAL PROMPT
VIC= VISUAL CUE   D = DEMONSTRATION
VBC=VERBAL CUE   WA=WITHOUT ASSISTANCE

Before one can set out to accomplish goals and objectives, it is necessary to identify impeding behaviors that may interfere with the achievement of the specified objectives. A teacher should always be aware of the distinction between a child's inability to perform a behavior versus an unwillingness to perform a behavior. The unwillingness to perform a behavior may be categorized as a behavior problem and must be addressed as an independent issue.

One of the more difficult decisions a teacher has to make is to choose which from among a number of skills to teach. One criterion for such a decision is that the child has the prerequisite skills in place that are necessary to learn the skill. For example, before a child can learn to ride to a specific location in an arena, that child must learn to focus on a specific point in space. A measure of such ability would be the teacher gaining eye contact with the child. Therefore, gaining eye contact would be a prerequisite skill for learning to ride to a specific point in the arena. Another criterion is that the child has at least one or two of the component parts of the skill to be learned. A child will not learn to sit at the walk until sufficient trunk control is in place to sit on a standing horse. An additional criterion is determining what the child is interested in learning or finds motivating to learn. Failing to engage the interest of the child will make the job of teaching much more difficult.

Applying Rewards
A reward is anything that follows a behavior and increases its frequency. The selection of rewards is critical in motivating a child to learn a new skill or behavior. The more powerful a reward is, the more willing a child will be to participate in the learning process. The only measure one can use to determine what is rewarding to a child is experience. While some children may be motivated by praise and attention, others may actually be deterred by such rewards. A teacher needs to maintain an active inventory of consequences that are likely to increase learning. Consulting with those who have worked closely with a child can be very helpful in determining what is rewarding and what is not. For example, mother may be aware of certain so-called

"primary reinforcers," such as a favorite food, which will increase her son's willingness to attend to riding instructions. Another rider's school teacher may be quick to suggest ignoring a rider's inappropriate hand gestures as a means of discouraging such behavior.

What is the difference between a reward and a bribe? All behavior is motivated by rewards, whether it is the employee working for a salary, the entertainer who performs for applause, or the missionary who labors long hours for the good feeling of knowing that others are being helped. Rewards are payment for tasks well done. In contrast, bribes are offerings that attempt to entice an individual into taking action, and come *before* the action.

There are several considerations that will make for the successful use of rewards:
- According to the Immediacy Principle, the sooner a reward follows a behavior, the more likely that behavior will be to re-occur.
- Avoiding satiation, the overuse of a reward, will help to maintain the reward's motivating power. Doling out small quantities is more effective than the delivery of larger quantities.
- Varying the rewards will help to maintain the learning process.
- During the initial phase of learning a new behavior, it is important to reward every successful trial. Once the behavior has been learned, rewarding intermittently is more effective than reinforcing every trial.

Getting down to teaching

Shaping

Jimmy is a five year-old boy who demonstrates moderate to severe autistic behaviors. His intellectual function borders on normal. Jimmy has never seen a horse before and has expressed some fear of riding. The first consideration is to prepare for Jimmy's arrival so that the circumstances are conducive to learning behaviors. Distractions are minimized by having no other riders in the immediate area. All necessary tack and safety equipment are laid out for easy access. Only the instructor greets Jimmy so that he is not overwhelmed by many new faces. Autistic children are more likely to display typically autistic behaviors when faced with new and overwhelming stimuli.

It is important to take careful note of how Jimmy responds to the new experience. The instructor's demands on Jimmy will be calibrated to Jimmy's ability to appropriately respond. Asking Jimmy to put on a helmet may be too demanding and may result in resistance or even tantruming. Using a procedure known as "shaping" makes it possible for Jimmy to experience new stimuli without fear. Allowing Jimmy to hold and inspect the helmet for a period of time enables him to get ready for the next step of putting on the helmet. Telling Jimmy that he will be wearing the helmet just for a moment will allay his concerns about the difficult experience of transitioning to wearing a strange new device. Depending upon his response to the momentary wearing of the helmet, the instructor may end this learning opportunity at this point, or proceed to the next step. If Jimmy shows mild resistance, this may be an indication that he is ready to have the helmet on for a number of such momentary trials. On the other hand, if Jimmy appears to show stronger resistance by his facial expressions or body language, persisting further may be counterproductive. In this case, the instructor could elect to introduce Jimmy to the horse he will eventually ride. A similar procedure can be employed to teach Jimmy to be willing to approach a horse.

Modeling

Jill is a fourteen year-old girl who was born with moderate cerebral palsy resulting in low muscle tone. She is able to sit on a horse but slouches and lists to one side. Through a procedure known as *modeling*, another rider who sits properly on a horse demonstrates correct posture and position on the horse. Jill is verbally rewarded for her attempts to imitate the more experienced rider's posture. As in Jimmy's learning to wear a helmet, Jill will be rewarded for successive approximations to the correct posture. At first, the instructor will verbally reward Jill for any attempt to replicate the more experienced rider's position. Each trial provides the opportunity to reward incremental improvements in Jill's posture. The crucial aspect of this method of teaching involves the instructor identifying how much improvement will be necessary before rewarding the rider. Too great a demand will result in failure. Too little demand may result in boredom. On occasion it may be necessary to provide Jill with physical guidance to properly position her.

Backward chaining

Nancy is a twelve year-old girl who has a learning disability that makes it hard for her to follow a series of commands. Traversing an obstacle course can be frustrating for her because she can never remember more than one or two steps at a time. *Backward chaining*, or learning the last step in a sequence of steps first, allows her to experience success every time, and reduces the anxiety that interferes with her learning. Nancy will be guided on horseback to the very last of the steps in the obstacle course. Having learned this last step, Nancy will then be led though the next-to-last step in the obstacle course. Once Nancy completes the next-to-last step, she quickly recognizes the last step (the one she has already learned) and eagerly moves though this last step. The secret of this procedure is that completion of the last step serves as a reward for learning the next-to-last step, and so forth. In this manner, Nancy is always able to end on a success -- another very important principle in teaching.

Rewarding desirable competing behaviors

Dustin has cerebral palsy with left spastic hemiplegia. He is reluctant to use his left hand and arm, and instead uses his right hand to help his left one whenever he is asked to use the left hand. By teaching Dustin to ride using English style direct reining, he necessarily uses his left hand as well as his right, and is instantly rewarded for doing so by the control he exerts on the horse. By rewarding a desirable behavior that competes with an undesirable behavior, the instructor can encourage the unlearning of the unwanted behavior.

Record Keeping

Record keeping serves two purposes. It enables the instructor to know that the instructional plan is moving forward. It also serves as a reward to the instructor by providing a concrete representation of the rider's success. The method of record keeping should be simple and clear. Most measures of rider's success involve the measurement of frequency of success or the duration of success. For example, the instructor may chart the length of time a rider can maintain an upright posture, or how many times the rider correctly turns his horse to the right. Record keeping can also demonstrate to the parents the effectiveness of the therapeutic riding.

RATING SCALE CUEING	0=CANNOT PERFORM 1=PERFORMS WITH MAXIMUM ASSISTANCE 2=PERFORMS WITH MODERATE ASSISSTANCE	3=PERFORMS WITH MINIMAL ASSISTANCE 4=PERFORMS WITH OCCASIONAL ASSISSTANCE OR 5=PERFORMS INDEPENDENTLY			
BEGINNING SKILLS:		1/3/96	3/5/96	6/2/96	DATE
Gets helmet		0	2	4	
Puts on helmet		0	1	3	
Climbs the mounting ramp		3	5	5	
Mounting		1	2	5	
holds reins and mane		0	1	4	
puts foot in		1	3	5	
sits		2	3	3	
puts other foot in		1	3	5	

Troubleshooting

The most successful teaching program will inevitably run into occasional obstacles. Troubleshooting is the process by which the instructor identifies the most likely cause of the problem. Suppose that the rider suddenly stops attending to the instructor during the riding lesson. The instructor needs to ask a number of questions to determine the cause for this loss of attention.

- Is the reward no longer motivating?
- Is the instructor not providing enough assistance to guide the rider through the learning experience?
- Is the riding lesson too long?
- Are there too many distractions?
- Does the rider have the necessary prerequisite skills to continue the lesson?
- Does the skill being taught exceed the child's level of interest?
- Is the instructor starting at an easy enough level for the rider?
- Are the instructions simple and clear?
- Is the lesson scheduled at a time when the rider is likely to be motivated to learn?
- Has the instructor moved too quickly to a too difficult skill level?
- Is the instructor moving too slowly in developing the skill?
- Is the instructor ending each learning experience with a success?

Achieving Success

The purpose of behavior modification is to provide a series of steps that, when followed, lead to success. The instructor first identifies the behavior or task that needs to be attained. An achievable goal is then set. The series of steps required to achieve that goal are planned. Careful records are kept to monitor the success of the program. Changes are made as needed, and finally, success is achieved. As the rider is rewarded for achievement, so is the instructor. There is no greater reward for a therapeutic riding instructor than to experience the success of the riders.

Ronald Fischbach, Ph.D.
Nora Fischbach
California, USA

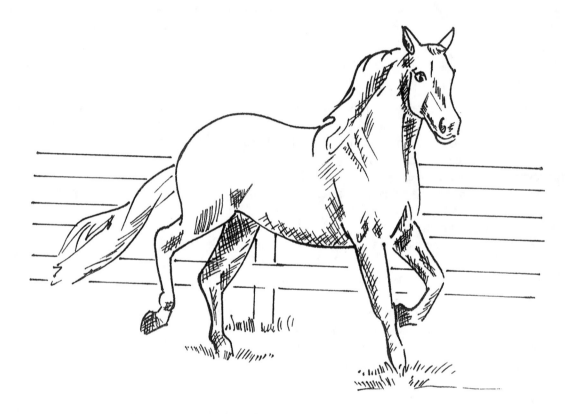

THERAPEUTIC HORSEBACK RIDING:
A SCHOOL DISTRICT PROGRAM

Chris McParland, BS

BACKGROUND

The excitement and success enjoyed by therapeutic riding programs in the United States throughout the past thirty-plus years can realistically be achieved within a school district. Special education students are served in a variety of ways including pull-out programs (students are seen individually or in small groups outside of classroom), partial integration into their regular class, full inclusion in regular education program, and in special day-classes.

Educationally, therapeutic riding can provide a wide spectrum of learning opportunities for special education students. It enhances existing services by complementing and extending other special learning programs such as speech and language, adapted physical education, occupational or physical therapy, and psychological services.

An example of a school district's success in utilizing a therapeutic riding program to provide expanded learning opportunities for special education students can be found in Elk Grove, California. The Elk Grove Unified School District (EGUSD) has integrated such a riding program into its curriculum--Project RIDE (Riding Instruction Designed for Education). Modeled after the nationally and internationally recognized Cheff Center for the Disabled (founded in 1970) in Augusta, Michigan, EGUSD's therapeutic riding program combines the background of an established center with the stability of a progressive school district to create a firm foundation for lasting success.

Project RIDE began in 1979 and served thirty students at Jessie Baker School once a week as part of their adapted physical education program. Soon after those modest beginnings, other special education classes throughout the District expressed an interest in adding horseback riding to their curriculums. Consequently, the case load of riders at Project RIDE increased considerably from one session a week to three times a week. After ten years and continued growth, Project RIDE became a full time teaching position staffed by an EGUSD adapted physical education specialist and an instructional assistant. And, in direct response to the program's acceptance and expansion, the District has included Project RIDE in its master plan for education. Underscoring the program's importance is the inclusion in the master plan of a fully enclosed riding arena scheduled for construction at Jessie Baker School in the very near future.

Professionally, the riding program has benefitted from the beginning as well. The credentialed, district teacher, an adapted physical education specialist, became the riding instructor. As Project RIDE'S instructor, she not only brought current knowledge of classroom and physical education curricula, but also a formal background in English and Western horsemanship. In addition, she accepted responsibility for program organization and coordination.

COMMUNITY INVOLVEMENT/VOLUNTEERS

From the onset, the history of Project RIDE represents one of America's finest traditions - community members coming together to help a worthwhile organization develop and become a solid and integral part of community. It was in 1979 that EGUSD and the Jessie Baker School, a school for students with severe disabilities, became the core around which community involvement could form and flourish. Adult volunteers provide the manpower to haul the horses to Jessie Baker for classes. An outdoor arena was built on the Jessie Baker campus for the riding program. They also feed and care for the horses at the ranch leased to house the horses, as they cannot stay at the school. Other volunteers assist with the daily classes as program volunteers, and organizing and holding fund raising events, demonstrations, competitions, and other special activities.

In 1980 the scope of volunteer involvement broadened as Project RIDE became an incorporated, non-profit organization (501(c)(3). With this legal status, the board of directors (comprised solely of volunteers) assumed additional responsibilities. Project RIDE, Inc. relieved EGUSD of financial support for horses, tack, truck, trailer, and other equipment. The District continues its educational support, however, by monetarily sustaining the instructor's salary and benefits. Also, EGUSD provides in-kind support by maintaining the campus arena, utilities in the tack room (lights and phone), processing student forms, and coordinating Project RIDE with other special education support services included on the students' Individual Education Programs (IEP'S).

There are two secondary schools within walking distance of Jessie Baker School. These secondary schools provide student volunteers to Project RIDE during school hours as well as after school. The Project RIDE Club is comprised of students from Joseph Kerr Junior High and Elk Grove High School whose parents, administrators, and instructors have given permission for the students to be released from a minimum of three classes one day a week to volunteer for the program at Jessie Baker School.

The integration of regular education students into this special riding program has had positive results for all students. The regular education students gain disability awareness and an understanding of special education students, in addition to receiving instruction in equine safety and equestrian skills. The riders are given a tremendous opportunity to interact educationally and socially with regular education students; thus the riders and student volunteers learn from each other and the educational opportunities for all students are expanded considerably. Related equine activities such as riding demonstrations, field trips, competitions (horse shows), and fund raising events provide other ways to integrate special education and regular education students.

DISTRICT COMPONENTS/FEDERAL LAW

Components of a program within a school district can be described by recapping the federal law which set the stage for developing adapted physical education programs. The definition of Adaptive Physical Education is: a diversified program that incorporates a variety of individual programs including developmental activities, games, sports, and rhythms. All the activities are considered to be suited to the interests, capacities, and the limitations of the students with disabilities who cannot safely or successfully participate actively in a regular physical education program.

In 1975, physical education was included in the Education for All Handicapped Children Act (Public Law (PL 94-142). This was the first piece of legislation to recognize physical education as an important component in the education of children with disabilities. The federal law defines handicapped children as those who are mentally retarded, hard-of-hearing, speech and language impaired, deaf, blind, and multi-handicapped. The law helped to regulate what was previously defined by AAHPERD,* that physical education is to include adapted physical education, special physical education, motor development, and movement education.

CHRONOLOGICAL PLAN FOR PROGRAM ORGANIZATION

The steps taken to develop a therapeutic riding program within a public or private school system are quite similar in many respects to the creation of a program through a privately funded group, public agency, horse-related group, or riding stable. The development of a program within a school district must be coordinated administratively first. The individual or group who has the best chance to sell the idea of a therapeutic riding program would probably come from within district staff. The idea might develop through the adapted physical education staff, special education teachers, occupational or physical therapists, speech and language specialists, or other district individuals knowledgeable about riding for the disabled programs.

Planning a therapeutic riding program for a school district contains many factors that make it unique; thus the proposal should be written by someone with an extensive background in horsemanship, stable management, veterinary care and hopefully, special education or disability awareness training. It would be quite difficult to develop a thorough proposal without a solid background in the previously mentioned areas.

Community support for the program will demonstrate to the district administration that financial responsibilities will not totally rest with the district. If the district allows one of their credentialed employees to teach the program, then the district's responsibility will probably be very significant in terms of salary and financial demands. Bussing the riders to a center will have a definite financial impact on the school district; therefore, the coordinators of the riding program may have to consider trucking the horses and ponies to a school site.

The next step, once an individual or small group has developed a proposal, is to seek support for the idea from the director or coordinator of special services for the district. That special education administrator will play a key role in presenting a therapeutic riding proposal to the superintendent, other district administrators and the school board. The proposal should include a brief history of riding for the disabled, information on the North American Riding for the Handicapped Association, and a review of state and local riding-for-the-disabled programs.

When developing a proposal, qualifications of instructional personnel, target population of students, entrance and exit criteria for service, funding sources, location of facility, bussing considerations, sources for volunteers and a board of directors, accident insurance and liability coverage, and sources for locating mounts and riding equipment are all areas to be researched and included in the proposal.

The proposal must be well-planned, concise and complete with funding alternatives. Those alternatives can be researched in the special projects office in the district. The funding options may include grant possibilities, public agencies, private funding sources, sponsorships, service groups, and perhaps, third party insurance reimbursement for occupational or physical therapy.

An information-sharing session, with invitations sent to all support agencies, parent groups, horse organizations, school district administrative personnel, and others from the community who may become involved with the therapeutic riding program, should be held prior to submitting the proposal. It is important

---

*AAHPERD: American Association of Health, Physical Education, Recreation, and Dance.
AAHPERD (1952) defines adapted physical education as "diversified program of developmental activities, games, sports, and rhythms, suited to the interests, capacities, and limitations of students with disabilities who may not safely or successfully engage in unrestricted participation in the vigorous activities of the general physical education program.

to have a support group organized before the proposal is formally presented to the district administration. There should be many private schools or public school districts in the United States who would endorse or support, as much as possible, a therapeutic horseback riding program just as the Elk Grove Unified School District has for the past ten years. It takes leadership, coordination, cooperation, pride in services and staff, and community support to create and sustain a quality program. Let's hope that other school districts will give therapeutic riding a place in their curriculum for special education students.

References
Seaman, J.A., DePauw, K.P. (1982). *The New Adaptive Physical Education*. Mayfield Publishing Co.
U.S. Congress. Education for All Handicapped Children Act, PL 94-142, 1975.

Chris McParland, BS
Clements, CA

SPECIAL EDUCATION WITHIN THERAPEUTIC RIDING

Virginia G. Mazza, MS

Special education is charged with providing education to children with special needs and with bringing them into the mainstream of life as much as humanly possible. Children of all disabilities of varying intensities are served. Special education can take place in a variety of settings ranging from the normal classroom setting to special schools. Therapeutic riding is a natural partner in special education.

It is important for the riding instructor to understand thoroughly the particular problems facing the children in a given class, as the more severely disabled are often grouped by disability as well as age. In particular, he or she must understand the problems of each individual child as well. Therefore, a good professional relationship needs to be established between the special education classroom teacher and the riding instructor so that together they can review the mandated IEP (Individual Educational Plan) for each child and develop appropriate riding goals. It is vital that the director of the riding program develop the necessary pathways to access this confidential material and, of course, this confidentiality must be respected. Parental authorization can be a very speedy and effective means of obtaining this important information. One of the critical roles of the riding instructor, as well as the special education teacher, who are both generalists, is to interface with the other professionals as they deem necessary, e.g., physical therapists, occupational therapists or speech/language pathologist. The whole child needs to be observed and appropriate teaching goals and strategies developed. These plans should include specific lessons for carry-over to the classroom as well.

Depending upon the age of the child and the disability he or she faces, a wide variety of activities exist that use the horse educationally. Reading, writing and arithmetic can be incorporated into riding lessons painlessly. The critical talents needed for professionals working in this field are an understanding of disability, a solid knowledge and experience in teaching riding to "able-bodied" riders and the ability to be creative. A sense of humor and tireless energy also help. The classroom teacher can often help in adapting academic material. It also falls to the riding program to let the many teachers out there know that remedial riding exists and to help them access this field on behalf of their students. Most teachers make wonderful volunteers and are very much interested in anything that can make a difference in the lives of their students.

Conclusion:

Good planning, specific goals, and incorporating happy times can give the riders a new look at life that is both therapeutic and exhilarating. It is a demonstrated fact that well-developed lessons do provide remedial value. Provide remedial work in a way that it is enjoyably. It is powerful. Fun is healing. Success breeds confidence. Having something to look forward to and talk about is a positive influence. Riding can provide all of this. Using the horse incorporates all of the senses, and all of the modalities, and that helps learning to take place. Riders should learn all there is to know about the horse world and be helped to aspire to be their best. To understand the many areas that can be integrated into a special education program in an equine setting, an information list has been provided.

SOME SPECIFIC ACTIVITIES FOR THE RIDING LESSON AND CLASSROOM

These activities can be adapted to fit the appropriate level from beginner to advanced student riders. The activities can incorporate special education skills that are needed in daily living:

- Balance exercises (the flag, bear stand, riding backward)
- Coordination exercises (all of the above activities in addition to ring tossing and other games)
- Concepts such as under, over, behind, in front
- Language development (group story telling, singing songs)
- Creating a horse story. Putting it on tape and finally writing it out
- Creating a trail course and acting out a horse adventure
- Scavenger hunts on horseback
- Learning relays using letters or sentences
- Grooming skills and learning to identify, read, spell and write the names of tools
- Learning riding skills by taking direction, sequencing tasks and maintaining attention
- Beginning trail class
- Advanced trail class
- Learning to canter
- Finding out what a horse show is
- Taking part in a horse show for persons with physical disabilities, 4-H club members or Special Olympics
- Planning a horse show
- Helping to develop a horse show
- Gymkhana games
- Joining a 4-H or Pony Club
- Scout Badge

This list is just the beginning--it is endless, so begin with your program ...to develop the education experience!

Virginia G. Mazza, MS
USA

THE IEP: WHAT IT IS AND WHAT IT MEANS TO YOU

Gigi Sweet, M.Ed

At an operating center that works with school-age riders, the therapeutic riding staff has probably heard teachers or parents talk about the **IEP (Individual Education Plan)**. Every public school student who qualifies for special services has an IEP in the US. The IEP is a product of the **Education for All Handicapped Children Act**, passed in 1975. It ensures that the needs of each student will be addressed on an individual basis. Annually, a staffing is held to establish each child's goals and objectives. The staffing team consists of a parent/guardian, teachers, therapists and clinicians with whom the student comes in contact, a special education representative from the school district and the student, if so desired. Support personnel, such as adaptive swim teachers, therapists, and others who have responsibility for many students may not be present at the staffing, but will submit objectives pertinent to their area. The minimum at a staffing will be the special education teacher, parent/guardian and special education representative.

Immediately upon a student's admission to a school, the staffing is held and a written IEP is the product. There should be no lapse time without a current IEP until the student graduates (which will occur on or before the student's 22nd birthday) or is discontinued in the program for other reasons.

The IEP is printed in quadruplicate, with copies given to each of the following: parent, classroom teacher, special education /support personnel, and the student's cumulative record file. Most school districts use three pages for the IEP; the items on each page vary between districts. Information provided includes: the student's pertinent record data, checklist of special services, present levels of performance, consideration of placement options as they relate to **least restrictive environment** (the student should be mainstreamed into the regular setting as much as possible), date of implementation, and signature lines for all those involved in the staffing.

Also in the IEP will be the yearly goals in any or all of the following areas: affective (behavioral), academic, vocational and recreational/physical. Goals are broad general statements summarizing targets for the year. A sample goal in the vocational area for a moderately mentally retarded high school student is, "Harold will function in the sheltered workshop independently on piecemeal tasks contracted to the school."

The remaining portion of the IEP (some districts use an addendum instead) will delineate one or more objectives that support the established goals. Objectives are written in behavioral terms with action verbs, and are measurable in some way, usually through quantitative data. Teachers may work on other objectives not on the IEP, as long as the objectives support the goals. Objectives are updated yearly or more often as they are either totally met (TM) or determined not suitable. Examples of objectives for the previously stated vocational goal are:

l. Using a template, Harold will package and seal items with 1OO% accuracy

2. Harold will clock in and out and deliver his packaged goods to his supervisor on each workday

What is the relationship of the IEP to a therapeutic riding program? Directly, absolutely none unless the therapeutic riding program is part of the school curricula . An IEP reflects a contractual agreement within the school setting. An exception to this is the school that includes therapeutic riding on the IEP, either generally listed as a support service, or more specifically with itemized objectives. Individually, the IEP goals and objectives will help a riding center integrate and coordinate activities with the classroom.

Sometimes a school district will not wish to include a therapeutic riding program on an IEP because of the difficulty and legality of blending federal regulations with a private industry that is not regulated by the government. It is helpful, nevertheless, to have the therapeutic riding program on the IEP, probably as an adjunct to adaptive education. One should be very careful, however, having therapeutic riding activities as specific objectives on the IEP. **Remember this is a legal contract that provides documentation of the educational program.** It is subject to continuous monitoring and evaluation. Even though the instructor is monitoring the riding activities, one does not want to lose control of what is happening at the center. What the teacher can include are behavioral and social objectives to be achieved through cooperation with the therapeutic riding staff. It would be unusual for a teacher to want to include specific riding objectives in the IEP. By doing this, she has made the responsible person (the instructor) someone who is not part of the school staffing team or district personnel.

What are the rights of a therapeutic riding instructor regarding the IEP? He or she has none. A teacher may wish to share the IEP with the instructor as it benefits both the school and the riding program. Establish with the teacher that each parent has agreed to release the information to the center staff. Respect the school's rights not to make such information available, and the confidentiality of the document if it **is** offered. Do not make it available to volunteers, but extract information that is pertinent to the program and summarize it for them. It is not appropriate to go over the head of an teacher who is unable to provide the instructor with a copy of the IEP by seeking parental permission. This is an excellent way to sabotage all the good will that has been created. For those school-aged riders brought to the program by the parents, one may ask them for permission to contact the teacher or preferably, request an introduction. Even though the parents can provide the instructor with a copy of the IEP, it is in bad form to accept it without the knowledge of the teacher, the main author of the document. One's primary contact however should be with the person who brings the rider to the center, be it teacher, parent or agency.

What does one do with the information provided in the IEP? Working with the teacher, the instructor can provide follow-through that is highly motivating on behavior programs, consistency in therapy goals, and practice of educational and vocational skills. Academic objectives from math to social studies maybe incorporated into the riding lesson. Vocational objectives are a natural way to address unmounted activities. If the instructor cannot gain access to the IEP, one can still do all the things that would be included in an IEP. Provide the cooperating teacher with a form on which she can briefly describe the student's academic functional level, current behavior plan, particular strength and areas of interest. Share this information with the volunteers who work with the rider.

IN CONCLUSION

The IEP can be a tool that helps the instructor align the therapeutic riding program with goals and objectives developed within the rider's educational setting. Consistency within the child's life maximizes the opportunities for success by providing structure, increasing familiarity and reducing frustration. Do not feel unable to achieve the same benefits without access to the IEP. As a therapeutic riding instructor one has had vast experience adapting equipment to fit the many needs presented by riders within the program. With initiative and expertise, one can create the necessary tools to get the job accomplished!

Gigi Sweet, M.Ed
USA

PSYCHOLOGICAL TREATMENT WITH THE HORSE
USING VAULTING LESSONS AS "REMEDIAL-EDUCATION"*

Antonio Kröger

Preliminary Remarks
1.1. Definition

The concept of *addresses the educational, psychological, psychotherapeutic, rehabilitative and socially integrating aspects of the use of horses to help individuals of all ages with various disabilities and disturbances.

The focus is on using horses to benefit individuals developmentally, emotionally and behaviorally rather than to teach riding as a sport. The individual is addressed holistically in his or her interaction with the horse, whether riding or vaulting. Holistically means physically, mentally, emotionally and socially.

1.2. Group Size

An ideal group size is six children or adolescents. This:

- Allows for various subgroups of two or three for specific lessons.
- Guarantees each participant the opportunity to recognize the limits of his or her abilities and thereby provides a basis for realistic self-assessment.
- Makes abandoning favoritism possible.
- Provides opportunities for cooperation.
- Kindles the participants' courage to try new things by allowing them to observe and then imitate each other.
- Allows group members to increasingly differentiate between horse and vaulter by counting the rhythmical movements of the horse's gaits. This requires the riders to hold still during the exercise.
- Gives the individual participant enough time to recover his attention and concentration and to overcome the fear after having exerted himself to his maximum ability.

A smaller group size may be preferable:

- When the experience of the vaulting instructor is so limited that if difficulties of a social nature were to arise, the riding instruction would be abandoned
- If the disabilities of the participants are so severe (i.e., their ability to participate as members of a group
  is so limited) that in the beginning, remedial-education riding and vaulting could only be done effectively either individually or in a correspondingly smaller group.

* (Healing Instruction) is a literal translation of the German term Heilpaedagogik. Since the concept is distinct from that commonly described in English by the word, it is here given its literal form (Translator). The term used in English is "remedial-education riding and vaulting" and will be used in this paper.

Translated from German by Eberhard W. Teichmann

1.3. Staff
The primary actors in an effective program of healing instruction in vaulting are:
- The group of participants
- A specially trained and reliable horse with a soft and easy canter
- A trained vaulting teacher whose constant concern is to teach in a professional manner

Anyone else who wants to be present in order to help can do so only by not being actively involved in what is going on in the program. The helper must only observe and privately take note of what is happening in the group and with individual participants.

This person (helper) can reflect back to the vaulting instructor how the vaulter's actions and reactions move him or her toward his or her goal. This feedback can be used to better plan future lessons, (cf. section III ff.). A bystander or helper must never do things such as entertaining those children who are not vaulting, or lifting participants onto the horses or intervening in conflict situations. (cf. section II.2)

Parents are seldom able to perform the functions of a helper described above, and for that reason, if they want to be present during the lesson, they should only be observers from a distance away from the group.

II. The Vaulting Lesson in Remedial-Education Riding and Vaulting

II. 1. Preparation (grooming and saddling) of the Vaulting Horse.
The participants help in caring for, grooming, and saddling the horse. However, they alone must decide how near or far from the horse they want to be, which activities they want to be involved in, and when and how much. The vaulting instructor should respect their choices. Otherwise, their natural interest in living things might be smothered and their motivation to make contact with the horse, extinguished.

II. 2. The Warm-up and Suppling of the Horse and the Vaulter
Especially in the beginning phase of therapy, the stability of the instructor is most important to children with social and emotional difficulties.

In order to maintain the horse as the primary medium for correcting the participant's personality development, the connection between horse and rider during the vaulting lesson should not be restricted in any way. The vaulting teacher is the person who maintains the participant's attention on the horse. Through appropriate initiatives, he controls the horse, and this is his means of education. That is the reason for excluding other reference persons (i.e., helpers).

The first task for the participants in a lesson in remedial-education riding and vaulting is for them to establish, by themselves, their starting order for that lesson. Any child or adolescent is capable of learning this process of creating order in his or her group. It always needs to be done in relationship to the horse. While this is happening, the instructor is warming up the horse in the ring near the group so that the participants can become involved in suppling the horse immediately after they have established their riding order.

It is good to involve the whole group in suppling the horse. The movements of the horse form the basis for all the demands made on the participants--both inside and outside the ring. This activity around the horse can be conceived of as multiform "games" played around the horse. Noteworthy is Bernhard Ringbeck's description of these in the book, *Heilpaedagogisches Reiten und Volti* (1990).

II.3. Exercises on the Horse

II.3.1. Exercises for individuals

The individual participant does his or her exercises on the horse in the order determined by the group; the person just finishing helps the person next in line onto the horse. Even more effective from the point of view of enhancing group process--if also more difficult--is to have the participant helped onto the horse by the person following him or her. If the group can also agree that the consequence of a person not helping is to miss his or her turn for that round, the participants' self discipline is quickly established.

If there are difficulties in helping someone onto the horse, others from the group may help. It does not matter whether help is asked for or given without asking. If help is not given or it is ineffective, the instructor can model giving help in an exemplary way.

Depending on the level of concentration in the group or the general spirit of the participants, the exercises for individuals are done in order and each exercise is repeated two or three times. The exercises are based on the six obligatory vaulting exercises. Those exercises that are accomplished in stride are soon attempted--often in the first hour--at a canter. In that way individuals can be kept at the edge of their capability at the moment, whether that capability is in concentration, in bodily attention, in physical strength, or in overcoming fear. Since the ability to make this maximum effort in healing instructional vaulting is so limited in these participants, and their turns so brief, typically everyone in a group can have two turns on the horse in a period of about fifteen minutes.

II.3.2. Exercises with a partner

In the very first vaulting lesson, exercises for individuals should be followed by simple exercises with a partner. The purpose of this is for relaxation and for the participants to begin to establish social and emotional ties with each other. Exercises for three soon follow those for two. These exercises are carried out for a longer period of time. They help the participants in many ways, and especially: to focus on another being (both horse and rider); to concentrate; to accept the boundaries of other participants; to further the ability to accept close physical contact; and to comprehend the good nature of the horse.

During this group phase of the lesson when group harmony seems difficult to maintain, the vaulting instructor has a good opportunity to keep all the participants actively involved by having them make observations. The three bystanders might observe:

- How long the exercise lasts?
- Which of the participants carries out the vaulting exercise correctly?
- Who begins to speak first on the horse?
- What sequence of exercises the vaulters invent?
- Whether the following group does everything correctly?
- During how many paces of the horse does the hind person stand?

- Which hand does the front person put on their head?
- With which hand does the front person praise the horse?
- And much, much more. . . !

With time, remedial-education riding and vaulting becomes calmer and more creative. Also the motivation of the participants increases.

II.3.3. Requested Exercises
Toward the end of the vaulting lesson, each participant may request to do an exercise or exercise sequence of his or her choice. He or she may choose the gait of the horse, if he or she is do the exercise alone, with one or two others, or even whether or not to do an exercise at all.

II.4. Care of the Horse
The care of the horse at the conclusion of the exercises is a way to acknowledge its contributions. This care includes:

- Praising the horse after the vaulting lesson by patting and stroking it.
- Feeding it small treats such as apples, oats, and so forth.
- Cooling it down in the arena by walking it in hand.
- Removing the tack.
- Taking the longe line, the whip and the saddle to the tack room.
- Leveling the surface of the ring.
- Leading the horse to its stall, removing the bridle and cleaning the bit.
- Spreading shavings in the stall and blanketing the horse, if necessary.
- Taking leave of the horse and the trainer.

III. After the lesson, preparing for the next lesson
If an observer was present for the vaulting lesson, his or her help is invaluable in preparing for the next lesson. In this regard, the following might be taken into account:

- Was the management of the horse proper--when was something missing--?
- Were the goals for each individual children achieved?
- Were the agreed upon arrangements upheld?
- For whom should a goal be changed?
- How might a change be introduced and developed?
- Were the corrections, i.e., the reinforcements appropriate to and for the conceptual level of the participants?
- When and how did the instructor engage in a power struggle with a participant and thereby abandon the partnership?
- What was obvious during the lesson regarding mutual attraction or rejection within the group members as it affected the partnership interaction?
- Should a consequence for frequent misbehavior be arrived at democratically within the group?

THE STUDY: U SING "REMEDIAL EDUCATION RIDING AND VAULTING" TO CHANGE THE BEHAVIOR OF ELEMENTARY STUDENTS

Project History

This project involved children from an elementary school who were in the first three grades. The school doctor identified eight out of seventy first grade children whom he felt needed special attention, i.e., their motor functioning was unusual and conspicuous. Seven of these eight children were in one class. The author would like to note but not elaborate on the observation that motor deficiencies in children often have behavioral consequences. The author also noted that four out of these seven children were so severely disturbed socially that classroom instruction with them was very difficult. At the end of the first semester, the school principal offered to give the classroom teacher an hour a week free from her regular duties in order to work with these most socially disturbed students to develop their social skills. The teacher, in searching for something to strongly motivate these students, came across my work in teaching vaulting as the head of a school for special children and asked me to work with the four most affected boys. The parents of these boys were informed about the proposed instruction which was to take place in a series of four sessions, each for a month. And arrangements were made regarding which parents would transport the children to and from the riding arena at what times.

Course of the Project

The author held the first social training session on February 7, 1990. In it he explained vaulting to the children. The author received the expected result that all four children wanted to try it. They were also willing to accept my conditions for beginning each of the four possible series of sessions (each lasting a month) until summer vacation began. These conditions were as follows: "whoever `hits' another person no more than eight times in each of the Wednesday sessions of a given month may participate in the next month." The point of this arrangement was to indicate unacceptable behavior in an objective way. The idea was that if these children could merely be made aware of their asocial behavior without being judged for it, it would be easier for them to work on changing it.

In the session on February 14, everything went according to plan. Three of the boys went on to canter during their first lesson. Only the most disturbed boy, whose aggressions were unpredictable, wanted only to walk the horse. He is the one labeled **S** in Table 1. The results of this vaulting lesson in terms of the boys' motivation and behavior in their regular classroom was nothing short of unbelievable. The student labeled as **P**, who regularly was involved in an average of eight major physical altercations each class day, abruptly stopped fighting and continued not to fight for the following five school days.

The tension engendered by this maximum effort in self-control broke into chaos on February 21. However, before this happened, the author took **P** for a private vaulting lesson as a reward for his accomplishments. In his car on the way back to school after the lesson, **P** remarked, "I don't think I can do it again next week." Since the other three students wanted the same privilege of a private lesson, individual standards of social behavior for achieving it were set for each of them. If any of them met these standards for five days, they would have an additional private session. Each student was given a card on which their teacher would note the days on which they had achieved their standard. However, each was responsible for giving the card to his teacher for the notation; if he forgot to do it, he lost that day.

On February 28, two of the children had earned a private session. On the next Wednesday, three had earned one. On March 14, a planned show was held in which, by the way, no fights occurred. On March 14, all the boys had met their requirements so that the classroom session in social behavior was canceled. In the following week, only two of the students earned an extra session. But one of them was **S**, for whom this seemed to be the first time that any kind of therapy had worked. **S** had been continuously in either group or individual therapy since the age of four, none of which had shown any results until the present. After an Easter vacation of three weeks, all of the children forgot to pick up their cards from the teacher. They did not notice until there was no vaulting lesson on April 25.

Since these four children had managed to rapidly increase control over their behavior (as evidenced by the proportion of them earning extra lessons: 50% in the first interim period, 75% in the second, and 83% in the third), their parents definitely wanted the sessions to continue. Thus, these sessions became a regular arrangement in the next school year, this time with six participants (five boys and one girl). We expanded the group not because I could fit six children into my car, but because adding two more to the original four seemed important to us in a group dynamic sense. It seemed an important step in integrating the first four difficult students into a wider group.

---

*Startfolge = Starting Order
*Einfuehrung = Introduction
*Osterferien = Easter Vacation
*Projektwoche = Project Week

*TRANSLATION FROM GERMAN TO ENGLISH

STARTFOLGE															
	7	14	21	28	7	14	21	28	25	2	9	16	23	30	6
	2	2	2	2	3	3	3	3	4	5	5	5	5	5	6
NAME															
P m		⊙	△	△		⊙	△			⊙	△		△	⊙	△
A m		⊙			△	⊙	△			⊙			△	⊙	
C m		⊙		△	△	⊙	△	△		⊙	△		△	⊙	△
S m		⊙			△	⊙	△	△		⊙	△		△	⊙	△
		1	2	3		4	2					3		4	3
			50%				75%						83%		

FIGURE 1.

MOTIVATIONAL REMEDIAL-EDUCATION RIDING AND VAULTING
FOR ELEMENTARY SCHOOL STUDENTS AS A BETTER WAY TO CONTROL BEHAVIOR?

REMEDIAL EDUCATION

<u>Anzahl</u>=number <u>V. Lehrer Verhindert</u>=prevented (from attending) by teacher <u>Herbstferien</u>=fall vacation <u>Schulfrei</u>=no school <u>Ferien</u>=vacation <u>Osterferien</u>=Easter vacation <u>Feiertag</u>=holiday	Anzahl der starts = number of special sessions a - Schulische Vorbedingung nicht erfuellt = academic conditions not met St - Verweis im stall = reprimand in the stall Sa - Sandwerfen = throwing sand Arabic numbers--arab. ziffer--Taetlichkeiten = acts of assault Roman number--roem. ziffer = verpasste starts = missed starts
Translation of German terms into English as they relate to Figure 2.	

FIGURE 2.

REMEDIAL-EDUCATION RIDING AND VAULTING AS A VOLUNTARY ASSOCIATION IN THE FIRST AND SECOND GRADES OF AN ELEMENTARY SCHOOL.

Figure 2 graphically displays the number of vaulting starts for the individual children in the period from the beginning of August, 1990 to the end of May, 1991. Thirty four events are tabulated in chronological order. The project continued as a voluntary working relationship outside of the required hours of instruction. Six children out of a class of twenty-four were involved. Conditions for participation that were not related to vaulting were retained in the second year of the program since they had been so effective during the first year. In doing that, however, we instituted something that I had formerly rejected. I will come back to that later.

In Figure 2 the dots indicate that student participated at that time. **K** means that the participant missed the session because of illness. **A** means that the student did not participate because he or she did not meet the conditions set by the school in order to be able to do so. For **P** that was so twice, for **A** three times, and for **C** not at all. **St** means non-participation because of a warning in the previous hour by stable staff. **S** did not meet the conditions six times, **D** two times, and **M** once. The last column gives the sum of the A's.

The Arabic numerals give information about serious physical altercations during the vaulting. That was hardly observed among the four children during the first school year. During the second year, some of it might be explained by the increase in size of the group, although the two new children did not trust themselves to become socially active during that time. In addition, **D** showed strong motor disturbances. I see further explanations in the fact that the sessions were no longer new and unusual and also in that in the larger group, the participants had to establish their starting order at the beginning of each session. The problems that arose could only be solved by force in the beginning. Telling the children that the horse could not stand being around this kind of violent problem solving because it would become afraid of the vaulting only helped for awhile. They then fought away from the horse so that it could not react to them. That at least was a step toward becoming more considerate, which was something the children were not able to be at all in the rest of their lives.

In order to make some progress in tackling this issue, I recruited a student teacher to secretly make a checklist of serious conflict and how often a and who was involved during the next hour. In doing that, the severity of the blows, the length of the fight and the instigator were all to be ignored. All she was to register was the frequency of the conflicts because this was what the children could most easily relate to. On September 9th, seventeen incidents were secretly recorded on the list. At the end of the hour, each participant was asked how often he or she thought they had participated in a conflict. The result of questioning them had little to do with what had been recorded.

Before the beginning of the next session, I asked each participant to guess how many times he or she would be involved in a conflict. That guess was also recorded by the student teacher and at the end of the hour that number was compared with the number on the checklist, which was now being recorded openly. Over time and without exception, all the children developed a certain pride in their ability to predict what they would do. From November on, the guesses were no longer registered because the children could relatively reliably count the number of conflicts they had been in. They did this regularly in the car on the trip back to school. The vaulting proceeded with fewer incidents and became progressively more performance oriented.

The Roman numerals indicate missed opportunities for starting a vaulting round. Each participant was responsible for noting his or her starting order for that day. Whoever did not approach the horse in the ring at the end of the previous rider's turn without being reminded, was passed over without either having an extra turn
or being admonished for missing one. It was made clear to the children that they were free to pass on their turn if they were afraid or if they did not feel like going at the moment.

For lack of space, an analysis of the last row will be foregone: the frequency of physical assault. I do want to mention that the group was able to democratically arrive at certain arrangements on occasion. A warning from the stable staff and throwing sand while the horse was in the area resulted in the loss of one session and the loss of five "points." Leaving the arena building without permission during the vaulting lesson meant being without supervision. The consequence for that was loss of the session. During the last three months a further rule was established that whoever lost his or her point card also lost the privileges contained in those points.

session	participants	0	=	0%	session	participants			
1	participants	0	=	0	4	participants	2	=	6%
2	participants	0	=	0	5	participants	11	=	32%
3	participants	1	=	3%	6	participants	20	=	59%

FIGURE 3. PARTICIPATION DURING 34 WEEKS OF SCHOOL

This graph displays the number of participants in the individual vaulting lessons. For fairness sake, those participants who missed because of illness (which happened eight times) are marked as being in attendance or a total of 34 occasions:

20 times	all 6 children took part	= 59% of the time
11 times	5 children took part	= 32% of the time
2 times	4 children took part	= 6% of the time
1 time	3 children took part	= 3% of the time

The results speak for themselves! A further point is clear. Out of 200 possible starts only 14 (7%) could not be used because the conditions for doing them had not been met. The author finds this last result rather puzzling since he had totally abandoned using conditions for participating in vaulting some time ago as the result of negative experiences. In thinking further about the question of why the setting of conditions in this project was so helpful, the author made the following conclusions:

- My earlier conditions were probably not concrete enough.
- The author did not give enough consideration to the principle of small steps in necessary changes.
- The timing of the conditions in relation to the desired changes was insufficient.
- Often the conditions were substantially and too rapidly changed to respond immediately to variations in misbehavior.
- Last but not least: the conditions were not directed enough at the reasons for the misbehavior; only when one knows the reasons for a misbehavior is a real behavior change possible.

The author finds the foregoing remarks confirmed by the following example. During vaulting, a participant totally deficient in group skills, began for the first time in his life to take requests that were directed at the whole group as being relevant to him as well. In addition, the more his interest in achieving was awakened, the more he changed his behavior. His conditions for participating were not to hit others in the classroom and not to take others' things away and then destroy them.

After summer vacation, these rules soon were applied to his behavior in the whole school building. Six weeks later they applied to his instruction in all his subjects. By the end of December, any fighting on the school property was grounds for denying him "points." The chart shows that even after his interest in achievement suddenly declined in October after fall vacation, his hitting and breaking of others' things was relatively contained. From that time on, he resisted participating in any instruction other than vaulting and was involved only in things that had nothing to do with school. He became increasingly animal-like, inflexible, and inadvertently got into physical altercations with his classmates more and more often, thus the five absences during this period until the end of January. All the efforts of his teachers, his parents and the principal to get him to participate again seemed to make him all the more determined to swim against the current. He was about to be transferred to a special school for Developmental Assistance which his parents had agreed to but had not yet undertaken because his mother had been in the hospital and had not yet returned home.

At this point I need to talk about the timing which I mentioned earlier. In January, when I confronted him about not working, he said, "Why should I? I didn't fight and I didn't take things away from people and break them, so I'm allowed to do the vaulting." As a result, on the first of February I decided to risk totally changing the conditions for his participating in the vaulting. I did this in the classroom in front of a number of his classmates. I made it clear to him that his next vaulting lesson was his last unless he decided to work in all his school classes in four out of five days. How he behaved was irrelevant. Therefore, today was his final vaulting lesson. All his classmates, all his teachers and even I believed (about 90% certain) that today was his last lesson.

SUMMARY

In a video showing the "last" vaulting lesson with S on the horse, it shows how he almost immediately follows my requests twenty three times in a row. On the ride back to school in the car with the others, he quietly added the following remark to the chatter of the other children: "You'll see."

Suddenly on the next day of school, he began to work continuously from class to class. He was allowed to participate in the vaulting five weeks in a row. Then he had to take a break because of throwing sand but after that he started regularly eighteen times until the end of school. He behaved unobtrusively, radiated inner contentment, traded tender behaviors with his father (which he had not been able to do before), and was promoted to the third grade without comment.

Finally, here are a few words about the other five children, all of whom overcame similarly tense situations.
- **P** and **D** demonstrated first in vaulting and later in the classroom that they are with certainty not learning disabled.
- **A** was also spared being sent to the special school for Developmental Assistance.
- **M** stopped sucking his thumb, is more self confident in his schoolwork and expresses his own ideas and wants.

FINAL OBSERVATION
Remedial-education riding and vaulting (Healing Instructional Vaulting) is an exceptionally productive educational tool not only for special schools but also for regular school children. It is indispensable for any elementary school from a preventive point of view.

Reference: Ringbeck, B. (1990). *Heilpaedagogisches Reiten und Volti.* edited by Marianne Gaeng, Munich and Basel: E. Reinhard.

Antonio Kröger
Germany

EQUINE WORK-ABILITY EDUCATIONAL PROGRAM

Pegi Ryan, Director HWAC

One purpose of the Helen Woodward Animal Center in San Diego, California, is to bring animals and people together in a cooperative work/learning environment to enrich both man and animal. With this principle in mind the Center staff set out to explore the environment in and around the barn to see what programs could be offered and for whom to develop this cooperative learning concept.

Three high schools in the San Diego area contacted the Helen Woodward Animal Center regarding their "*work- ability*" programs (work training) to see if students could be trained in marketable job skills. The work-ability program, sponsored by the vocational education division, is a state-wide cooperative solution to assist students with disabilities to enter the work world. Schools screen applicants to work and be trained at particular job sites. The schools also pay the students a wage. This seemed like a viable program for the Center so for the past five years four students have been in training here each semester. Southern California is an area rich with horses, from backyard stables to public facilities to multimillion dollar race track training sites. It seemed there was a sure market needing properly prepared applicants.

In the Center's program students are trained primarily in barn skills so that they may enter the job market with good, safe, competitive skills. Each student is introduced to the barn animals, the equipment and safety procedures. They start out learning the skills of cleaning stalls since this is a major barn job. Every two students have a job coach, either a trained volunteer or one of our staff. The coach verbally goes over each task to be completed with the student. The coach then physically performs the task for the students. Next the coach and the students do the task together. Finally the coach watches the students and is there to answer questions that arise or to assist the student should a problem develop. Once basic skills are learned the coach then works on performance quality; finally he or she emphasizes quality work within a reasonable time frame. Students learn not to chat on the job, not to interrupt lessons, to ask questions when they need help, to put tools away correctly and to conform, as required by the job, in dress and attitude.

In the program, students come for 2 to 2½ hours at a time. Within that time frame they are given one fifteen minute break. Approximately one third of the time is spent on actual animal hands-on exploration. What is a horse, goat, sheep, burro? How are they alike? Different? We discuss how to safely move around the animals, to lead and handle them. Students practice these skills weekly. Grooming skills are learned and practiced. Weather permitting, students may also assist in bathing a horse. If the hot walker is working, students learn how to place the horse on it. In the last half hour of the student's stay, things taught are reviewed and how and why they are done at the center. During the semester appropriate behaviors are taught, and employment applications, forms, interviews, and dress codes are discussed. The program has worked well for the Center. Two to three times a week, four extra workers come. Many of the students have gone on to other "real" jobs from here. One, in fact, went on to work at Charlie Whittingham's race training facility.

In evaluating the program, it was felt that exposing the students to the various animals--burros, goats, and sheep--along with the horses, was good because many farms have a variety of animals. In fact, when the Center's equine hospital gets an occasional llama in for observation the students are exposed to the llamas as well. Continuing the evaluation it was found many students had the interest and desire to learn and work with horses, but many were extremely fearful and unsure around larger animals. They had very little prior exposure to horses, and farm animals. The very size and movement of the animals was intimidating and confusing. Therefore, it was decided that perhaps a pre-vocational class was necessary to expose students to various animals and their movements and behavior <u>before</u> the student reaches the "work-ability" age of junior and senior in high school. With such a class students would (hopefully) better understand and know for themselves if they would want to work in such an environment and if they would feel safe and comfortable. Also such a class would cut down on ultimate training time.

At present the Center is working with a middle school for children with severe learning handicaps. Five students come two times a month with three assistants to work for two hours with one of the staff in just such a pre-vocational program. The students are shown all the animals at the center, barn animals as well as rabbits, guinea pigs, birds, ferrets, dogs, cats. In each visit they are to introduced to work with a new animal--touching, feeling, leading (if applicable). If students show an interest but are frightened, then they work with the same animal for several visits to establish a comfort zone. Once a comfort zone is reached, related job skill is introduced. At first the task tends to be very removed from the animal, i.e., cleaning out the automatic watering troughs for the horses. This can be done through the pipe corrals without having to get near the horse, raking shed rows, or helping to mix a bran mash are other examples. The vocational skills, however, are not the main intent of this pre-vocational class, rather developing an interest level is sought.

The pre-vocational program for younger riders with learning disabilities has begun, during holidays and vacations. Not only do they receive more exposure to the horses but they can see and do jobs with the other animals as well. With such an overall exposure one student went on to volunteer at a pet store. For students working in this pre-vocational atmosphere it was found they have developed more confidence, and are more apt to approach and interact with people. Their communication skills have improved. At the same time, the Center receives extra help in regular maintenance chores. Eventually some of the riders have gone on to assist as big brother or sister with other youngsters during our summer camps. Others are now volunteers in the riding program. As for the children of the middle school, the same group of children are now coming for the second year. They too are more confident, much less fearful and take a much more active role in working with the animals.

The results of these vocational programs have encouraged the Center to work with Partnership With Industries (PWI), made up of clients from San Diego Regional Center and funded by the Department of Rehabilitation and Habilitation. There is now a contract with PWI to hire five disabled workers for year-round full-time employment. They clean stalls, watering troughs, keep the grounds raked and neat, level stalls, clean the goats' and burros' pens, the chicken coop, and duck pond. They feed the chickens, ducks and horses. They walk the horses, groom and bathe horses and in general perform all the duties a barn worker would. They have a PWI job coach (trained by the center to direct the workers) to assist them should they run into problems. They do the work well and always within the required safety standards.

In this arrangement both parties have benefitted. The Center has competent help paid at a rate that does not overly tax its budget, and a group of people who did not work before are gainfully employed. Before PWI clients are hired they must go through an interview with the director of the Center's therapeutic programs. If they "pass" the interview they must call in to the office to let the department know they have passed the interview and are ready for their jobs. Then they receive on-the-job training. If they repeatedly practice unsafe techniques that are dangerous to themselves, others, or the animals, they are subject to termination. Happily, however, many of these workers have gone on to placement in individual jobs in a competitive market.

The Center feels its vocational and pre-vocational programs definitely fulfill the stated goal of bringing animals and people together in a cooperative work/learning environment. The staff have learned how to be creative and flexible in their teaching. The Center has received assistance at a fraction of usual cost while students learn job skills, giving them confidence to compete in the job market. All parties have been enriched.

Helen Woodward Animal Center, P.O. Box 64, Rancho Sante Fe, CA 92067

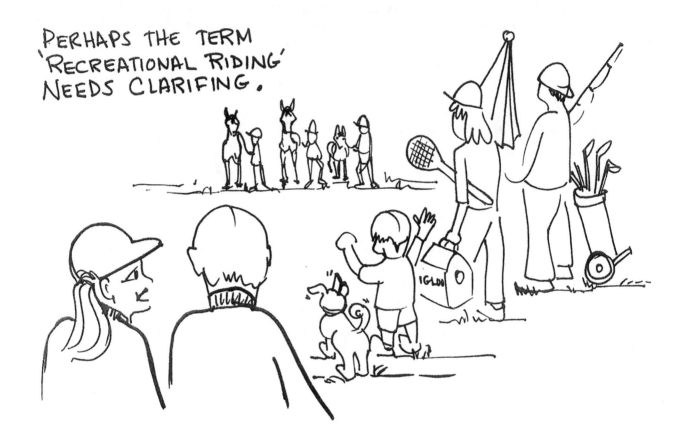

SENSORY INPUT THROUGH RIDING

Anita Shkedi, HV., SRN., Obs.

We need the company of animals. Animals serve to remind us that we are a part of nature. For many, without animals there is loss of intimacy and interest. People who live with animals are known to live longer, suffering less stress, often show a more stable neurophysical state. Man has created this contract with animals that has often become challenging and personal. No better example of this contract can be given than the relationship with a therapeutic riding horse.

Riding a horse can surpass many other methods of kinesiotherapy or neurophysiological treatments. Horseback riding is the finest method of coordination training. It is unsurpassed because of the challenging factor of motivation (Prof. D. Riede, 1990). The horse is a huge tactile moving surface. It is covered with millions of receptors stimulated by its own sensory interpretations. These receptors can give powerful sensory information through touch, vestibular and proprioception that are vital for motor development. When the human brain receives the correct sensory information, magic can often happen, stimulating endorphins, which allow our body to function as a whole.

Our senses are the very center of our being. If we lose the function or facility of one or more senses, then our body begins to lose certainty. To lose sense may mean to lose a fundamental organic mooring of identity. This means the loss of body ego, which is the basis of self (Oliver Sacks, 1983). The sensory stimulation from the horse passes through to all the human body receptors, sending corrective signals to the higher centers in the brain, improving speech, concentration, changing emotions and behaviour. Sensory impulses pass from the periphery, initiating the voluntary motor control loop that is the periphery to the cerebellum, parietal and frontal lobes and back to the periphery. This means that we can use the sensory stimulation from the moving horse to help people improve their memory, and to help them make judgements. This stimulation can also improve balance, equilibrium, coordinating and body awareness. These improvements lead to raise their self-esteem.

It has been well documented in sensory integration literature that the tactile, proprioceptive and vestibular stimuli are factors in motor development. (J. Ayers, 1983). The stimulation of tactile, proprioceptive and the vestibular impulses can easily be achieved by riding horseback.

TOUCH

The sense of touch can be explored to its limits when a rider contacts the horse. Touch receptors are within the skin which covers our body. Skin is so important that it is one of the first to evolve in uterine life. Touching a horse can motivate all types of responses, such as love, power, warmth, friendship, sexual fantasy and fear. When a rider sits on top of a horse, he or she uses more of his or her tactile skin receptors at once. Increasing the area stimulated by the skin receptors accentuates all of the feeling responses.

Recently, I have been working with a blind and deaf child. While teaching Joey how to ride a horse, I saw him become powerful and motivated. As he progressed, we increased the pace and speed of the horse, he became euphoric with the feeling of fast movement. Joey, with his severe sensory loss, had poor posture, balance and was introverted. His idea of movement was often wrong. The improvement came when Joey took up the reins and started to ride. He found that if he squeezed the horse with his legs it would move forward.

Joey became attached to the horse's mouth with his hands that held the reins. He found that when he pulled the reins, he could stop the horse. This discovery motivated him to develop riding skills and to understand what it was to move forward. Joey began to feel powerful with this new control. He began to sit balanced, to coordinate his movements, and feel confident with his raised self-esteem. It was because of what he had gained through riding that I had the pleasure of seeing this little boy run fast across a large field to reach his horse.

VESTIBULAR

The vestibular system is extremely complex since it interacts with all the other sensory systems. It gives us the mechanism that makes it possible for us to stand up against gravity and to orient us in space. The vestibular system is particularly sensitive to bone vibrations. It, therefore, interacts very closely with the proprioceptive system. Today we see many people with disabilities who have become motor-inactive and, therefore, their brains may not be receiving sufficient or correct vestibular impulses. When this occurs, the systems, which depend on vestibular information may show additional deficits. We now know that if we stimulate the dysfunctional brain with the correct sensory impulses given through different, new and uncommon forms of exercise, the brain can find new pathways, and new motor programs. When the person with a disability rides a horse, he or she may feel the three dimensional rhythmic movements of the horses. This is a new and excellent way for a motor-inactive person to be stimulated by the vestibular system.

A young man, John, received a severe head injury caused by a car accident. Three years later he began horseback riding for therapy. Before he started riding, he was unable to stand alone or to sit up unassisted. He suffered from muscle spasms and tight adductor muscles. We used the technique of hippotherapy, a method that allows the rider to move with the rhythm of the horse. We can achieve considerable success with this technique.

John rode on a large German-bred horse. He sat directly on its back and held on by two handles fitted to a leather strap in front of him (a vaulting roller). This allowed the close contact with the horse and its movement. The close contact had many effects, one of which was to release the spasms in his hips and legs. The three-dimensional movements stimulated and strengthened his back and neck muscles. Continuing the therapy, John began to balance without using his hands. The benefits away from the horse were as pleasing. He began to move his legs and started trying to walk to his wheel chair. He was attempting to develop a functional gait, thus making him less reliant on others. Family members responded to this progress by adding rails to the walls at home so he could walk around the house alone. John is still receiving riding therapy and the whole family loves the horse.

PROPRIOCEPTION

Proprioception, which is sometimes called the "secret sense," comes from all the sense receptors in the bones, muscles, and joints. It is the sensory information from the receptors in contracting and stretching muscles, and the bending, straightening and compression of the joints between the bones. This gives us a constant awareness of the position of our trunk and limbs. Without proprioception the body becomes, so to speak, blind and deaf to itself. Often a person with paraplegia will describe the experience of sitting in the cinema and putting his or her hand on the wrong leg - the leg of the person in the next seat. Without proprioception our bodies become clammy, slower, disembodied, and without ego.

As the horse moves in rhythmic movements at all paces, the rider picks up a continual flow of information through all the movements and speed. Downward transition through the paces adds to the sensory exercise, improving posture, balance, coordination, concentration, and equilibrium reactions.

Riders who have suffered traumatic head injuries may be suffering from movement deficiency or perhaps are lacking the correct concept of movement patterns. To make this point, I quote Professor Reide, saying they would have passed through the stages of low performance, intuitive consciousness of the disorder, strategy of avoidance - lack of training resulting in insufficiency. Motivating psychic and motor stimulation are needed to break the vicious circle. We need interesting motor tasks that will challenge our brains and underutilize motor programs (D. Riede, 1990).

When these people begin horseback riding, they become motivated. The motivating psychic and motor stimulation break the vicious circle of low performance. Horseback riding creates motor tasks that do exactly what is wanted in asking the brain for the revival of motor programs. As the rider progresses, he learns riding technique and skill. He or she tries to improve his or her style. The horse will respond positively to this sensory contact and correction. The results are not just seen while riding. Away from the horse, the person has personality changes, losing many of their unconventional behaviors.

This success with riding therapy applies to many other types of disabilities, especially to our children with spastic cerebral palsy or those with learning disabilities. Experts in modern kinesiotherapy techniques would say "The correct riding position asked for is in line with all the well-known techniques for balance exercises that stabilize a person's trunk and improve posture."

Riding therapy adds to the Bobath technique by using the exciting factor of motivation. A fourteen year-old girl came to therapy four years ago. She had quadriplegia cerebral palsy and she was deaf. She dribbled a great deal, had poor communication skills and a poor attention span. At the age of ten years she had no ability to balance. Riding therapy involved an army of volunteers to keep her on the horse. Nevertheless, with continual perseverance by everyone, she gradually found balance. After two years she was riding alone. At this point, she had to return to the orthopedic surgeon to arrange for an operation to lengthen adductor muscles. The orthopedic surgeon said it was no longer necessary, due to the successful stretching taking place while riding. The girl began to take part in riding competitions. This increased her motivation to ride well. The results have motivated her to continue to show improvements. She can now canter independently and wins in competitions.. She has learned to concentrate, to express her self, and to walk, and now she feels good about herself. Her family is proud of her. She has become an independent person.

MOTIVATION

I would like to take the theory of sensory information through riding a little further. Sensory receptors develop in all forms of life from the time the creature evolves. In humans this development begins within the first weeks of uterine life. Therefore, sensory receptors are clearly essential for the survival of all forms of life. Deep in the ocean the nautilus sea snail has managed to survive in its original form since prehistoric times. It has survived by adapting its sensory system to its harsh environment.

Primitive man had a high ability of sensory awareness. He was well balanced in his neurophysical state. This was essential and kept him healthy. Primitive man had limited needs. His activities were concerned with collecting food, looking for shelter and reproduction. Life progressed at a slow pace, was based on his instincts and was controlled by his sensory awareness. Later the call for adaptation came. Changes had to be made more rapidly. The power of reasoning took over from the slow instinctive behavior. An imbalance began to occur between the neuro and physical state. This was the end of our fine physical specimen. We became a thinking creature - many of whom are out of shape (F.M. Alexander, 1923).

The motivating therapy of horseback riding can cross the reasoning mind and apply itself to our instinctive behaviour. The horse relies on its senses for survival. It responds to clear sensory information given by a keen rider. In turn, the rider responds well to the feeling of successful riding. This positive communication finds its way to the rider's feeling of love, power and fantasy that are within the subconscious. As instructors or therapists, we can use this knowledge to help many people with various types of disabilities, especially the mentally confused, or the child with delayed development. Sensory stimulation from the horse passes through the primitive brain to activate a person's instincts.

A three-year-old child came for riding therapy. Sarah had obvious delays in her development. The primitive reflexes prevented her from crawling and standing. She had no eye contact nor did she show any obvious signs of communication. The child was always screaming, and if not, she was playing with her fingers. During the first lessons, it was difficult to keep her on the pony. Everything went to her mouth including the reins, volunteers' arms or the odd sun hat. At first, I had to fix her hips, to sit her on the felt saddle over the pony's back. We walked the pony up and down the hill and through the grove. The results began to happen. At first, she started to rock with the horse's movement. After a few lessons she stopped screaming and began to smile. Now when she came to the pony, she showed excitement with her whole body. There are definite change in her neuro-physical state. She began to stand and then after a few months, she could walk with her parent's help.

Sarah does not use words but uses primitive social communication skills that were developed using food rewards by the parents. As riding therapy continued, she began to recognize her pony and the riding school. The child continued to increase her balance and coordination. Abnormal reflex activity began to decrease. After one year of riding, Sarah can sit independently on the pony. She can hold the reins when requested. Eye contact can be maintained and she follows simple commands. Sarah can walk alone, enjoys music and takes an interest in the world around her. Screams and finger play has stopped.

Man will never achieve a better partnership than the one he or she can have with animals. Man still has to reach a higher standard of reasoning before he or she can understand this. After years of service to man, the horse may be leading the way in showing us that it has the unusual ability to unlock and release new pathways in our brain. New pathways are essential to rebalance and improve the quality of our life.

References:
Alexander F.M. (1923) *Constructive Conscious Control of the Individual.* Gollancz Paperbacks, London
Ayres, AJ. (1983). *Sensory Integration and the child.* Western Psychological Services, Los Angeles, CA.
Riede, D. (1990). *Physical therapy on the horse.* (distributed by The Delta Society, WA., USA.
        Originally published in German as *Therapeutisches Reiten im der Krankengymnastik,* 1986.
Sacks, 0. (1985). *The man who mistook his wife for a hat* Picador Edition, published by Pan Books, London)

Anita Shkedi,
Israel

CHAPTER 25

RECREATIONAL THERAPY, RECREATION AND LEISURE

THE APPLICATION OF RECREATIONAL THERAPY PRINCIPLES IN THERAPEUTIC RIDING

Gloria Hamblin, RRT

Recreational therapy uses participation in leisure activities to improve functional behavior and physical condition in clients while giving them the opportunity to acquire skills and knowledge. Therapeutic riding blends elements of therapy and education into a fun recreational activity which includes a living creature - the horse. Ultimately, the goal is to use horses and riding as a vehicle by which clients challenge themselves to achieve their potential. The objective could be improved physical fitness, better socialization skills, or independent recreational riding. Ideally it could be all of these together, producing an increase in self-esteem, control, and freedom.

Therapeutic horseback riding is but one aspect of recreational therapy, which includes a wide variety of pursuits from bowling to painting to drama. According to the National Therapeutic Recreation Society, "The purpose of therapeutic recreation is to facilitate the development, maintenance, and expression of an appropriate leisure lifestyle for individuals with physical, mental, emotional, or social limitations" (NTRS, 1982). To do this, the therapist designs programs with one or more goals:
1. Therapy--to improve functional behaviors.
2. Leisure education--to expose the client to activities allowing them to gain new knowledge and skills.
3. Recreation participation--to generate voluntary involvement in recreational activities.

These goals, while generally pursued simultaneously, are emphasized to different degrees at different times, depending on the needs and abilities of the client. In therapeutic riding the goals of each session will be tailored to each client by talking with parents, caretakers, doctors, teachers or other therapists, and, most importantly, with the client himself. An appropriate treatment program can then be set up, implemented, and periodically assessed.

A recreational therapist in a therapeutic riding program, may work with clients who are at the lower levels of functional ability, such as persons with brain injuries who live in a group home setting. In this situation the therapist may need to work on appropriate group interaction and socialization skills in order to conduct a productive group lesson. This would be in addition to teaching basic riding, grooming, and stable management skills. The client will learn to participate in a group lesson, and to visit with the volunteers in a socially acceptable manner. He may also work to increase physical stamina and balance by gradually increasing the time spent on horseback and the number and difficulty of the exercises he performs. As he continues to ride, an improvement in his control of the horse may also be observed.

As the client progresses and possibly is discharged from the group home to his family or to live independently, the goal of leisure education comes into focus. Now the client may have questions about equestrian events in his new neighborhood or need a referral to another riding program or regular riding stable. Where can he continue to learn about horses, horse shows, clinics, trail rides, or horse clubs that are available to him? He may well need continued guidance.

The last goal area mentioned is recreation participation, and would here refer to recreational riding or riding as sport. This includes participation in horse shows, trail rides, or lessons. These can occur in a therapeutic riding program or can be found at a regular training stable. The disabled client who is high functioning may come to a program just to learn to ride. He then progressively challenges himself to ride better and gain more knowledge.

It is clear that the three goals: therapy, leisure education, and recreational activity overlap a great deal and are often sought concurrently. A client who has had a stroke illustrates the model of the three areas of service well. A 55 year old man began riding eight months after a stroke left him with hemiplegia. He was naturally withdrawn and depressed about his condition. He had been forced to sell the business he had run all his life. He began to ride at weekly intervals with a leader and two sidewalkers, and to speak of his early twenties when he rode frequently and received a good bit of instruction. He progressed to riding independently and no longer needed a cane to walk. He learned about a horse science program at a local community college where he enrolled. The stables and horses became his avocation. He assisted the program where he rode by training new volunteers and often oriented new disabled riders. He purchased his own horse which he now cares for independently and has received an AA degree. It is easy to see that he has adjusted well to his disability and his leisure time is full and rewarding.

Ken Mobily (1985) in the *Therapeutic Recreation Journal* concludes that therapeutic recreation practitioners should "induce in their clients perceptions of control, responsibility and freedom". Showing clients the choices available and encouraging them to become self motivated, the recreational therapist who works in a riding program can offer the rider a myriad of benefits, from improved physical enhancement to social skills. Using therapy, leisure education and recreational activity, people with disabilities can be helped to achieve their fullest potential, increasing not only their own physical abilities and riding skills, but also their sense of self-esteem and independence.

References:
Mobily, K.E. 1985. A Philosophical Analysis of Therapeutic Recreation: What does it mean to say "We Can Be Therapeutic"? part 2, *Therapeutic Recreation Journal*, 18, no. 2, 2.
Approved by the Board of Directors of the National Branch of the National Recreation and Parks Association May 1982. NTRS. (1982)

RECREATIONAL RIDING

Barb J. Brock, PhD

Lance, disabled from a parachute jump six years ago, had not been involved in <u>any</u> physically challenging activity since the accident. He rode for six months in a therapeutic riding program. After gaining the skills to ride, he then quit the program, began to attend weight-lifting classes and signed up for white-water rafting trips. For Lance, the riding had been a means to another end .

Chin, disabled with polio, was told by many doctors that he would lose his ability to walk. To conclude his six months of riding, Chin led his horse to the arena, mounted, and with only a small amount of assistance, galloped away. He did not continue to ride with the next program. He had proven something to himself, and walked away with a grin on his face.

Pat, Chip, Diana, Lori, Steve, Lonnie, Jay, and many others also needed exercise, therapy, and confidence, but continued to harbor an interest in riding. The most important reason they continued to ride was "just for the fun of it." They enjoyed horses and the freedom felt from being in command, having the wind in their hair and the dust in their boots. They always arrived a little early to watch and assist with preparation and stayed a little longer to pet and groom their horses.

There are no statistics in the literature on the number of disabled persons who are recreational riders, "just for the fun of it." However, participation statistics have been extrapolated from the records of outcomes with disabled winter skiers with some agreement among equestrians. Approximately 2% to 5% of disabled skiers choose to enter into some form of competition, 25% drop out of the program, and 70% continue to ski for a variety of reasons (Cogley, 1989). Similar estimates might be made among disabled riders. Of one hundred riders, five may go on to seriously compete, 25 may go on to other recreational pursuits, and about 70 may continue to ride, if the opportunity exists, "just for the fun of it."

The beauty and benefits of **recreational riding** for persons with disabilities should not be taken lightly nor overlooked. In teaching an activity, i.e., riding, cooking, camping, swimming, sewing, or reading, if one teacher becomes caught up in the singular goal of "accomplishment", students may miss out on a wealth of positive side effects from the activity. For example, to teach cooking, aside from basics of measuring, heating, and combining ingredients, one should also teach how to arrange a plate, how to combine colors, how to use textures, how much fun it is to sneak a taste, and how great one will feel when others benefit from the learned skill. Likewise, to teach a fitness activity such as running or swimming, one must be aware of not just teaching the skill, but also the dozens of benefits associated with that skill.

Benefits in therapeutic riding may not only be mastery of riding and fitness, but also freedom, weight loss, relaxation, social skills, fresh air, a change of pace, competition, self-confidence, stress relief, or many others. The positive side effects of learning to ride are many and varied. Some of those "other" benefits from horseback riding are documented from as far back as 5th century B.C. It is written that Greek athletes would place those with disabling conditions on the backs of champion horses following the Olympic Games. It was reported to cheer their spirits, and improve mental and physical well-being. (Encyclopedia of the Horse, 1973). Physical, intellectual, and emotional benefits have been reported and documented by riding therapists.

intellectual, and emotional benefits have been reported and documented by riding therapists. Speech, sensory integration, social skills, strength, coordination, verbal skills, and self-esteem have improved as a result of riding programs (Brock, 1987).

After the skills of riding a horse are gained, after strength and coordination improves, after self-esteem and confidence have grown, and after many doors have been opened for the rider to expand his talents, the singular motive that keeps most participants riding is not the benefit of therapy or the ecstasy of successful competition, but simply the joy of riding.

> *"Those who continue to ride, win...even if ribbons are not the reward,*
> *something greater is. One thing that all disabled riders will attest*
> *to is this: any limitation experienced in daily living is lost in the*
> *thrill of commanding the movements of a 1,000 pound (plus) animal of*
> *grace, beauty, and power" (Williams, 1985).*

Aside from gaining strength, coordination, and muscle control from use of the horse purely as a therapeutic tool, and aside from the keen confidence developed in advanced levels of horsemanship and competition, there is something more that attracts most of the disabled riders. The lack of limitations and barriers, development of friends among fellow riders and volunteers alike, feelings of control, love and warmth of the friendly beast underneath, and the powerful sense of freedom of direction and movement are usually enough incentive for most disabled persons to continue to ride.

There are many wonderful and "right" ways to teach and offer therapeutic horseback riding programs. The beauty of creativity and the fun of spontaneity need to play a part in each class as well as expert instruction and therapy. Don't forget, ALL riders need to have fun!

> *"Sometimes the best thing for us to do is*
> *to "get them out there" and let the horse take over!"*

Reference

Encyclopedia of the Horse. (1973). New York: Viking Press. 130-131.

Brock, B. (1978). *Effects of Therapeutic Horseback Riding on Physically Disabled* Adults. Dissertation. Indiana University.

Cogley, J. (1989). Personal Communication. October 20.

Williams, M. (1985). Personal Communication. June 30.

CHAPTER 26

DEVELOPMENTAL RIDING THERAPY

DEVELOPMENTAL RIDING THERAPY: HISTORY AND EVOLUTION

Jan Spink, MA

HISTORY AND EVOLUTION OF THE NEW HARMONY SYSTEM

Riding therapy (health care or treatment focus) in rehabilitation has an interesting and complex history. This chapter describes how therapeutic riding has evolved nationally and internationally over the past twenty five years. An understanding of the historical foundations, the strengths and the limitations of various approaches, is necessary to appreciate the need for and the components of Developmental Riding Therapy (D.R.T.[Sm]).

THE FIRST 25 YEARS: THE UNITED STATES, BRITAIN, AND WEST GERMANY

The first twenty-five years of therapeutic riding in North America were characterized by enthusiasm, dedication, and devotion to the often quoted phrase, "The outside of a horse is good for the inside of a man." (Ogilviy, 1869). In response, numerous programs and philosophies of riding therapy were developed and offered to a wide range of clients. Like most evolutionary fields, however, it was also characterized by an overall dearth of definition, use of loosely applied terminology, and evidence of high variability in areas of quality control, professional training, and competence.

In response to these circumstances, a comprehensive review and comparative analysis of therapeutic riding in the United States, Great Britain, and West Germany was conducted (Spink, 1982). All three countries had been using the horse specifically to benefit the person with disabilities for about twenty-five years. The review focused primarily on medical and psychological treatment techniques that used horseback riding as a therapeutic medium. Also investigated were the elements of educational and sport programs and whether client placement within these programs was appropriate for client needs. Five western German programs from the Kuratorium of Therapeutic Riding (1985) were studied thoroughly to identify characteristics and dimensions of interest in riding therapy. Also included were on-site reviews of Britain's two most recognized riding programs for the disabled. A similar review of five long-standing and representative American programs was also conducted. A total of twelve programs were included in the review.

The reviewer assumed the importance of defining competency-based models to guide professional development and structured approaches to client evaluation and treatment. It was apparent from this study that only the Germans had developed a set of structured educational standards to guide the activities of professionals in the field of riding therapy. In fact, as early as 1970, a basic model delineating three areas most relevant to their country's operation had been defined. These areas were Medicine, Education, and Sport.

Because sub-specialty areas linked to clearly defined treatment approaches were described early, the Germans attracted to the field many professionals (physicians, psychologists, special educators and physical therapists) who were interested in integrating equestrian activities with rehabilitation. Systematic study of the outcomes of riding therapy ensued, as many of these professionals used their associations with universities and teaching hospitals to conduct studies to further a scientific understanding of the method (Laban Centre). This enabled therapeutic riding to be recognized in Germany as a valid treatment option in medicine, psychology and education. As a result, the emerging field in that country was operating successfully under a standardized structure by 1982. It had also yielded a variety of replicable treatment methods for specific disorders such as multiple sclerosis and scoliosis, to name just two (Heipertz, 1981).

The United States and Great Britain appeared to have no structured visual schematic to help frame or guide the early development and organization of riding therapy. The initial appeal of equine use to benefit the disabled seemed to be greater for lay-horsemen and riding instructors than for professionals in medicine, education and psychology. Consequently, therapeutic riding in these two countries developed more as a recreational or adapted group sport activity rather than as a specific remedial or treatment activity.

Even in view of the lack of structure, a handful of professionals in both Great Britain and the United States entered the field initially out of a desire to blend their clinical training with their personal interests in equestrian activities. Unfortunately, these individuals did not have the benefit of specialty training in using the horse as

Original German Model

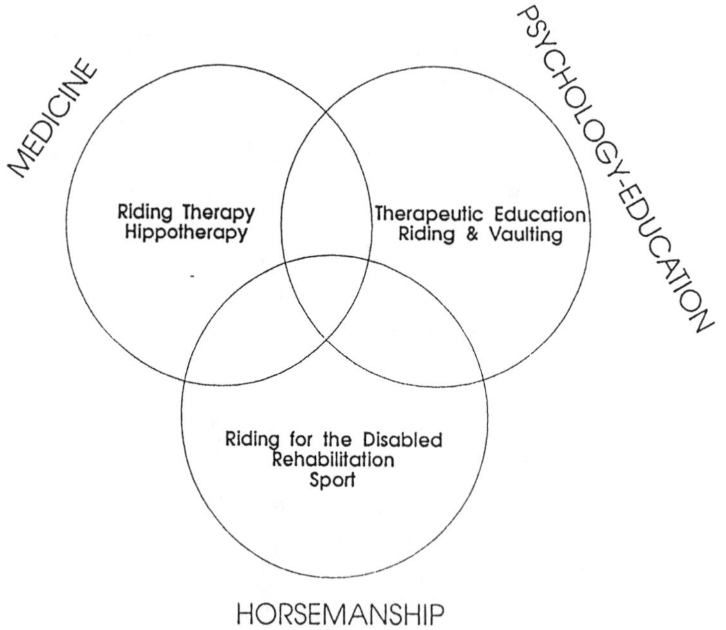

Heipertz, 1981.

FIGURE. 1
THREE-CIRCLE GERMAN MODEL

a therapeutic agent. In most cases they were working in isolation and without support from a substantive, national knowledge base. However, in spite of the lack of available training programs, relevant clinical literature, and mentors, innovative and creative approaches were developed. These simply were not substantiated by systematic study, training or research.

The 1982 review yielded several specific areas that potentially could improve the quality of programs in the United States and Great Britain. These directions for improvement were projected to foster structure for training programs and competence of professional personnel. The following goals were recommended:

a) Creation of competency-based training curricula with definite structures for professional development.
b) Promotion of specific treatment choices and techniques based on legitimate rationales.
c) Development of strategies for reliable clinical evaluation and data collection.
d) Specification of protocols for horse selection, training, and development as related to specialty areas (Spink, 1982).

A concerted effort was initiated in order to promote competency-based, organizational approaches similar to the German model. This desire to educate professionals prompted a series of technical papers and presentations across Europe, Canada, and the United States including:

- Hamburg, Germany: American progress in therapeutic riding was reported at the Fourth International Congress On Therapeutic Riding (Glasow and Spink, 1982).

- Milan, Italy: A presentation regarding progress in the vaulting field was given at the Fifth International Congress On Therapeutic Riding (Spink, 1985).

- Vancouver, British Columbia. An overview paper promoting specialization and competency-based approaches was given at the Delta Society Annual Meeting (Spink, 1987). This paper supported adopting a new, specifically defined four-phase model for therapeutic riding. This model included the areas of Medicine, Education, and Sport as identified by the German Kuratorium of Therapeutic Riding in 1977. It also included one more area, psychomotricity, an area previously unknown in therapeutic riding in the United States. However, it enjoy a respected history in France and Italy.

- Toronto, Ontario: This paper supported the same theme and recommended that American and Canadian therapeutic riding organizations adopt the expanded, four-phase construct in order to attract a wider array of clinical professionals. It was presented at the Sixth International Congress On Therapeutic Riding (Spink, 1988).

- Houston, Texas: The final paper in this series presented more detail about the creation of theoretical structure and methodology that embody the systems approach called Developmental Riding Therapy. It was presented as the McCulloch Memorial Lecture at the Annual Meeting of the Delta Society. (Spink, 1990). Although most American programs had become familiar with the basic three-phase German construct by 1988, the need to develop and incorporate other professional disciplines to expand the organizational construct was emphasized in the later presentations. A structured model for integrating other disciplines into a schema of riding therapy was the result.

The overall goal for these presentations was to inform practicing and incumbent professionals of the potential treatment scope and broad applicability the horse offers to clients with special needs. A more comprehensive model and treatment system were expected to facilitate significant understanding and recognition of specific equine-assisted therapies such as Developmental Riding Therapy as a legitimate rehabilitation approach. By

equine-assisted therapies such as Developmental Riding Therapy as a legitimate rehabilitation approach. By standardizing treatment techniques and quantifying the objectives and goals of client intervention, the field hoped to attract the interest of researchers and clinicians alike.

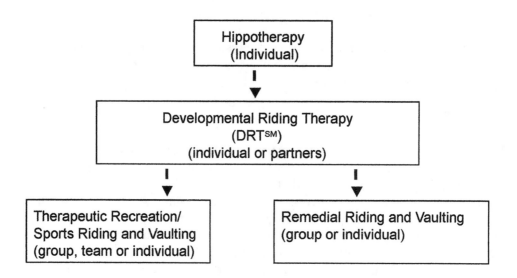

FIGURE 2.
FLOW CHART APPROACH FOR CLIENT PLACEMENT IN PROGRAM

The need for credible, empirical research focusing on the therapeutic application of the horse is acute in North America. The organizational model proposed was expected to influence a positive trend toward more systematic study and more formalized, university-based, training. The increasing demand for training and certification programs in the medical, psychomotor, and educative use of the horse reflects an appreciation for the diverse applications. Attracting a wide array of skilled professionals from medicine, physical, occupational and speech therapy, rehabilitation/ psychomotricity, psychology, clinical social work, special education, and adapted physical education would strengthen the foundations of the entire field and help ensure its future viability.

The addition of psychomotricity as the fourth specialty area is intended to stimulate further professional expansion and client treatment opportunities. In D.R.T.^{Sm}, the basic tenets of psychomotricity have been synthesized to yield an innovative and eclectic systems approach. The approach incorporates treatment techniques previously unavailable in either classic hippotherapy or remedial riding and vaulting. It invites the participation of six health or education professions which previously had limited formal involvement or recognition within the field. These specific fields are occupational therapy, rehabilitation or psychomotricity, speech therapy, special education and psychology.

Attracting occupational therapists who are trained in sensory integration as well as in developmental and psychological domains is important to the process of D.R.T.^{Sm}. This system also provides a properly defined area of practice for psychomotorical or rehabilitation specialists who have graduate level training in psychology, movement, and mind/body integration techniques. Speech and Language pathologists are included here because of their advanced training in language development, speech production, and cognitive re-education. Special educators and psychologists, with their training in affective and cognitive development as well as therapeutic intervention strategies, are also integrated. The following schematic illustrates how all the various professions can be viewed within one broad field.

AN ESTIMATION OF SUB-SPECIALIZATIONS IN THE THERAPEUTIC RIDING FIELD

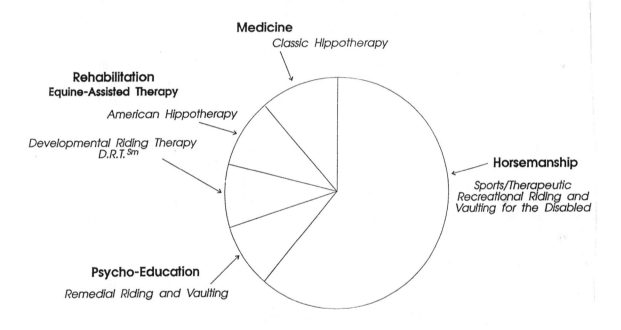

Copyright 1992 Spink.

FIGURE 3.
THE PIE GRAPH

The contribution of each specialty area has been estimated for this illustration. Currently, there is no information available to accurately assess current (or desirable) contributions from individual professions. An important direction for the future might be to identify the optimal mix of these professions to ensure quality programming. Until then, it is assumed that the needs of each client dictate the prescription for an individualized mix of contributing professional expertise. The next section of this chapter details the concepts of psychomotricity and rehabilitation. Traditional theory and methodology which influenced the development of this specialty use of the horse are chronologically described. Finally, the new American treatment approach termed Developmental Riding Therapy (D.R.T.[Sm]) is outlined. This therapeutic approach is organized within a comprehensive framework that New Harmony Foundation refers to as the New Harmony System of D.R.T.[Sm].

PSYCHOMOTRICITY: HISTORY AND DEFINITION

Psychomotricity is a psycho-medical specialty area which was developed in the late 1940'S in response to the need to treat motor disorders that were not caused by neurological trauma or lesions (Barwick, 1986). Official recognition was granted in 1963 when the French Ministry of Education began to require training at the graduate level and certification for psychomotor therapists. Psychomotricity has evolved significantly since that time.

Sylvie Barwick, a French psychomotor therapist practicing in England, clearly describes the theoretical basis of psychomotricity when she writes:

> "Unlike most other medical or psychological professions whose approach tends to consider either physical or psychological symptoms, psychomotricity concerns the progressive development of both the psyche and the soma and their interaction under the influence of organic maturation and social stimuli. It considers the individual in his psychosomatic entirety thus rejecting the traditional dichotomy between "mind" and "body" stemming from Cartesian philosophy. It reunites man within himself and observes him in action with his environment. It aims at building an individual whose healthy psychomotor development reflects his mental and physical ease and harmony." (Barwick, 1986)

There are many therapeutic applications and modalities used in the field. Related expressive therapies employed by psychomotor or rehabilitation specialists include art, dance and drama approaches. Psychomotricity also incorporates various popular approaches to movement such as those developed by Laban (Laban Center, England), Alexander (1985), Feldenkrais (1981), and Ayres (1974). Clearly, this comprehensive specialty which integrates emotion with language development and movement experience/education can be applied to the field of therapeutic riding.

HISTORY AND PHILOSOPHY

In the developmental phases of riding therapy, especially in the United States and Great Britain, it appeared that selected types of clients were not receiving optimal benefits from group recreational riding sessions, hippotherapy, or remedial group vaulting or riding. Most of these clients experienced specific deficits in the following areas: learning, language, behavior, sensory integration and visual perception and movement quality. What is now formalized as Developmental Riding Therapy (D.R.T.[Sm]) began as an effort to blend movement principles from classic hippotherapy with developmental positions and sequences.

It also incorporated specific perceptual-motor, cognitive, and affective development skills in order to meet the needs of these particular clients. A surcingle was used as it allowed the client more freedom of movement on the horse. Initially, the approach was referred to as developmental vaulting, a form of riding therapy. The objectives of the approach were strictly therapeutic and therefore quite different from those established in programs of sports or gymnastic vaulting (Spink, 1985).

In the early 1980's, programs throughout the United States began to include developmental vaulting as a method. Instructors and therapists incorporated various isolated movements and exercises and began to use a surcingle and pad instead of a saddle to facilitate movement while astride. It appeared, however, that the concepts on which developmental vaulting was based were not being as thoroughly integrated as the specific techniques.

This left practitioners ill-prepared to coordinate and combine these specialized techniques to create individualized programs for clients. There also appeared to be incomplete rationale for equipment selection and modification of activities. The overall tendency was to develop an emphasis on the isolated motor tasks which most resembled traditional vaulting. In addition, there seemed to have been a breakdown in practitioners' abilities to interpret and integrate techniques which specifically addressed cognition, affect and perceptual-motor skills. Subsequently, the original holistic theory and complex methodology of developmental vaulting had been unintentionally fragmented and not applied as an integrated treatment system.

In order to correct any confusing resemblance to gymnastic vaulting and to clarify the goal of rehabilitation through riding therapy, the specialty approach was re-named the New Harmony System of Developmental Riding Therapy (D.R.T.[Sm]) in 1987. New Harmony's primary project focus is to develop and test methodology and techniques in therapeutic riding and treat clients with specific central nervous system disorders. The Foundation's multi-purpose, non-profit educational programs also serve to provide national and international exchange in various fields of study such as psychomotricity and the human-animal bond.

A FOUR PHASE MODEL FOR US THERAPEUTIC RIDING:
a progressive model for physicians, therapists,
educators, and riding instructors

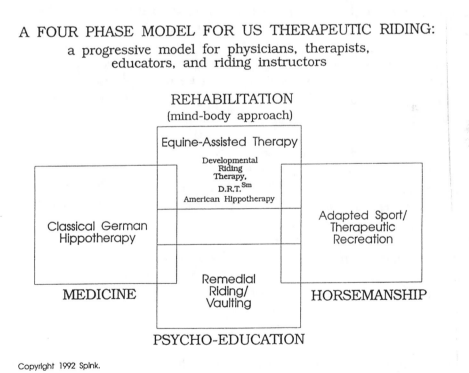

FIGURE 4.
THE NEW HARMONY FOUR-PHASE CONSTRUCT

This newly integrated approach is an evolutionary hybrid which preserves its psychomotoric integrity but extends its attention to other client systems as well. New Harmony utilizes the U.S. Patent and Trade Commission's protocol for service marks (Sm) which signify and protect methodological uniqueness of service areas. Figure 4. represents the New Harmony four phase construct for therapeutic riding. Here, D.R.T.Sm lies within a continuum, between the medical application of the horse (hippotherapy), psycho-education (remedial riding/vaulting), and horsemanship (sport/therapeutic recreational riding/vaulting for the disabled). The New Harmony system is distinct because of the population it serves and the inclusion of six mandatory elements which embody its definitive approach. The movement and horse handling components are derived in part from the movement principles of classic hippotherapy.

The fundamental, prerequisite elements are as follows:
1) Individual or partner sessions with active therapist input.
2) The use of developmental positions on the horse which directly correlate with specifically controlled movement challenges from the horse.
3) Development of the inter-relationships of the client, therapist and horse.
4) Specific adaptations in selection of equipment.
5) Selected components of riding and vaulting skills.
6) The use of equine-adapted, purposeful activities.

(Spink, 1990).

Hippotherapy is a method which focuses on benefiting clients who have mild to severe movement dysfunction from a purely medical or physical rehabilitation orientation. D.R.T.Sm is different in that it is distinctly designed to address clients with deficits in learning, language, behavior, cognition, and/or general movement competency. D.R.T.Sm can be a complement to hippotherapy or a much needed transition between these specific medical techniques and the group work which characterizes psycho-education and sport or therapeutic recreation. It also serves as an entry point for clients whose skills are not yet developed enough for remedial group riding or gymnastic vaulting.

To become a capable developmental riding therapist, one must demonstrate accurate clinical judgment, keen awareness, and a strong equestrian background. A text called *Developmental Riding Therapy: The Horse in Psycho-motoric and Psycho-education*Sm will be available by 1992 which will specifically detail the use of the specialty system. Candidates for training in the system must already possess entry-level professional credentials at the graduate level in one of the following five fields:
1. Psychomotricity/rehabilitation therapy.
2. Special education with training in movement approaches.
3. Educational, clinical, counseling psychology or neuro-psychology, and/or licensed clinical social work, with training in movement approaches.
4. Speech therapy.
5. Occupational therapy (O.T.R. or O.T.R.\L).

Developmental riding therapy requires significant skill in the areas of dressage, specialized horse handling techniques, and basic vaulting. Mastery of a standardized set of horsemanship competencies is mandatory to qualify as a developmental riding therapist. It requires considerable professional dedication to devote the time necessary to understand the complex marriage of theory, ideology, and methodology embodied in this specialty approach. A significant amount of personal recreational time must be devoted to dressage, as necessary riding skills need to be maintained and/or developed to a minimum of **first level dressage**.

New Harmony aims to provide systematic, competency-based training programs for professional specialists who want to use the horse as a treatment agent. More thoroughly trained professionals yield better treatment opportunities as well as improved treatment results for clients. Selectively developed horses also greatly enhance quality control as the field evolves. Finally, it is projected that the combination of all these factors will attract increased interest in the study of outcomes achieved from combining carefully screened clients, systematically trained therapists and selectively developed horses within a structured system of treatment in which horses are the medium.

A DEVELOPMENTAL RIDING THERAPY SESSION
Profile #3
Name: Felicia
Age: 7

General Diagnosis: Central Nervous System Dysfunction
Present Level of Performance

I. **Sensation, Perception, and Motricity**:
Felicia has a mild decrease in tone (hypotonia) mostly in her trunk and upper extremities. She has a very subtle hand tremor in some fine motor activities. She appears dyspraxic when running, skipping, and hopping. There is evidence of proximal instability throughout her shoulder girdle during movements involving upper extremities. Equilibrium reactions are slightly delayed. [Sm]

II. **Cognition:**
Felicia has above average verbal skills but has delayed performance skills. Standardized testing reports indicate hat she has visual perceptual problems in the realm of spatial relationships and form constancy. She appears to have some attention deficits. She also has some mild articulation problems in a structured, screened environment.

III. **Affect:**
Felicia displays some mild impulsivity and verbal inappropriateness during physical activity. This may be an adaptive avoidance technique she employs in order to control her environment and some underlying apprehension about physical challenges. She has considerable difficulty with staying in the moment. She is constantly talking about what is next or later versus what is being done right now, even if her safety depends on her awareness of what is happening currently.

Treatment Outline
    I. Sensation, Perception, and Motricity:
        A. Target Goals
            Bilateral Control
            Static and Dynamic Balance
            Motor Planning

B. Strategies
1. Improve upper body strength and hand stability in fine motor tasks.
2. Improve motor planning or praxis areas via organizing and controlling her body movements as she performs D.R.T.^{Sm} position sequences. Start with slow, graded movement challenges from horse. Then proceed with basic dynamic variance progressions within walk using straight lines, in curved figures progressing to slow trotting shifts. Trot work should be graded back down to straight lines during the transition phase. Use the T.T. initially, then move to C.C.L. for trot work once she is ready for a higher level of challenge to her equilibrium.

First establish correct postural alignment and good balance reactions sitting upright and forwards on horse. Incorporate the dynamic variance progression, gradually adding in more challenging figures and more abrupt rhythm changes. Grade up to some low level sitting trot work including walk/trot/walk transitions. Then, build in activities that focus on improving upper body strength with D.R.T.^{Sm} position sequences such as quadruped and full kneel forwards and backwards, horse sit-ups, prone prop backwards, ball work, all at walk again. For eye/hand control, use placement of colored clothes pins in the horse's mane, lace horse cut-out cards, or place felt cut-out animals on rump of horse with double sticky tape.

Grade up challenge in D.R.T.^{Sm} positions by manipulating movement of horse to increase her sense of adaptability and competence. This may include slow, steady sitting trot work on a large circle. Add rein use in component parts after evidence of good control and alignment in upper body areas and when emerging confidence is consistent with movement performance. Use a moderate to wide horse with a flat, low amplitude trot.

II.   Cognition:
A. Target Goals
Concentration and Select Attention
Problem Solving
B. Strategies
1. Improve ability to focus attention for one hour session with progressively fewer prompts while decreasing impulsivity.
2. Utilize small components of guiding horse, halt/walk/halt and steering in and out of obstacles to reinforce praxis areas.

Felicia has the ability and the proclivity for responding to technical language and an instructing voice. Take advantage of her cognitive strengths (language processing, vocabulary, memory, causal relationships) to prepare her for physical challenges. Verbally define a task or movement pattern as it is demonstrated. Use highly descriptive language that defines very specific and finite steps of the task. Then repeat the verbal input as she practices the movement. After repeated practice, remove the excess words from the prompts until only key words or phrases remain. Eventually eliminate all verbal cues except for the initial request.

To help her practice clear articulation, first work on the enunciation of individual words directly related to her therapy routine. Once she concisely pronounces the words individually, have her describe her actions as she is doing them. A more motivating exercise is to have her explain to the horse what she is going to do on its back. This helps her stay in the moment by matching her verbal expression with her motor output. She can also use her mastered pronunciations to "instruct" the therapist or an assistant through a familiar task by allowing her to assume the role of teacher.

III. Affect:
    A. Target Goals
          Self Image
          Risk Taking
          Perseverance

    B. Strategies
        1. Decrease avoidance tendencies and empower her self esteem
        2. Improve fluency of emotional range from one of being totally stuck to moving on through resolve of frustrations and anxiety.
        3. Increase her introspective abilities to monitor her feelings about self in regard to things she perceives as potentially difficult or threatening

Task analyzing and discussing an activity before it is performed should relieve a lot of Felicia's avoidance tendencies. Focus on her abilities to do each step of an exercise. Discuss rational consequences of typical difficulties in performing said task. Acknowledge what she is feeling and why she may feel that way. Emphasize the positive feelings of accomplishment, pride, happiness, and even mild relief when an activity perceived as risky is successfully completed. Provide her with the opportunity to be a role model for a peer and/or to demonstrate her abilities to a parent or friendly audience.

PRECAUTIONS: STANDBY GUARDING IN ALL TASKS

Terms unique to Developmental Riding Therapy:
Dynamic Variance:
New Harmony created the term "dynamic variance" to describe the unique variable process which harnesses the horse's movement character and scope within a chosen gait pattern. In a dynamic variance progression the horse's movement is regulated to fit the individual client's needs by adjusting, and sometimes interrupting, the horse's striding tempo, and rhythm. These adjustments in turn affect the amplitude or arc of the motion transmitted from the horse's back. A developmental riding therapist must understand how to apply the dynamic variance progression as it is an essential ingredient in the overall movement formula. It contributes significantly to the guided, progressive development of movement competency in the client.

The horse must be able to increase and decrease its length of stride smoothly, without losing its balance or carriage. Lengthening of the stride specifically elicits a flexor response. Shortening the stride conversely elicits an extensor response. For a slight higher level of gradation, walk/halt/walk transitions are incorporated. Halting, reining back smoothly, and walking forward again is perhaps the most demanding sequence to elicit an interplay between flexion and extension control.

Client Centered Driving (C.C.D.):

What many people refer to as "long lining" is more accurately a form of driving in hand. In order to eliminate any confusion, when the horse is being driven by long reins for the purpose of client treatment New Harmony refers to it as "Client Centered Driving" (C.C.D.). The terminology is a more accurate reflection of the focus of the adaptation for therapy purposes. C.C.D. is also more in keeping with the typical level of skill competency of most practitioners. Generally, it has been the experience that most horse-oriented therapists can be taught this basic method in a relatively short period of time. This is much more realistic compared to the time it would take to teach classical long lining, which is a slowly evolved process.

New Harmony Therapy Triangle: (N.H.T.T.)

In this specifically configured handling technique, the horse, the head developmental riding therapist, and the assistant therapist form the "therapy triangle" during a treatment session. The horse is controlled by the therapist and assistant by means of light, woven canvas lines of approximate eight feet. The excess line is neatly folded and held in the outside hands of the therapist and the assistant. These two lines make up the sides of the triangle and allow the therapist his or her assistant to make very specific adjustments to the quality of the horse's movement throughout the session.

The therapist and the assistant are positioned directly at the client's side so they are able to maintain constant contact with the client. This three-point bond (therapist to client to assistant) makes up the base of the triangle. In this arrangement, the therapist and the assistant can use their free hands to constantly guide and support the client within the "movement moment." The triangle is a "closed circuit" system because each member of the team can have a direct effect on every other member. When this circuitry is used appropriately, there is a strong sense of connectedness, both physical and emotional, that develops within the group.

Indications:

It is only used for clients with good head/trunk control, consistent behavior control and is never used as a substitute for someone who would require a leader and two side-helpers for maximum security if posturally challenged. Generally, this is a highly specialized technique which New Harmony requires to be taught to practitioners during a curriculum/seminar training session. Practitioners using this method are expected to have a minimum competency level of first level dressage to use it properly.

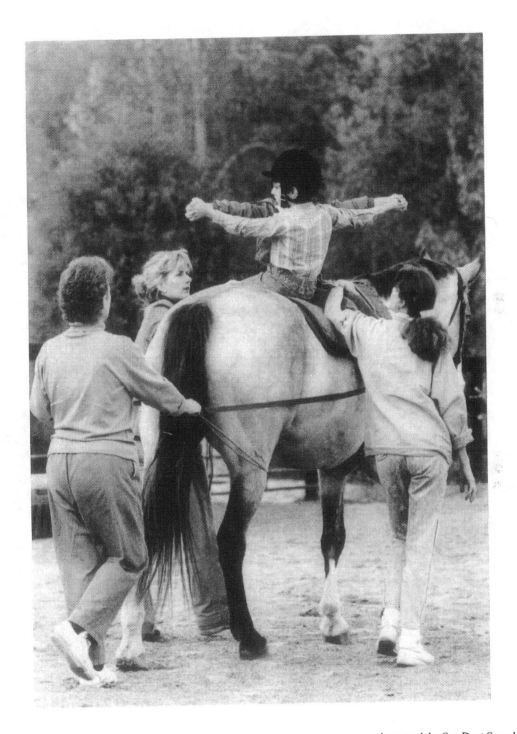

photograph by Sue Dent Sounder

FIGURE 5
A TREATMENT SESSION

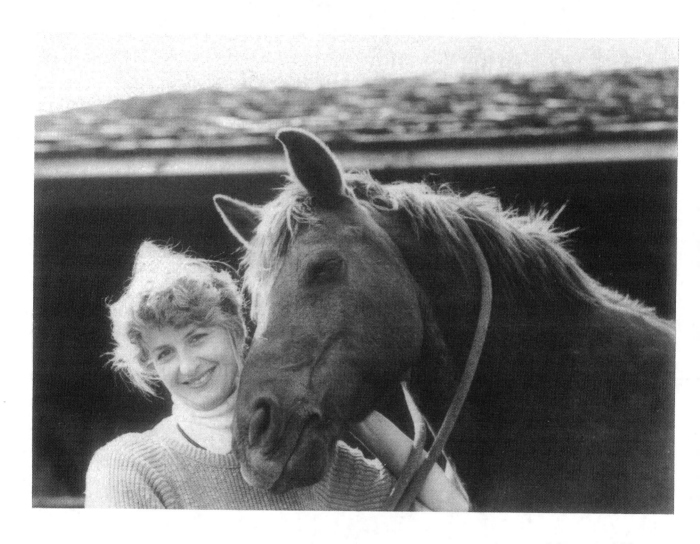

photograph by susan feldman

Jan Spink and her Horse

REFERENCES

Barwick, S. (1986). Psychomotor therapy. In **Therapy through movement**, edited by Lorraine Burr. Nottingham, England: Nottingham Rehab Limited.

Glasow, B., Spink, J. (1982). Therapeutic riding in the United States. Report presented to the *Fourth International Congress on Therapeutic Riding*, Hamburg, West Germany.

Heipertz, W. (1977). **Therapeutic riding, medicine, education and sports.** (English translation), Greenbelt Riding Association, Ottawa: Canada.

Ogilviy, W. H. (1869). A Scottish poet. Referenced for New Harmony by Alexander McKay Smith and Peter Winnants of **The Chronicle of the Horse**.

Spink, J. (1982). A comparative review of medical and psycho-educational techniques in therapeutic riding. Unpublished master's thesis, Goddard Graduate Program, Vermont College.

Spink, J. (1985). A categorical approach to vaulting for the disabled. Report presented to the *Fifth International Congress on Therapeutic Riding*, Milan, Italy.

Spink, J. (1986). *The adjunctive use of the horse in therapy: A progression.* Unpublished seminar reference material.

Spink, J. (1987). *Rx: The horse.* Presentation to the Delta Society Annual Meeting, Vancouver, British Colombia.

Spink, J. (l988). A four phase construct for therapeutic riding. Report presented to the *Sixth International Congress on Therapeutic Riding,* Toronto, Canada.

Spink, J. (1990). A model application for the horse in riding therapy: the Michael McCulloch Memorial Award lecture, *Delta Society* Annual Meeting: Houston, Texas.

Kuratorium for Therapeutisches Reiten. (1985). German film converted to U.S. video format. **The horse in medicine, education and sport.** Available from the Delta Society, Renton, Washington. (See suggested contacts)

SUGGESTED READING:

Spink, Jan. (1993).*The Therapy Horse: Developing Standards and Competencies* Barbara Engel Therapy Services. Avaliable from Spink.

Spink, Jan. (1993).*Developmental Riding Therapy.* 3830 E. Bellevue, PO Box 42050-B, Tucson, AZ: Therapy Skill Builders.

Brown, O., Tebay, J. (1991). "Standards and accreditation for therapeutic riding centers - A model". The proceedings of the *7th International Therapeutic Riding Congress,* Aarhus, Denmark. (See chapter 3.03 in this book.)

SUGGESTED CONTACTS

Delta Society
P.O. Box 1080
Renton, Washington 98057
Tel. 206/226-7357

New Harmony Institute (N.E.A.T. Project)
Contact Person: Jan Spink, M.A.,
Morven Park International Equestrian Institute
Route #4, Box 43 (Rt. #740)
Leesburg, Virginia, 22075 U.S.A.
*written information only

American Hippotherapy Association
Contact: NARHA

North American Riding for the Handicapped
Association, Inc.
P.O. Box 33150
Denver, Colorado 80233
Tel. 303/452-1212

United States Dressage Federation (USDF)
(Training Level and First Level Test Series)
1212 O Street, P.O. Box 80668
Lincoln, Nebraska 68501
Tel. 402/474-7632.

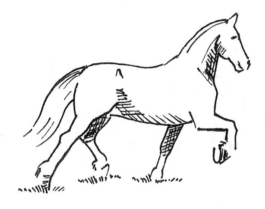
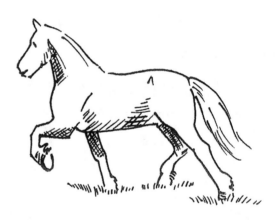

CHAPTER 27

Directory of major college courses in therapeutic horseback riding(effective 1997)

Centenary College, Hackettstown, NJ. Octavia Brown , Director of Development, Equine Program.
Clemson University, SC
Penn State University, 323 Ag Administration Bldg, Therapeutic Riding Programs, State College, PA
Feather River Community College, CA
Findlay University, Findlay, OH, Robin Koehler
Philadelphia College Pharmacy & Science, Occupational Therapy Dept, Philadelphia, PA
St. Andrews Presbyterian College, Laurenburg, NC, Lorraine Renker
Tarleton State University, Stephenville, TX
Texas Tech University, Lubbock TX
University of New Hamshire, Durham, NH.
University of Main at Farmington, Farmington, ME. Ms Ruby Tracy, Professional Development Center.
University of Texas Health Science Center, Physical Therapy Dept. San Antonio TX

Western Michigan University Occupational Therapy Department, Kalamazoo, MI 49008-5051
   with the Cheff Center: contact Mary Bush, Occupational Department, Western Michigan University.

Related Associations

North American Riding **for the Handicapped Association Inc** .... 303-452-1212 PO Box 33250 Denver CO 80233	**American Vaulting Association, Inc.** ..... 206-780-9353 **Alford Place** **Bainbridge Island, WA 98110**
American Hippotherapy Association ..... 303-452-1212 **% NARHA** PO Box 33250 Denver CO 80233	**American Horse Show Association (AHSA)** Main office----4047 Iron Works Pky. Lexington KY 40511..................................606-231-2472
American Horse Council .... 202-296-4031 1700 "K' Street, NW Suite 300 Washington D.C.	Headquarters------220 East 42nd Street New York, NY 10017-5876 212-972-2472
Delta Society .... 202-226-7357 PO Box 1080 Renton, WA 98057	United States Pony Club, Inc. (USPC) .... 606-254-7669 The Kentucky Horse Park 4071 Iron Works Pike Lexington, KY 40511
Canadian Therapeutic Riding Assoc .... 519-767-0700 PO Box 1055 Guelph, Ontario N1H 6J6 Canada	National Association for Driving for Disabled (NADD) 87 Main St. Fort Plain NY 13339
Sensory Integration International .... 310-533-8338 1402 Cravens Avenue Torrence CA 90501	United States Dressage Federation (USDF) .... 402-434-8550 PO Box 6669 Lincoln , NE 68506-0669
	Neuro-Developmental Treatment Assoc. .. 312-386-2445 PO Box 70 Oak Park, IL 60303

INDEX